REBEL KETO

The Totally Awesome Girlz Guide To Losing Weight, Breaking the Rules, and Having a Life Outside the Kitchen (With 100+ Easy Low Carb Recipes)

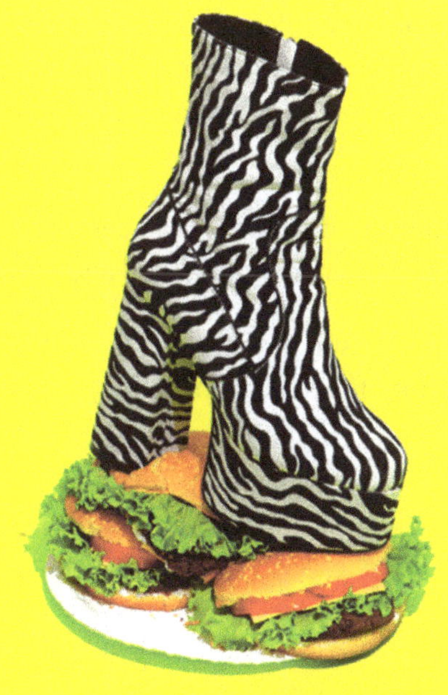

HEATHER STRICKLAND

Rebel Keto: The Totally Awesome Girls' Guide to Losing Weight, Breaking the Rules, and Having a Life Outside the Kitchen (With 100+ Easy Low Carb Recipes)

Before starting any new diet and exercise program please check with your doctor and clear any exercise and/or diet changes with them before beginning. We do not claim to help cure any condition or disease. We do not provide medical aid or nutrition advice for the purpose of health or disease, nor do we claim to be doctors or dietitians.

Any product recommendation is not intended to diagnose, treat, cure, or prevent any disease. Our statements and information have not necessarily been evaluated by the Food and Drug Administration.

We expressly disclaim responsibility to any person or entity for any liability, loss, or damage caused or alleged to be caused directly or indirectly as a result of the use, application, or interpretation of any material provided to you as the reader.

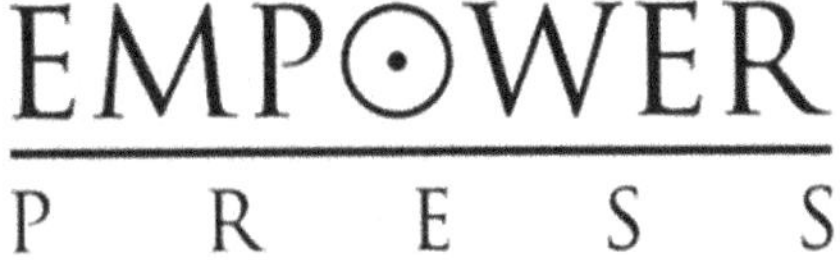

GracePoint Matrix, LLC
624 S Cascade Ave. #201
Colorado Springs CO 80903
www.GracePointMatrix.com
Email: Admin@GracePointMatrix.com
SAN # 991-6032

Library of Congress Control Number: 2021901856

ISBN-13: (Paperback) # 978-1-951694-68-5
ISBN-13: (Hardback) # 978-1-955272-02-5
eISBN: (eBook) # 978-1-951694-67-8

Rebel Keto Reader's Agreement

I'll make this experience as entertaining as possible if you solemnly swear to the following …

But me first. **ahem**

My promise to you:

I, Heather Strickland, solemnly swear to give you the most accurate info about a low-carb diet without boring the crap out of you with too much medical jargon and worthless bits of information nobody truly needs.

I promise to get you in and out of the kitchen as fast as humanly possible because losing weight does not mean you have to love to cook.

Now, it's your turn:

You agree to be kind to yourself along this journey, which means no standing in front of the mirror talking smack about your body.

When reading this book, you promise to give it your undivided attention.

No play reading while you're trying to avoid eye contact at the airport or scanning while you search for the best online promo codes to use at Pottery Barn.

You agree to understand that while you're *technically* an adult learner, you have to be patient with yourself along the way. (You also agree that "adult learner" is a little offensive, but you're not sure why.)

You solemnly swear you will not sabotage yourself: AKA, seek out or pay attention to the Keto Police, or Alice from accounting *(*barf*)* who thinks she's a diet guru after losing 15 pounds on a cleanse.

You promise to set small achievable goals for yourself that will set you up to win every day, and you promise to call all your friends at the end of every chapter to tell them they MUST read this book!

You understand that following this totally awesome guide will change your life by walking you down memory lane—the good one—and challenging everything you thought you knew about dieting.

Do you agree to these terms?

Good! Now sign your name on the line below!

Name: ____

Date: ____

You are now invited to sit with the cool kids at lunch, add your name to the list of Rebel readers, and open The Vault at **rebelketo.com/The-Vault**.

*******Psst, it'll help and it's free! Pinky promise***

Scan here or go to rebelketo.com/the-vault to access the Rebel Keto vault!

Rebel Keto features your favorite '80s jams. Scan below to access the totally radical modern-day mixtape or access it in the Rebel Keto vault!

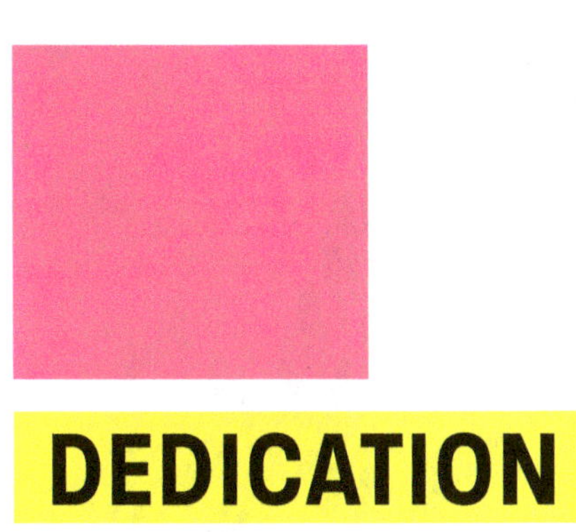

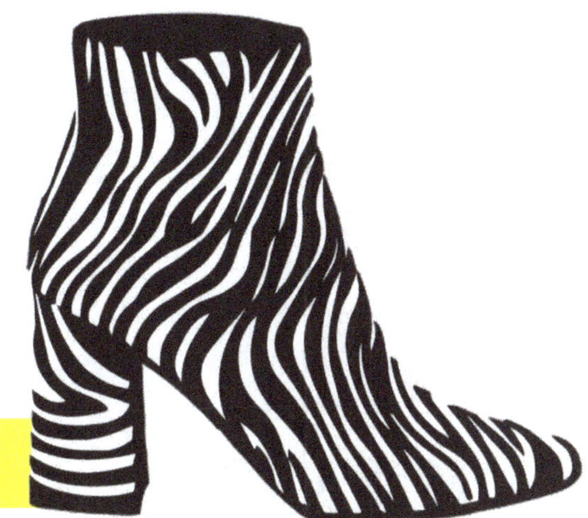

DEDICATION

For Savannah, Lylah Kate, and Na,

Thank you for always being your unique, back-talking, brilliant selves. You are the heroes of my life, and you were born to make an impact. Keep their heads ringin'.

And

For every girl who has thought she'd never be good enough and who has ever awkwardly attempted to casually cover her belly with a throw pillow because she believed she needed to be perfect to be loved—I see you because I've been you.

Don't believe the hype. You are amazing right now. Don't ever forget that.

"If I ever let my head down, it will be just to admire my shoes."

—Marilyn Monroe

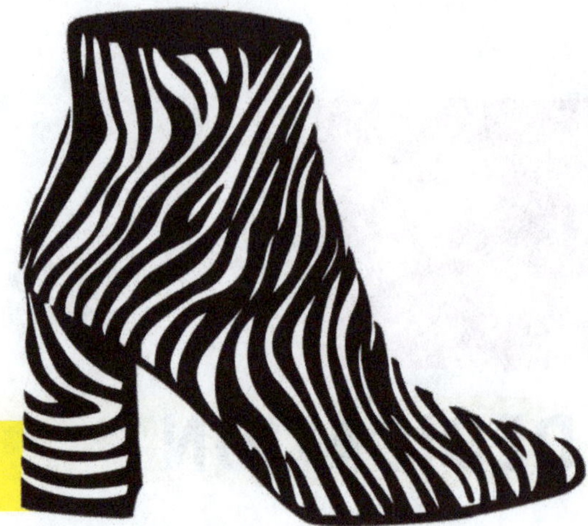

CONTENTS

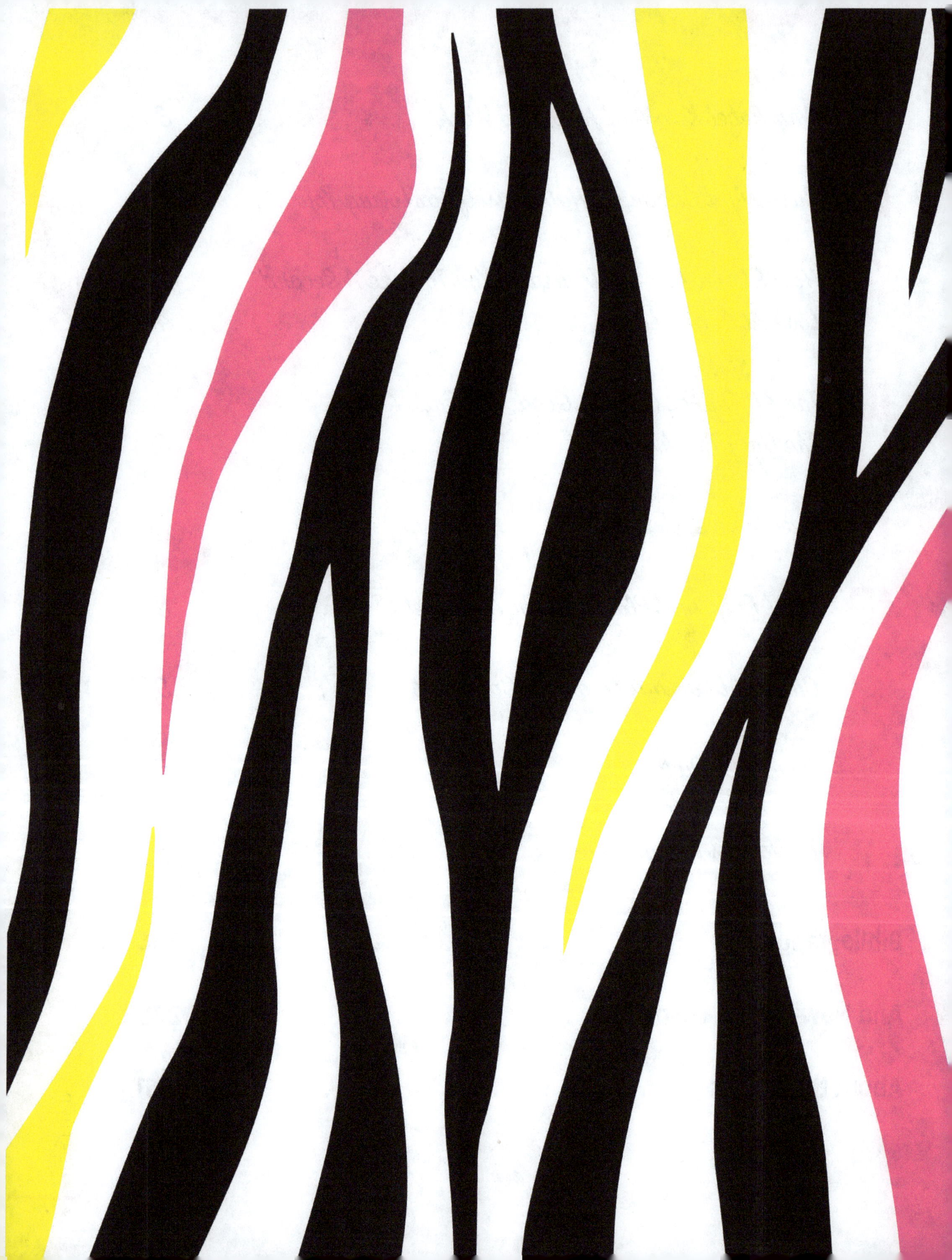

INTRODUCTION

I don't know if I'll go straight to hell for admitting this, but when my grandmother didn't recognize me, I prayed she had dementia.

I had been living in a hellish denial about my weight for months.

I blamed the camera angles for making me look fat. I blamed gravity or the unsteady ground when I attempted to walk in anything other than crocs. I blamed the fashion industry for effed up sizes because the only pants I could squeeze into were stretchy *As Seen On TV* PajamaJeans. I pointed my unmanicured finger at everyone but myself.

In other words, I failed to take responsibility.

I blamed my excessive sweating on some oddball gland problem I read about online.

And my back and knee pain? Well, I chalked that up to massive boobs and genetic predisposition.

But it was my fault. I had put on so much weight that I was unrecognizable, and my grandmother—the woman who helped raise me—was about to call the police because a random woman was in her home. Now, how in the hell was I going to get out of that?

"Um, no officer, the thing is, I'm not a criminal; I'm just unrecognizable at this size. Please carry on with your day and thank you for your service."

Just no.

What's worse than my grandmother not recognizing me? How about introducing yourself to a group of people you have known for twenty years who have no idea who you are after you've lost the weight?

I thought of getting a t-shirt that says, "Hey, it's Heather. Just one hundred forty pounds lighter." You know what always comes next, right?

"NO WAY! How did you do it?"

That's one of those two-minute elevator pitches I have yet to master because the truth is, there are a couple of things I did to lose weight that cannot be summed up in two minutes.

I can tell you what I don't say.

I never tell folks, "Oh, you know, I just went on a diet, like no big deal," or, "Oh, it was super easy. I just had a shake for breakfast, a shake for lunch, and a sensible dinner."

I cannot and will not tell people "Hey, I did this, and it was easy" because anybody who's ever tried to lose weight knows it's not easy. Anytime someone tells you that losing weight is simple or no big deal, they are lying to your face.

Another thing I cannot say is "I just did keto" because the truth is, it took a lot more than just one diet to do what I did, and it wasn't just one thing. It was a combination of choices I intentionally made each day.

I did what I refer to as Rebel Keto. My version of keto is a more sustainable version that has kept the pounds off for over six years. I've told the story, or tried to … I don't know, a gazillion times?

The short answer is, I took the parts of keto that work, and I took out the parts that really suck. And then I added a few things about mindset because if your head and your heart aren't in the game, you're going to lose.

I'm writing this book so that it will be easier to explain. Otherwise, I'm going to be boring you with a long story about carbohydrates, and annoying people is not my jam.

As I was writing this book, I kept thinking of all the boring-ass diet books that I have read over the past twenty years, and I came up with a couple of things I didn't want to do.

I knew I didn't want to sound like an encyclopedia—or like Mr. Lorensax from *Ferris Bueller's Day Off.* I didn't want to report basic information (even if it was helpful) in a monotonous, brain-numbing way. Is anyone with me on that? Anyone? Anyone?

It was also a big deal to me not to throw around foodie terms and sound like a poser in the kitchen. You know, like if you're not born with the knowledge that the lovely stalk of fresh asparagus pairs well with salmon, you're doomed. I'm not too fond of that. I don't love cooking, so I made the recipes easy. I spliced all the best ones together like an old-school mixtape.

Also, I wanted to make sure that I was entertaining, because have you ever tried to read a diet book? They're just straight-up boring. (Sorry, not sorry.)

So, I thought, what could have the power to keep women engaged in a diet book without making them want to throw themselves off a cliff or set themselves on fire?

I figured if the '80s can't do it, nothing can.

Look, I was born in 1975, so the 1980s raised me. It formed my opinions, in both good ways and bad.

Commercials programmed me to drink Diet Coke, just for the taste of it. Prime time sitcoms like *Family Ties* and *The Cosby Show* modeled free-thinking women with careers and respected opinions; movies like *Footloose*, *The Breakfast Club,* and *The Goonies* taught me how to think for myself.

What brings me joy and fun, on the regular, is music, movies, TV, and old school MTV—the '80s. I love the '80s. You love the '80s. We all love the '80s!

There are so many amazingly epic, fabulous things that happened in the Greed is Good decade. Punk rock. Hip hop. Slap bracelets.

Cross-dressing became a thing both on TV and the big screen. Remember Dustin Hoffman as Tootsie? Tom Hanks on *Bosom Buddies*? Joyce Hyser on *Just One of The Guys*?

The '80s brought us Stridex, Sun-In, Jenny's phone number, the Super Bowl Shuffle, the Running Man, the Moonwalk, the Moonman, the Safety Dance, MTV, CNN, EPCOT, *The A-Team,* The Clapper, *The Golden Girls*, the *Ghostbusters*, acid-washed jeans, the Walkman, mixtapes, and *Wayne's World.*

The '80s influenced what we wore—scrunchies, Swatch watches, jelly shoes, leotards, leg warmers, Members Only jackets, shoulder pads, and off the shoulder sweatshirts.

The eighties brought the love songs too, "Love Bites," "Love Stinks," "Making Love Out of Nothing at All," just to name a few!

Along with all those lovely '80s influences came a bunch of BS about our food and our health. The way we thought about how to lose weight screwed us all over.

I'm going to make this as simple as possible, as fun as possible, and as liberating as possible. I didn't lose weight by playing by the rules.

Rebel Keto is my gift to you. Think of it as cracking open a time capsule—going back to the '80s to uncover the truth about the lies you were told about weight with splashes of '80s-style wisdom and fun along the way.

Rebel Keto tells the story of how I lost the weight and kept it off, got my life back and my head on straight, and how you can too.

"If you obey all the rules, you miss all the fun."

—Katherine Hepburn

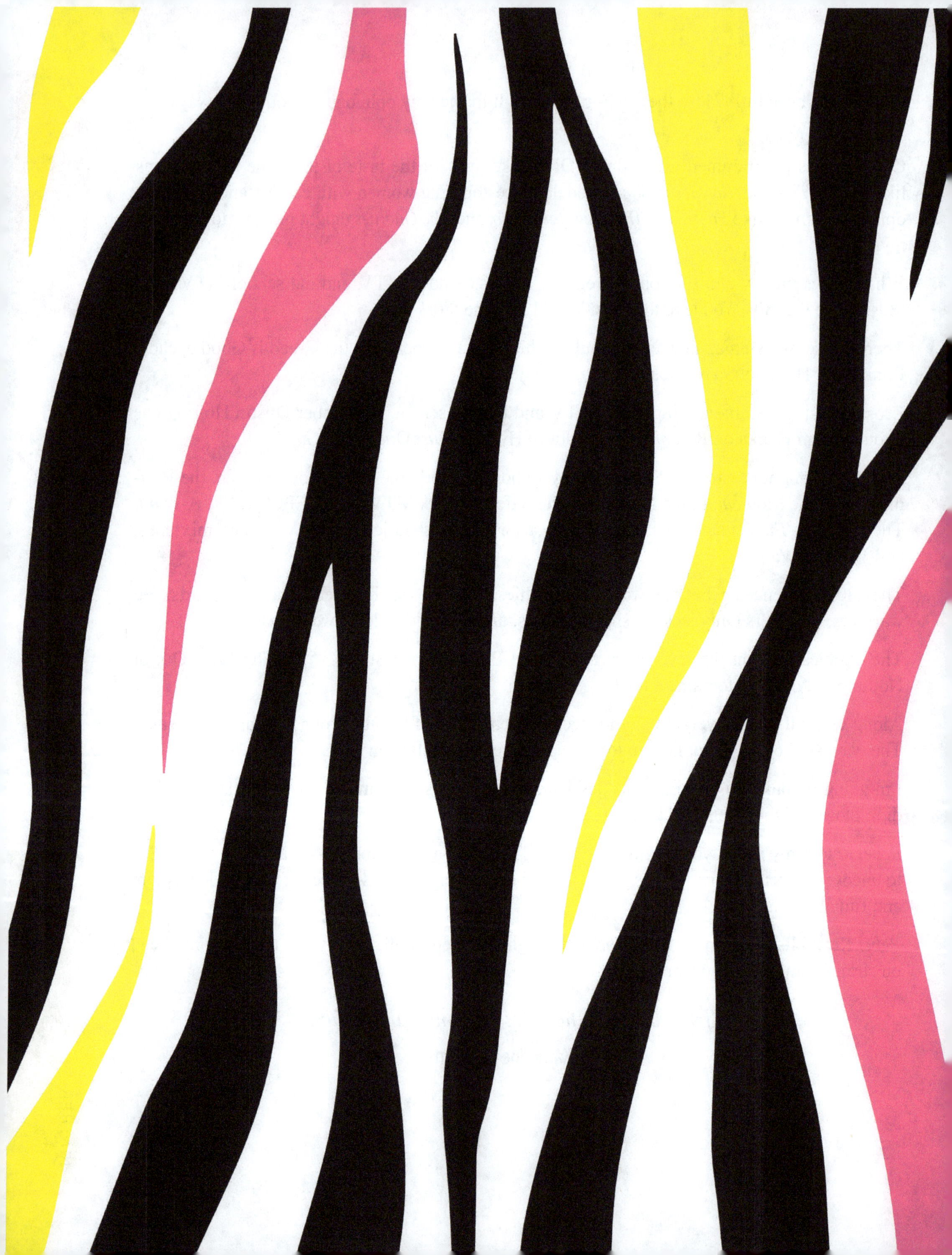

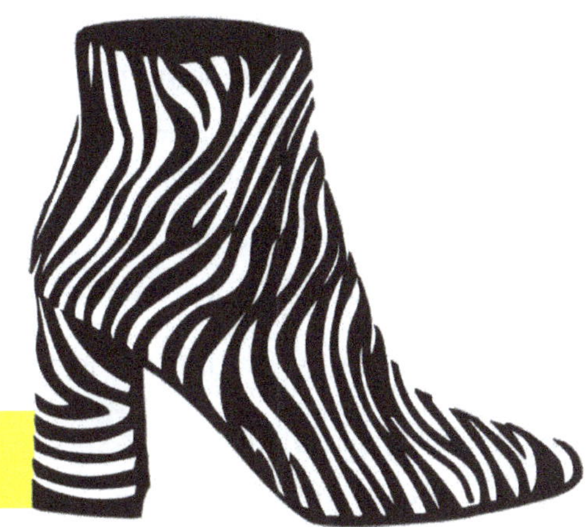

WTH is Rebel Keto?

Now, here's a thought—how long would you stay on a diet that didn't work? We're talking straight-up zero results. How much time would you allow for it to "kick in"? Two weeks? Maybe a month?

What if I told you that diet had the opposite effect you desired? It made you gain weight, feel lousy and tired? You'd stop it the moment you realized it, right? Of course you would because that's logical.

So, the question becomes why have we been following the forty-year-old Standard American Diet that fails us? We've got a deadly and costly obesity epidemic on our hands. Yet, we're still following the "standard" diet that got us here. Hold up a second.

Can we take a moment and talk about "standard"?

Standard? Seriously? When was the last time you bought the "standard" version of anything? Called up your best friend to tell her you just found the most "standard" outfit? Posted a very "standard" selfie? Or used #standard on Instagram.

Probably never.

When was the last time you read a weight loss success story brought to you by the Standard American Diet (SAD)?

Also, never.

There's a good reason for that. The results suck.

Your gut tells you that "standard" isn't the best—it's the status quo, and it is full of lies.

Do you know what happens when you follow a SAD diet? Over forty years of experience gives us the answer. America gets an obesity epidemic and a healthcare crisis. You stay stuck in your dirty, stained T-shirt, watching reality TV, trying hard to hold onto your dream of a fit body. As your fantasy of laying out on a tropical island with your new husband waiting for your server to bring you infused water and cocktails (every hour on the hour) gets dashed.

SAD recommends carbs should make up 45-65% of your daily diet. On a 2,000 calorie per day diet, that comes to 900-1300 calories from carbs, or 225 to 325 carbs per day.

The United States is one of the world's unhealthiest countries.

- Our "standard" is processed packaged and fast foods
- Our "standard" is too many low-nutrient, high-carb foods
- Our "standard" is too many trans fats via hydrogenated or partially hydrogenated oils
- Our "standard" is way too much sugar.

It's time we raise our standards.

Why The Sad Guidelines Were Created

Because inquiring minds want to know, I'll fill you in with the 411 on why we settled on the standard.

A senate committee that came together to focus on programs to eliminate hunger got off track. The evidence was rolling in that linked diet to the "Nation's killer diseases," so they took a closer look to determine whether or not the government needed to step in and advise us how to eat a healthier diet.

The committee decided that yes, Americans did need guidance regarding what to eat, and that eating healthier foods could promote health and potentially reduce healthcare costs. The government should play a role to encourage nutrition research and industry food reformulation.

U.S. Dietary Guidelines provide no limit for added sugar, and the U.S. Food and Drug Administration (FDA) still lists sugar as a "generally regarded as safe" (GRAS) substance. That classification means the food industry adds unlimited amounts of sugar to our food.

That first set of SAD guidelines came out in 1980.

Cut to today—2021:

Over 40% of American adults are obese (Craig M. Hales 2020). 20% of our kids are obese (Cheryl D. Fryar December). Do you know what happens to these kids other than early-onset diabetes? They grow up to be obese adults dependent on medications and our country's healthcare system.

The standard is not working. The rest of this book will look at what does work.

Rebel Keto

Let's take a few minutes and make sure we're all on the same page.

I'm going to talk about the definitions of Rebel and Keto, introduce the Rebel Rules, and tell you how to *Just Say No* to The Standard Way.

Rebel Definition

noun

noun: rebel; plural noun: rebels

/ˈrebəl/

a person who rises in opposition or armed resistance against an established government or ruler.

adjective

/ˈrebəl/

Rebellious, defiant.

verb

verb: rebel; 3rd person present: rebels; past tense: rebelled; past participle: rebelled; gerund or present participle: rebelling

/reˈbəl/

rise in opposition or armed resistance to an established government or ruler.

- (of a person) resist authority, control, or convention.
- show or feel repugnance for or resistance to something. (Oxford Languages 2021)

Keto Definition

The ketogenic diet, also known as keto, is a low carb, high fat, moderate protein diet that limits carbohydrates to 20-30 net carbs per day—which results in obsessing over macronutrients, crazy mealtime math, and complete confusion.

Rebel Keto is my non-mathematical version of the OG low-carb diet that is way easier to follow.

Rebel Rules You Knew In The '80s But May Have Forgotten

Other than being rad '80s movies you loved, what do *Footloose*, *Ferris Bueller's Day Off*, and *Dead Poet's Society* have in common?

Kevin Bacon's character, Ren, used the same source the city council used to ban dancing as an argument for dancing.

Matthew Broderick's Ferris Bueller used his creativity to brilliantly engineer a day off to remind us that every moment in life counts.

As Professor Keating, Robin Williams encouraged his students to take a stand for themselves in life and on their desks in class to gain a different perspective.

So, what does a biblical argument for dancing, skipping school, and an unconventional English lit class have in common? A group of rebellious leaders who refused the day's norms and dared to think differently. Not to blindly break the rules or destroy anyone, but to assert their individuality for others' benefit.

The rebel influences of the '80s weren't the bad guys. They were the game changers who helped us learn how to think, not what to think.

That's what Rebel Keto did for me. Think of it as a significant reminder of all the rule-breaking lessons you knew back in the day. Channel your inner Ferris and stop punishing yourself.

Rebels Think Differently

- Rebels don't give in, and they don't back down.
- We do not accept stereotypes; we fight them.
- We study the basics, then reinvent the rules.
- When everyone else is quietly falling in line, Rebels speak up.
- Rebels don't take someone else's word for it. Rather, we ask "Why?" and "What if?" and "Then what?" and "How do you know?"
- A Rebel doesn't allow anyone to define her limits.
- Rebels challenge the status quo. We ask, "If everybody else is doing it, why the hell should I?"
- Rebels never take conventional wisdom as fact.
- Rebels seek the truth.

Rebels don't break the rules because they want to be bad. They break them because they know that rules must be broken for lasting, positive change.

Forty years of diet rules have created a culture where food is a number, a point, or a stereotype, not a nutrient. We've allowed these diet rules to consume us, perpetuate perfectionism, and make us feel less than. It's time to start saying NO to one-size-fits-all mentality and say YES to trusting ourselves instead of what others tell us to do.

If you're a woman who has tried diet after diet and failed, if you're tired of rules, "don't" lists, calorie, macro, and keto math, you're in the right place.

Following Rebel Keto will result in an epic shift on the scale, fewer cravings, more energy, and more focus. Rebel Keto will put an end to deprivation … no more starving, no more shaming. You'll have a sense of control and confidence in your body.

Standard Keto vs Rebel Keto

How to *Just Say No*

Let's break down a few differences between the standard keto diet and Rebel Keto and learn how Rebels *Just Say No* to the standard set of rules.

Standard Keto Rule: Keep your macronutrients at 75% fats, 20% protein, 5% carbohydrates or go directly to ketogenic hell. No passing go; no collecting $200.

Rebel Keto: Monopoly and macro counters are for kids. We follow our instincts, not what a calculator tells us to eat.

Standard Keto Rule: No bread! No sugar! No pasta! No carbs—no excuses.

Rebel Keto: Chill. Out. We, as Rebels, know our bodies and that when a food group goes on a No list, we want it more than ever. Pick the battles you can win—and screw the shame.

Standard Keto Rule: No carbohydrates! Not now, not ever.

Rebel Keto: Not all carbs are the devil. Rebels know the difference between simple and complex.

Standard Keto Rule: No grains. No rice. No starch.

Rebel Keto: Rebels consult the glycemic index like a Magic 8 Ball.

Standard Keto Rule: No fruit! Don't you know that it has fructose? GASP!

Rebel Keto: Eat fruit—but check yourself before you wreck yourself.

Standard Keto Rule: Test your body to see if it's in ketosis by poking yourself with a needle or peeing on a test strip.

Rebel Keto: Feeling fabulous in your own skin is all the "Atta Girl" you need.

Standard Keto Rule: Spend every waking minute looking over your shoulder to see if the Keto Police are coming for you.

Rebel Keto: Give zero effs about the Keto Police.

Standard Keto Rule: Restrict all carbohydrates to 20 net per day to get into ketosis

Rebel Keto: Cut high glycemic, starchy carbohydrates. Go with your gut, not a number.

Standard Keto Rule: Follow a one-size-fits-all mentality for men and women. Obsessively stick to your macros and lose weight, living happily ever after in ketosis.

Rebel Keto: One size never fits all. Every woman knows that.

Standard Keto Rule: Everyone else is doing it this way.

Rebel Keto: Everyone else is following the leader. What if the leader is an idiot?

2

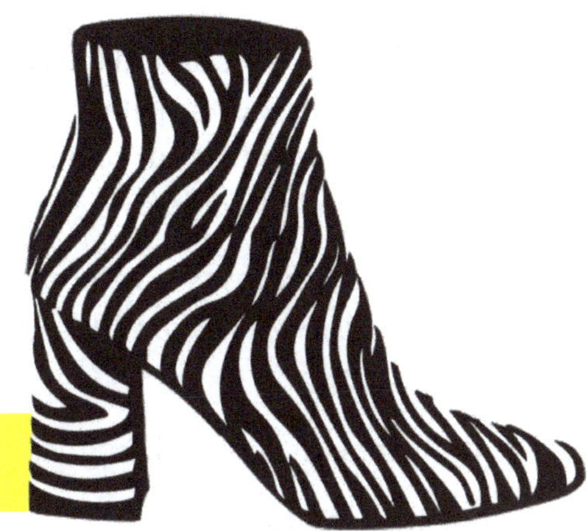

How You Got Here – The '80s Made You Do It

Have you ever looked at a picture of yourself from the '80s and thought, "What the hell was I thinking?"

At the time you thought your big bangs and blue eyeshadow was hella-cool. Your off-the-shoulder *Flash Dance*-inspired sweatshirt paired with tightly rolled Jordache jeans, Sabagoes, and a rubber band guard Swatch watch ruled. Riding in the back of your mom's station wagon (and flipping off traffic) ruled. Your caboodle full of Bonnie Bell lip smackers ruled. Heavy metal hair bands—Journey, Def Leppard, AC/DC, and Pat Benatar—ruled.

The '80s ruled. And that's why we can't get enough. But here's the deal. Just like every word of "Girls Just Wanna Have Fun" is permanently ingrained in your head, there are a few diet myths on your most excellent hits list that are holding you back.

I'll cut to the chase. You got fed a bunch of lies.

The '80s was all about excess. Michael Douglas told us greed was good. McDonald's said bigger was better. Conventional wisdom said that fat was bad. Low-fat versions of everything from crackers and cookies to yogurt and frozen pizzas dominated all aspects of life. You couldn't listen to the radio or watch five minutes of *Magnum PI* without being reminded to drink a Diet Coke—just for the taste of it.

Saturday morning cartoons turned into low-fat marketing opportunities. Smurfs were selling cereal, and Care Bears doubled as celebrity spokesmen—ahem, *spokes-bears*—for candy, cookies, and fruit roll-ups.

The lunch ladies did their part in the cafeteria by wearing the unfortunate, yet required, hairnets and following the first-ever dietary guidelines. They served up a mean sloppy joe with a large order of carbs on the side. Your science teacher may have even given you a copy of the Standard American Diet food pyramid to memorize.

The diet of the decade was low-fat and low-calorie. Weight loss gurus like Richard Simmons encouraged you to *Sweat to the Oldies*, and Jane Fonda convinced you that you could Jazzercise your way to a size 6.

But the problem is… it was all bogus.

When they told you to eat low fat, they didn't mention that meant you'd be eating more sugar.

When they told you to count calories, they made food a number, not a nutrient. When they made fat public enemy number one, they removed an essential part of the diet—one that up until the '80s had long been a staple necessary for good health.

Simply put, you got hoodwinked. You were brainwashed! The marketing machine's propaganda and false hope led to epic diet failure and a nationwide obesity epidemic which threatens to cripple our healthcare system and takes millions of lives every year. (World Health Organization 2021).

The Proof Is in The Non-Fat Pudding

In 1980, adults with obesity made up around 13% of the U.S. population (U.S. Department of Health and Human Services 2010). Today, in 2021, that number has grown to 40% of adults (Craig M. Hales 2020). That's over forty years of proof that low-fat diets fail.

Houston, errr, America, we have a problem. But you knew that, right?

Every year, as is shown in numerous studies and by the CDC (Centers for Disease Control and Prevention 2021), millions of women are diagnosed with obesity-related diseases, including cardiovascular disease related to high blood pressure (hypertension), high LDL cholesterol, low HDL cholesterol, and high levels of triglycerides (dyslipidemia). (I would list all sixty chronic illnesses related to obesity, but you'd get super depressed.)

Obesity is becoming the new normal.

What's worse is, instead of shining a light on the issue and discussing the serious health problems that go hand in hand with being overweight and what we can do about it, we sweep it under the rug.

Have we become a nation of cowards too afraid to speak out because we fear the court of public opinion? Seriously? People are losing their limbs and lives. The obesity epidemic is real and currently threatens to cripple our nation's healthcare system.

There should be outrage. It is officially time to sound the alarm. Ding, Ding, Ding! Why are we OKAY WITH THIS?

If you're reading this book, you are one of the millions of women impacted. You may have tried other diets and failed. And you are most definitely not okay with the conventional wisdom, also known as craptastic BS, that points the finger at you. In other words, you're sick and damn tired of being told it's your fault. You're over being talked down to by doctors who tell you losing weight is simple math. Eat less; move more. As if it were that simple.

Why I Call Bullshit on The Conventional Wisdom of the '80s

Here's what we know doesn't work—which is pretty much everything you learned about losing weight in the '80s.

Lie #1: Count Calories!

Nope. The fact is calorie counting is a grand distraction and a waste of your time. The source of the calorie, as in the food you eat, matters much more than any number.

Lie #2: Feel the Burn! Exercise = Weight Loss

Nope. The hypothesis that exercising is an effective way to lose weight is over one hundred years old; we have one hundred years of proof that it does not work.

Don't believe me? Consider this quote from The American Heart Association:

"It is reasonable to assume that persons with relatively high daily energy expenditures would be less likely to gain weight over time, compared with those who have low energy expenditures. So far, data to support this hypothesis is not particularly compelling"(William L. Haskell, et al. 2007, 7).

Holy crap, Batman! Seriously? The data isn't compelling? Um, that's a problem.

Lie #3: Lose Weight by Eating Low Fat

Nope. Does not compute. When you remove the fat and replace it with sugar, you get a diet so high in carbohydrates you don't have a snowball's chance in hell of losing weight.

Bottom line: it's time to stop counting on conventional wisdom and calories.

I know this may seem a little crazy. You probably have a few questions, like, why would our food pyramid direct us to eat the very foods that are sabotaging our health, and how did we get forty years into this Standard American Diet that led us to an obesity epidemic?

I'm going to cover all of that and more in the following chapters, starting with the biggest lie of them all: Eating fat makes you fat.

But first, I want to cover a few reasons you believed the hype or how they sold us on the lies.

Deregulation: Why Ronald Reagan Is Responsible for Papa Smurf Pimping Breakfast Cereal

President Reagan is famous for telling Mr. Gorbachev to "Tear down this wall," but he was also the dude that gave the Federal Trade Commission the go-ahead to self-regulate. Meaning, he lifted restrictions that had been in place to make sure junk food ads didn't target kids.

Now, why would Ronnie do such a thing? Well, it's pretty simple—the food lobby, the toy industry, and the TV networks wanted it that way so they could make more money. And when they teamed up, they became more powerful than GI Joe, Gargamel, and He-Man combined.

You don't have to be a marketing guru to know that kids are more likely to fall for sugar advertising than adults. As grown-ups, we see right through Ronald McDonald's tactics. But kids don't. They buy right into the Hamburglar's BS because they are children. They haven't lived long enough to be skeptical.

Time for A Startling Statistic

Between 1984 and 1985, cartoons featuring licensed characters increased by 300% (Goodam 2010). By the end of 1985, more than forty animated series ran with licensed products and active marketing campaigns.

Papa Smurf Becomes a Celebrity Spokes-Smurf

Deregulation meant free reign to market sugar to kids during peak times, like during *The Smurfs* or *Pee Wee's Playhouse*. (Ahem, the Word of the Day is *SALES*.)

That gave cartoons breakout opportunities to become mini commercials.

1982: E.T. Cereal "Made with E.T.'s favorite flavors, chocolate, and real peanut butter."

1983: Smurf Berry Crunch Cereal with blue and red "smurfberries."

1983: Donkey Kong Junior Cereal "Wild with fruit flavor."

1983: Pac-Man Cereal, with marshmallows!

1984: Kellogg's rolls out C-3POs a year after the first Star Wars trilogy wrapped up.

1985: Nerds Cereal, a two-in-one double dose of sugar, just like the candy.

1988: Nintendo Cereal System—another two-in-one concept with an incredibly catchy jingle.

Deregulation made it possible for toys to have TV shows. So yeah, basically, the entire thirty-minute Care Bears episode you religiously watched on Saturday morning was one gigantic ADVERTISEMENT.

The 8-Hour Perfume for the 24-Hour Woman and Other Ads that Targeted Women

Damn that Enjoli commercial. Do you remember that one? It featured a woman with perfectly feathered bangs, who went from business suit to evening gown to cook dinner, all while looking like a supermodel. All for the sake of her husband's manhood, dear God!

Because deregulation opened the floodgates for advertising targeting, guess who else they went after? Women. The food companies exploited family roles. Nearly every TV ad featured a woman, not a man, faithfully serving meals. Were you struggling to multitask as a working mom? Frozen pizza to the rescue!

Tab

Tab was for those of us who wanted to "keep tabs" on our weight. The commercial featured a curvy—ahem—freakishly endowed woman with a perfect body fresh out of the ocean in need of hydration. The problem? They left out the fact that Tab's secret low-cal sweetener was saccharin—which has been linked to cancer (Reuber 1978).

What a beautiful drink, right?

Coke

Want to talk about cheesy ads? Coca-Cola's "Can't Beat the Feeling" campaign featured women and children going from being bored out of their minds from monotony to total transformation. As in, suddenly being super stoked to do everyday tasks—stopping for the occasional spaz level dance break because they couldn't beat the feeling of Coca-Cola. Of course, they couldn't. They were all hopped up on high-fructose corn syrup.

Fun Fact: From 1982 to 1989, Coke held a controlling interest in Columbia Pictures (the motion picture and entertainment company) (The Editors of Encyclopaedia Britannica n.d.), which explains all of the product placement in movies. Thanks a lot, deregulation.

Sugar-Free Jell-O

Who can forget the catchy yet annoying Give In Jell-O commercial that celebrated surrendering to dessert with women and overly enthusiastic kids dancing with reckless abandon in leotards after giving into the taste? It appears to be heaven on earth.

The problem? The sweetener was NutraSweet, which is aspartame, which is linked to serious health problems (Malkan 2020).

Give me a break. And I don't mean a piece of that Kit-Kat bar or a low-fat Snackwell's cookie. Remember how their commercials asked if they could ever make enough?

Well, since they replaced the fat with addictive sugar, probably not.

Low-fat everything exploded in the early '80s, and as a result, fat became the villain. In the following chapter, I'll explain how this logic screwed up more than our waistlines.

Just the Facts, Ma'am – Takeaways

- We have forty years of proof that low-fat diets fail.
- 40% of American adults are obese (Craig M. Hales 2020).
- Obesity is linked to multiple chronic diseases, including cardiovascular disease related to high blood pressure (hypertension), high LDL cholesterol, low HDL cholesterol, and high levels of triglycerides (dyslipidemia).
- You were sold a bunch of lies in the '80s that are affecting your weight and health today.
- Calorie counting is a grand distraction and a waste of your time. The source of the calorie matters much more than any number.
- The hypothesis that exercising is an effective way to lose weight is over one hundred years old; we have one hundred years of proof that it does not work.
- When you remove the fat and replace it with sugar, you get a diet so high in carbohydrates you don't have a snowball's chance in hell of losing weight.
- 1980s deregulation allowed the food industry to start pitching their products on the large and small screens.

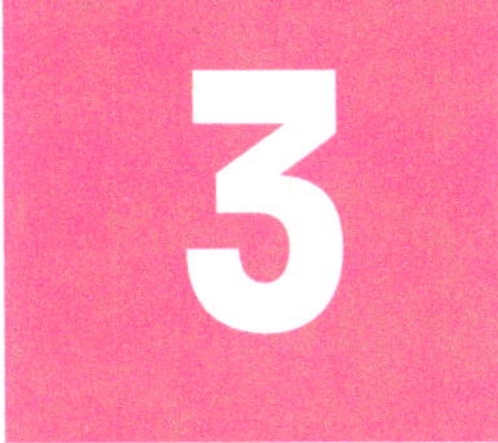

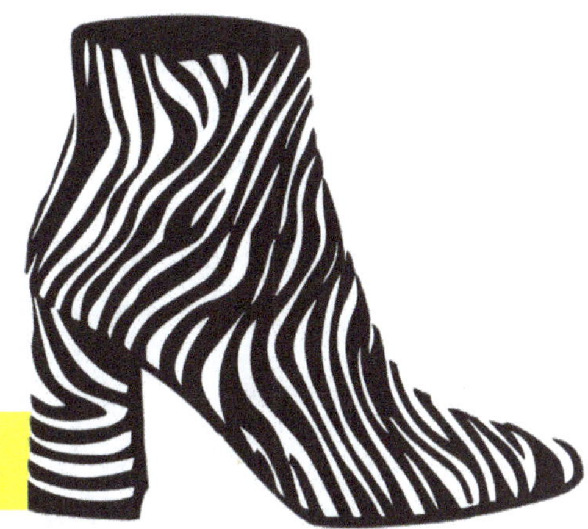

Fat Is Not Public Enemy #1

Am I evoking one of the most potent political rap duos ever to make a point?

Yup.

Because you deserve to know the truth about what a public enemy is, and I'll give you a hint: It's not fat, and it's not Flavor Flav.

You were fed a big FAT lie in the '80s. You were told low-fat food was the answer to all your weight loss prayers, that by eating low-fat versions of everything, from yogurt to butter, you'd be less likely to have heart attacks, and you'd lose weight without feeling deprived of your favorites.

Women across the country could celebrate! Dessert was officially back on the table thanks to guilt-free, low-fat cheesecakes, cookies, and pies.

Moms were told that now they could make healthy choices for their kids—thanks to low-fat Jell-O! The catch? It was all a lie. Low-fat food didn't make us healthier or weigh less; it did the opposite.

When the food companies started using "low-," "non-," and "no-" before "fat," they made fat the enemy.

Think about it. If all the labels put low-fat and no-fat on their products, then fat must be what we're avoiding, and if we're avoiding it, it must be bad.

They didn't tell you that when they took out the fat, they replaced it with sugar.

They also didn't do a hella good job explaining the two types of fat: dietary and body fat. I suppose that made it easier for the marketing companies to vilify fat, make it the enemy, and stereotype it as bad instead of going the extra mile to educate folks.

Of course, we are talking about sales, not school, so I suppose it also checks out that no one mentioned that up until the 1980s, it was common knowledge that carbohydrates and sugar were the driving forces of obesity, not fat.

> *"The amount of plain, starchy foods (cereals, breads, potatoes) taken is what determines, in the case of most people, how much [weight] they gain or lose."*
>
> — Dr. Spock (Spock 1946)

> *"Every woman knows that carbohydrates are fattening; this is a piece of common knowledge, which few nutritionists would dispute."*
>
> — *British Journal of Nutrition* (Passmore 1963)

Well, Damn. If It Wasn't Broke, Why Did We Try to Fix It?

That's a good question that I wanted to answer when I started writing this book. I'll warn you now: The truth is disturbing.

You see, in the 1950s, warning signs showing a connection between sugar consumption and coronary heart disease began to be reported by the Journal of the American Medical Association (JAMA).

If the general public learned of this connection, and journalists and scientists were free to report based on their constitutional rights, the sugar industry stood to lose a lot of market share—I mean, money.

And by money, I mean billions of dollars.

This fact was not lost on Sugar Research Foundation president Henry Hass who, in 1954, addressed the American Society of Sugar Beet Technologists in his speech, "What's New in Sugar Research."

Here's where you want to pay close attention if you briefly checked out because this is where things get super sketchy.

In Henry's speech, he identifies a significant business opportunity, which was to increase sugar's market share by getting Americans to eat a lower-fat diet.

"Leading nutritionists are pointing out the chemical connection between [American's] high-fat diet and the formation of cholesterol which partly plugs our arteries and capillaries, restricts the flow of blood and causes high blood pressure and heart trouble… if you put [the middle-aged man] on a low-fat diet, it takes just five days for the blood cholesterol to get down to where it should be… **If the carbohydrate industries were to recapture this 20 percent of the calories in the U.S. diet (the difference between the 40 percent which fat has and the 20 percent which it ought to have) and if sugar maintained its present share of the carbohydrate market, this change would mean an increase in the per capita consumption of sugar more than a third with a tremendous improvement in general health"** (The American Society of Sugar Beet Technologists 1954, 28,29).

That's when the sugar industry started banking on increasing sugar consumption. And by banking, I mean paying off scientists and journalists, funding studies to skew the scientific data in their favor and strategizing to undermine the United States public health policy regarding sugar. You can read all the sketchy details in the JAMA Internal Medicine article published in November 2016 (Cristin E. Kearns, Laura A. Schmidt and Stanton A. Glantz 2016).

The Original (Sort Of) Scientific Fat Lie

In the '50s, two conflicting schools of thought emerged. One spearheaded by Dr. John Yudkin, an honest man with a Ph.D. in biochemistry and years of independent research, asserted added sugar was the cause—a hypothesis that made him the enemy of The World Sugar Research Organization (Yudkin 1972) (Leslie 2016).

The other theory, backed by Ancel Keys, a clever man with a Ph.D. in oceanography, also known as the "original big data guy," indicted fat and cholesterol as the culprit, making him the sugar industry's poster child. It also scored him a massive grant from the United States Public Health Service that gave him the funds to set sail to study the correlation between diet and cardiovascular disease (Seven Countries Study n.d.).

All the "evidence-based" data pointing away from sugar and vilifying fat stemmed from oceanographer Ancel Keys's research, which would be considered criminal by today's standards.

Keys studied twenty-two countries and found that the people who ate lots of saturated fats had more cholesterol problems and heart disease. It sounds pretty cut and dry on the surface, and that's exactly how the FDA ran with it. The low-fat trend skyrocketed. The food pyramid guidelines told us to avoid butter and opt for margarine.

The problem was that Keys' study left a few things—I mean countries—out. His findings were based on the results of only seven of the twenty-two countries. The other fifteen did not back up his claims.

When Keys' epically weird science pointed to fat as the cause of obesity and cardiovascular disease, the U.S. government answered by issuing the first dietary guidelines in 1980. Food companies answered the call with an abundance of "healthy" low-fat products like I Can't Believe It's Not Butter and low-fat yogurts, low-fat chips, and low-fat frozen pizzas.

Proof That Low Fat Diets Don't Work.

Look around you. Can you spot the obesity epidemic? As of today, 155 million Americans are overweight, according to the U.S. Centers for Disease Control and Prevention (Centers for Disease Control and Prevention 2021). Obesity rates have doubled since 1980. In the '80s, 15% of Americans were considered obese; by 2007, that number had grown to 34% (David S Freedman 2011).

Before you go on a guilt trip because you bought into the hype, slow your roll. Pretty much everybody bought in, including heart surgeons and cardiologists who recommended a low-fat diet to prevent heart disease.

So How in The Name Of Richard Simmons Did We Get Here?

Here's the thing that screwed us all up—when they took out the fat, they had to replace it with something. They knew Americans would not go all-in on tasteless food, so they replaced the fat with sugar, and we got addicted to it. Of course, this didn't do anything but make the problem—and your waistline—bigger. The sugar was addictive, which is why nobody in the history of womankind has eaten just one reduced-fat Snackwell's Devil's Food cookie or reduced-fat Oreo. Or why nobody loses weight on a low-fat diet.

Too bad it has taken us over forty years to reveal the truth. Playing the blame game and pointing fingers at the Sugar Research Foundation, Ancel Keys, or the marketing companies that perpetrated the lie is a waste of time and energy. It's time to embrace the truth and move forward.

Just the Facts, Ma'am – Takeaways

- The sugar industry vilified fat to make money
- The scientific evidence used to create the low-fat hype was flawed
- Low-fat diets are not the answer—they are the problem
- Fat isn't public enemy #1—sugar is.

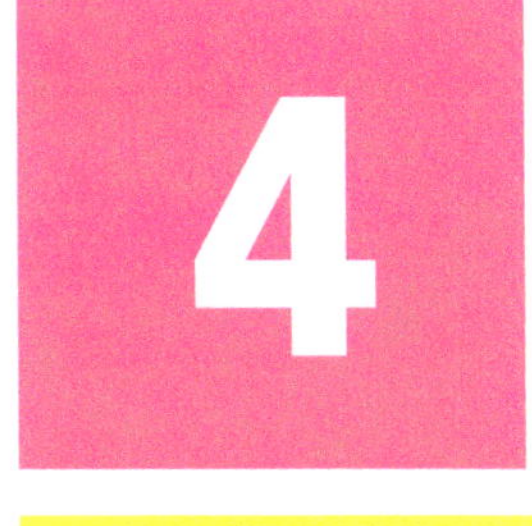

4

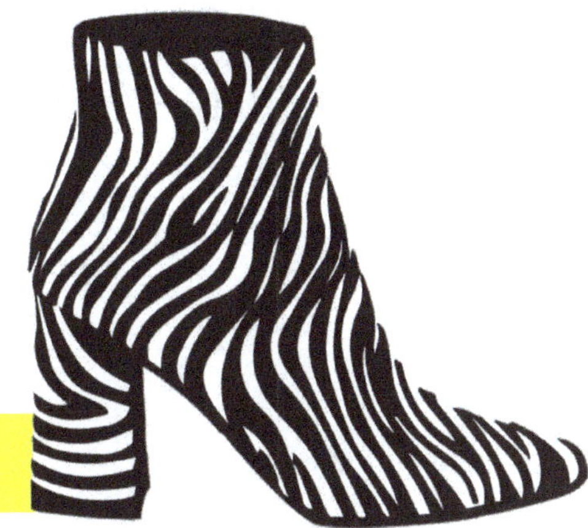

This Is Your Body On Sugar

Do you remember the "Just Say No" campaign? It was Nancy Reagan's platform as First Lady, and nothing said, "Say No to Drugs" like the horrifying parallel of frying one's brain like an egg in a skillet. The commercial was brilliantly created to scare millions of kids to stay drug-free. Damn, Nancy. That shit was harsh, but it got the job done.

Nobody wanted their brain fried over easy. So, if you don't want brain damage, don't do drugs. Message received.

It's a damn shame they didn't warn us about sugar while they were at it.

Chronic Illnesses Associated with Sugar Consumption

Just *look* at all of the chronic illnesses associated with sugar consumption.

- Heart Disease
- Diabetes
- Hypertension
- Obesity
- Insulin Resistance
- Non-Alcoholic Fatty Liver Disease
- Cancer
- Dementia
- Tooth Decay

(Centers for Disease Control and Prevention 2020) (Angelopoulos 2016)

More Sugar Side Effects

But wait, there's more! In addition to disease and tooth decay, anecdotal research shows that sugar impacts your skin, mood, immune system, and energy levels.

1. Premature aging and rapid aging
2. Weakened immune system
3. Loss of libido
4. Hyperactivity
5. Anxiety
6. Trouble focusing

Sugar, The Other White Drug

In 1986, you couldn't turn on the TV without seeing the National Pork Board Commercial for Pork: The Other White Meat. Well, think of sugar as the other white drug.

It's addictive, just like the other addictive white powder you might have come across in the '80s.

Consider a study from 2007 showing cocaine-addicted mice. Researchers gave them a choice: their daily dose of cocaine or sugar. They chose sugar over cocaine within two days (Magalie Lenoir 2007).

I don't know whether to laugh or cry when I hear women refer to sugar consumption like it's not a big deal.

They'll avoid pasta and dessert all day long, but when it comes to a tall glass of sugar, they don't think twice about ordering a sweet tea or stocking their fridge with Gatorade for the kids. They may laugh it off—say something about empty calories—because they honestly have no idea how freaking bad this stuff is. And I think that's by design, y'all.

I don't want to get too conspiracy theory on you, but there's a lot of money in the food industry, and billions are supporting Big Sugar. If the word about sugar gets out, gets too mainstream, major companies would go belly up.

Here's The Truth About Sugar

Consuming sugar leads to much more than empty calories, cavities, and acne. It puts you directly on the "Highway to Hell," also known as Type 2 diabetes and obesity. Sugar ages your skin, damages your immune system, causes hyperactivity and emotional outbursts, and it's crazy addictive (Magalie Lenoir 2007) (James J DiNicolantonio 2018). The worst part of the sugar story is that it gets downplayed as empty calories. Or a little sugar problem. But y'all, this is no joke, and don't feel bad if you didn't know until now. As I said, there's big money betting on you never finding the truth.

Why It's So Hard to *Just Say No* to Sugar

Sugar works in your brain like a drug. That's why it's more than a hard habit to break. Here's the lowdown on what happens after your first bite or sip of sugar.

Sugar gets down to business quickly by activating the sweet taste receptors on your tongue. It creates a chemical reaction that lights up your brain's reward center, triggering the feel-good neurotransmitter dopamine release.

Dopamine is part of the "reward circuit," the same system linked to drug addiction. Dopamine is responsible for the warm and fuzzy "oh, hell yes!" feeling you get when you take a bite of chocolate.

Who hasn't experienced a Meg Ryan moment after chocolate pie? You *feel* that pie. You *love* that pie. *You want to marry that pie.*

As crazy as it sounds, there's a logical reason for wanting to commit your life to a baked good. You've overstimulated your reward system, and now your brain associates this lovin' feeling with sugar, and it is going to crave it, just like a drug. Your brain adjusts every time you eat sugar and releases less dopamine, so the only way to feel the same Meg Ryan style "high" as before is to repeat the behavior with MORE. Over time, your body will need more and more sugar to achieve the same effect.

You'll experience sugar highs and sugar lows, or what I like to call the blood sugar roller coaster from hell.

The Blood Sugar Roller Coaster from Hell

This sugar-high-then-sugar-low phenomenon is also known as the blood sugar roller coaster. It's a ride that millions of people are on at this very moment, without even knowing it. You may be on it right now.

Buckle up, ladies. I'm about to break it down. You're about to learn everything you need to know about why sugar makes you lose control and what to do to get it back.

I grew up in a suburb of Memphis, Tennessee, home of the blues, the best barbeque known to man, and Elvis Presley. Even though Elvis left the building in the seventies, he is celebrated everywhere. His home, Graceland, is now a museum and major tourist attraction. And one of his favorite places, LibertyLand, a once fab amusement park, is now, sadly, a parking lot.

But back in the day (both his and mine), Elvis's favorite ride was the Zippin Pippin. The Pippin was super vintage, as in, old as hell and dangerous. Every time you took a ride, you risked your damn life—which is one of the reasons my mother made me swear I wouldn't ride it and one of the reasons I rode it every single time I went.

The truth is my mother was right. They should've torn down the Pippin in the '80s. It was too old, too creaky, and under repair every other hour because, bottom line, it was dangerous as hell.

The Pippin was all about death drops. You'd go up, up, up, and with every inch you climbed you'd hear a *creak, creak, creak* because, hello, we were riding on an original 1950s wood-tracked roller coaster. Once you had creaked your way to the top and breathed a sigh of relief that you weren't dead, yet, without warning, you'd free fall.

Let me just tell you, more than one kid pissed their pants on the Pippin—per hour. That's how freaking powerful this thing was. And why mothers everywhere feared the attraction. It was unsafe for everyone, but at least we were warned.

Believe it or not, the blood sugar roller coaster is more dangerous because nobody tells you the risks involved until it's too late. You find yourself with a mad sugar addiction; you're overweight, or worse, diagnosed with diabetes or heart disease.

Your Life on the Roller Coaster

Emotional outbursts. Mad cravings. Insane breakouts. You are going through hell every day, and your weight hasn't budged. Holy bleep, Batman, is this menopause? Advanced age? It gets so frustrating that you think it's time to hang up all your revenge body dreams, embrace Gawd-awful blousy tops, Pajama Jeans and Crocs and take up more appropriate ways to pass the time, like adult coloring books or basket weaving.

No. No. No. And yeah, I feel you on those Crocs. Look, up until this point, you may have thought you've been going crazy. But what if I told you that all your frustrations would be gone if you cut the sugar?

Let's say you are eating a big-ass salad for lunch. You skipped the dressing and went with olive oil, so you think you made a healthy choice. Then you ordered a sweet tea to drink. That's where you screwed up. The second that sugar hits your system, your blood sugar levels skyrocket before the sugar starts to give you a little buzz.

Meanwhile, your body has your back because it has a built-in system in place for dealing with this sudden spike in blood sugar: insulin.

Here's the thing. Your body can burn this sugar as energy—if you're active immediately after you eat it. So, if you're running a marathon after lunch every day, you're cool. The problem is you're not. None of us are.

We're working at our desks, sitting for long periods scrolling through Facebook and Livin' La Vida Sedentary. We are nowhere close to the active hunters and gatherers our primal ancestors were.

When you are inactive, your body isn't burning sugar; it stores it as fat. And while your body is busy storing that sugar, your bloodstream picks up on the auto-generated internal memo: Your blood sugar is down.

That's about the time the buzz from the sugar wears off. You get cranky. Deb from accounting is starting to get on your last damn nerve. You're like that dude who morphs into Betty White in the Snickers commercial. Suddenly you're starving, and you need another hit.

Time for another ride on the coaster...

The vicious cycle continues as you repeat the process multiple times throughout the day, and your body builds up its fat stores repeatedly.

A Not-So-Tubular 1980s Solution to Gauge Sugar Consumption

The glycemic index (GI) is an index that ranks carbohydrates from low to high. This number measures how much a food impacts blood sugar.

The glycemic scale concept came in 1981 to determine which foods were better for people with diabetes, and the idea behind it was solid. It was designed to be a tool to help people identify the foods that have the most significant effect on blood sugar, so they could make healthier choices.

I'll walk you through the three Glycemic Index categories, examples of each one, as well as the factors that impact the GI of foods.

The glycemic index (GI) is broken down into three categories that rank food on a scale of zero to 100. When it comes to GI numbers, lower is better. The lower the GI, the less effect it will have on your blood sugar.

There are three GI rating categories.

- Low GI: 1 to 55:

  Examples: Almonds, apples, carrots, chia seeds, cherries, grapefruit, hemp seeds, macadamia nuts, minimally processed grains, oranges, pears, peaches, pistachios, poultry, sesame seeds, strawberries, and seafood.

- Moderate GI: 56 to 69:

  Examples: Bananas, couscous, white and sweet potatoes, sweet corn, and white rice.

- High GI: 70 and higher:

  Examples: Bagels, breads, breakfast cereals, cakes, cookies, crackers, croissants, doughnuts, fruit juice, oats, muffins, pasta, sodas, and smoothies.

While knowledge is power, and the GI is a good source of information, there are several variables that impact the GI of a food that can make using it frustrating.

- Cooking: Cooking foods raises the GI because the body digests cooked food faster. The longer a food is cooked, the higher the GI will be.
- Ripeness: The riper the fruit, the higher the GI.

- Combinations of foods: GI values are based on the effect of food eaten alone not in combination with other foods. This can cause a huge amount of variation in the effect on blood sugars.
- Nutrients: Adding fats or proteins slows digestion and will reduce the glycaemic response.
- Type of Sugar: Not all sugars share the same GI. For example, the GI of table sugar is 63, while keto-friendly Stevia GI is 0.

Just The Facts, Ma'am – Takeaways

- Eating sugar isn't just bad for your waistline—sugar consumption is harmful to your overall health and can lead to cardiovascular disease, high blood pressure, insulin resistance, and dementia.
- Eating sugar ages your skin, weakens your immune system, causes hyperactivity, mood swings, and negatively impacts your sex life.
- Sugar is hard to quit because it's just as addictive as cocaine and heroin (Magalie Lenoir 2007) (James J DiNicolantonio 2018).
- Sugar causes you to ride the blood sugar roller coaster all day (the vicious cycle of blood sugar spikes, mood swings, and hunger).
- The Glycemic Index is a scale that tells you how foods impact blood sugar.
- High Glycemic Foods to Avoid: bread, baked goods, rice, cereal, pasta, starchy veggies, and sugar-filled drinks.
- Your best choices for a low-carb lifestyle are low G.I. foods like seafood, poultry, nuts, and seeds.

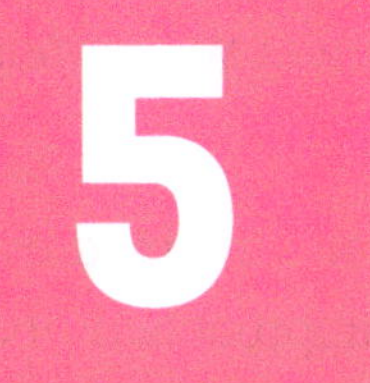

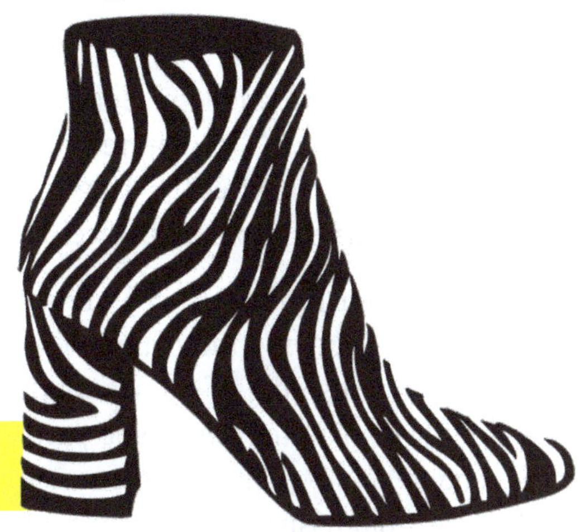

Turns Out, The GD Germans Have Everything To Do With It

(Or How Carbs Really Are The Devil)

Full disclosure, I'm fully aware that this reference to the legendary Burt Reynolds movie *Smokey and the Bandit* is technically from '77 but work with me on this one. It is 100% germane to our topic you need to know.

If we're thinking critically here, which we are, then the question we have to ask is, what changed? If we were healthy in the 1950s with our common-sense approach to weight, i.e., avoiding carbs and sugar, what have we done differently in the past seventy-some odd years that resulted in an obesity epidemic?

Did our iPhones make us gain weight? Netflix? New technologies? No. It was the carbohydrates.

When I say "carbs," I mean all starches and sugars. Sure, there may be a few subtle differences between the molecular structures, but I'll spare you the science lesson and cut to the chase—your body breaks down all carbohydrates into sugar. No matter what the source is.

So, if low-fat diets don't work, and counting calories is BS, what in the hell is making us so fat?

Well, that's a fabulous question, and, based on our major obesity crisis, you'd think it was a real head-scratcher. But it turns out we've known since 1908. And yes, the Germans did have everything to do with it.

Which was part of the problem. Before WWII, if you wanted the legit 411 on nutrition, endocrinology, and genetics, German research was the go-to, the respected gold standard for evidence-based medicine. After the war? Not so much. The anti-German sentiment was strong, as evidenced by Sheriff Buford T. Justice.

Here's the deal. In 1908, Gustav Von Bergmann came up with a theory that explained everything. Instead of shifting the blame of weight gain onto an individual, he approached obesity biologically as a disorder of fat accumulation. He even invented a term—lipophilia, meaning "love of fat"—explaining why some parts of the body get fat and others do not. And why some people tend to gain weight and others stay rail-thin no matter what they eat. That fat accumulation differed from tissue to tissue, depending on the person.

Just like some people are hairy, and some are not. Some guys have a hairy chest; some have two hairs on a nipple—it's a genetic thing.

Fat works the same way. Some women gain weight in their butt and hips; others get big arms. It all depends on the person.

By the 1920s, the lipophilia theory was catching on in Vienna, and by the 1930s, it was widely accepted in Europe and was making its way into the U.S.

Then World War II happened, and within ten years, the idea pretty much disappeared.

By the sixties, most psychologists were profiting from framing obesity as an eating disorder. But there was at least one who was thinking logically, Edwin Astwood, Rebel hero and President of the Endocrinology Society.

He wasn't buying the idea that obesity was the result of overeating. His explanation, given in his "Heritage of Corpulence" lecture (E. B. Astwood 1962), where he flexed his critical thinking skills, went like this:

If we focus on the evidence (what a fab idea) as in the fat and fat tissue, we could address it adequately without any preconceived notions (or blaming you).

He asked all the questions you and your girlfriends discuss at that book club meeting where nobody reads the book. First, he asked, "what about our genes?" It made sense to him to credit heredity for at least some of our weight problems—as in, it runs in the family—so, why not look into genetics? If we credit our genes for our hair color and how tall we are, why not credit it with weight?

Then, he dug into the science. He researched the hormones and enzymes associated with fat—some work to accumulate it, others work to move it out—and found it's a balance between these that determine whether or not your cells hold onto it or release it.

In the '80s, the researchers pretty much quit trying to work out this delicate balance and shifted the blame to you. It was a more straightforward message to sell. You overeat, you get fat—end of story.

Except that's not the end. The truth is, there is one primary hormone that plays a starring role in the accumulation of fat, and that hormone is insulin.

Insulin is the regulator of fat metabolism. Insulin is the fat-storing hormone, and we hate her for that, but she has a big job to do. She keeps your blood sugar levels from getting too high (hyperglycemia) or too low (hypoglycemia). She determines whether you use the carbs as energy or store them for a rainy day.

And what drives insulin levels? Carbohydrates.

As much as you may agree or disagree with genetic factors associated with fat, there's not much you can do about it. But there is something you can do about insulin, and that's cut carbs.

Just the Facts, Ma'am – Takeaways

- Your body breaks down all carbohydrates into sugar. We did not have an obesity epidemic in the 1950s when we avoided carbs and sugar.
- Gustav Von Bergmann's theory approached obesity as a disorder of fat accumulation that explained why some people gain weight more than others. The idea disappeared after World War II.
- In 1962, Edwin Astwood found it's balance between hormones and enzymes associated with fat that determine whether or not your cells hold onto it or release it.
- One primary hormone plays a starring role in the accumulation of fat, and that hormone is insulin.
- Insulin is the regulator of fat metabolism. Insulin is the fat-storing hormone.
- Carbohydrates drive insulin levels.

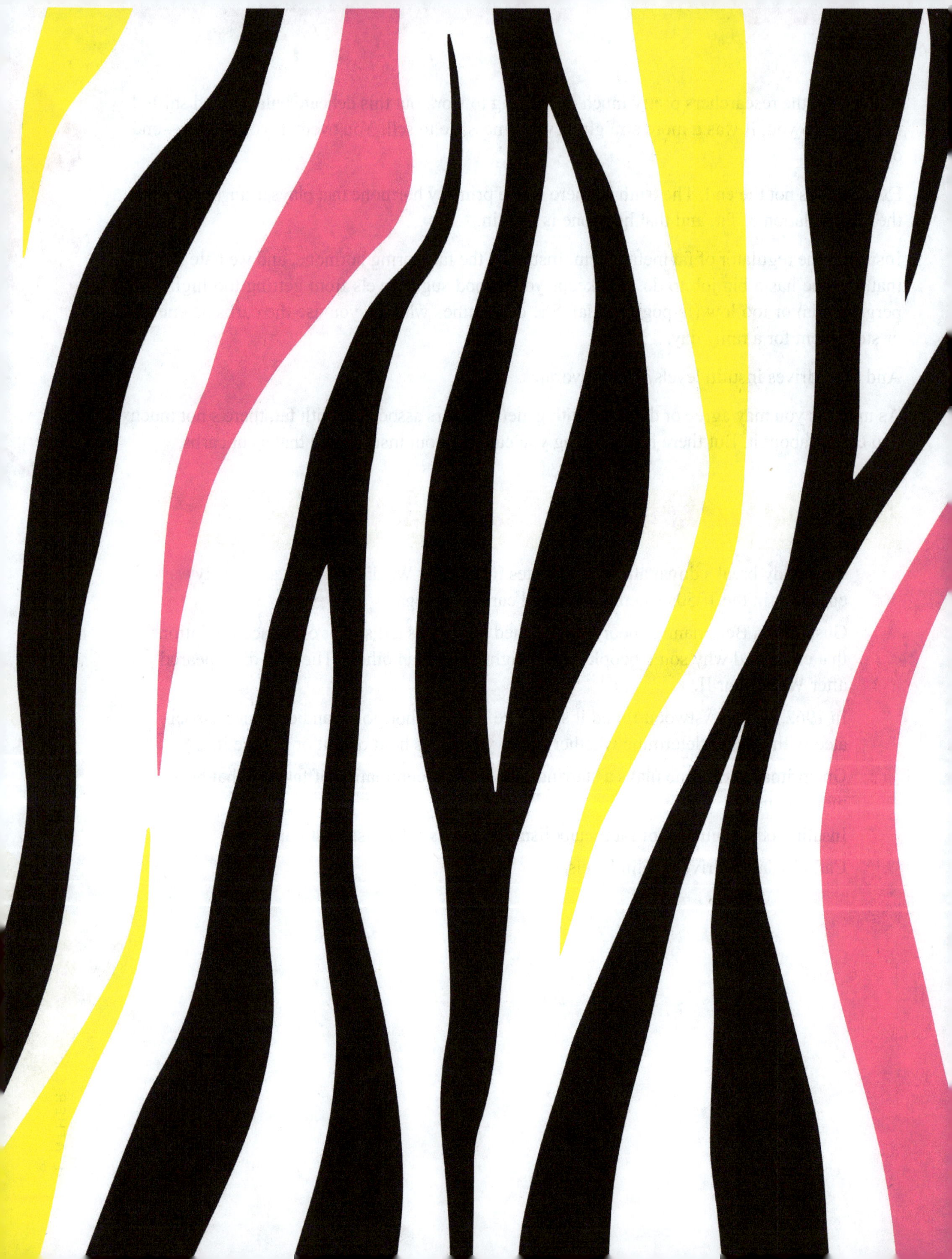

6

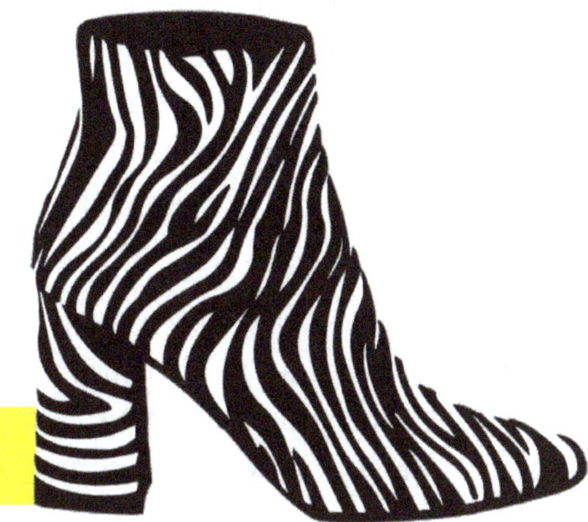

The "Calories In, Calories Out" Lie

When it comes to girls of the 1980s, there were two types: Those who sat up all night obsessed with finding the solution to the Rubik's cube, and those who said screw it and tried to manipulate their way to the win by rearranging the stickers. The cube craze was epic. Millions were obsessed by the original gangster of fidget toys, making it the best-selling toy in U.S. history.

So yeah, it was hip to be square for a while, working out one of the 43 quintillion possible combinations (that's eighteen zeroes in case you're counting) without a freaking guide (there was NO instruction manual) and NO options for shortcuts. Keep in mind this was pre-Google. In other words, you were on your own and most likely frustrated AF, which is why the mainstream popularity gradually faded; because it was Mission Impossible, and who wants to spend all of their time working on a hella frustrating puzzle?

Nobody.

Trying to lose weight following the status quo advice to "eat less, move more" is like attempting to master the Rubik's cube while hiking Mount Kilimanjaro naked in stiletto heels, especially when you've been following a totally bogus "guide." You end up feeling like a failure, hopeless and frustrated, blaming yourself for lack of willpower or shaming yourself because the number on the scale refuses to move.

It doesn't have to be this way.

The truth is you're not up against an impossible puzzle; you've just been handed the wrong solutions. This chapter will explain why counting calories and suffering through workouts you despise isn't just unnecessary, it's ridiculous. The "burn more calories than you consume" approach creates an unhealthy relationship with food and exercise.

More than one-third of Americans are obese—that's twice the amount from forty years ago. The proof is in the pudding, folks—just take a look at the results. In 1980, we were looking at an obesity rate of 12-14%, now it's 42% (Centers for Disease Control and Prevention 2021) (Craig M. Hales 2020) (David S Freedman 2011). After following the advice of trusted physicians and government-issued diet advice, we got fat and sick.

Look, I know this may sound shocking, but you've got to trust me that limiting and counting calories does not work. I know it's the standard operating procedure. I understand that it's tough to wrap your head around because counting calories is all you have known until now—and I realize that cutting and counting calories is how most doctors and "experts" tell you to lose weight. So, let me ask you something: If everybody's doing it, why should you?

Conventional Wisdom: *Obesity occurs when a person consumes more calories than he or she burns.* (Medical News Today 2020)

Truth: *Weight loss achieved in calorie-restrictive diets is "so small as to be clinically insignificant."* (S Pirozzo 2002)

You may be surprised that no amount of "feeling the burn" at the gym will help you lose weight. It sounds too good to be true, especially if you'd rather light yourself on fire than do another step workout. Rest assured, I'm not pulling your leotard.

Remember, Rebels don't take conventional wisdom as fact, especially when it doesn't yield results. We question it, we ask why, and we uncover the truth. Warning: The information you are about to receive will liberate you from counting calories and the gym. I kid you not.

"The truth will set you free, but first, it will piss you off."

— Gloria Steinem

If we lived in a perfect world where everything made sense, the logic behind the "use more calories than you consume" mentality works. Movement—any physical activity—burns calories. So, if we move more, we burn more, and as long as we don't replace those calories, we lose weight.

Unfortunately, we don't live in a utopia of logic and understanding.

The eighties decade's dogma was that weight loss success depended on cutting calories and jazzercising your way to a size 6 Gloria Vanderbilt blue jean. They told us it was simple math because, duh, the fewer calories you eat, the less you weigh. Eat less, move more, lose weight.

Ahem, bullshit! (cough)

Of course, we know this is like, lousy advice now.

What is a Calorie? Or Why a One-Size-Fits-All, Calories In/Calories Out Diet Fails

Let's break down what a calorie is so you'll understand why stressing about them is a time suck. A calorie is a unit of measure, just like ounces, pounds, or inches. The logic behind limiting calories is that if you eat a limited "prescribed" number of calories per day, minus however many you burn doing the Jane Fonda Workout, you'll lose weight. Simple enough, right?

Wrong. We know this one-size-(or calorie)-fits-all mentality is unrealistic for a few reasons.

1. All calories are not created equal. The source of the calorie, the quality of the food you are eating, matters much more than the number listed on the nutrition label.

2. No two bodies are identical. Your metabolism is not the same as your best friend's. Your digestive system isn't twinning with your OB/GYN either. So, if all of you made a pact to team up and go on a diet journey together, eat the down-to-the-letter same 1,200 calories per day diet, one thing is guaranteed: You will not get the same results. Why? Because your bodies are not identical. We are all unique, special snowflakes with various rates of metabolism.

3. It is ridiculous to convince yourself that you need to eat, let's say, 1,200 calories per day because you and I both know your day-to-day activity changes. Hell, some days, you'll be stuck at your desk for hours on end. You'll be stressed out, sedentary, and praying to God Janice from accounting won't try to sell you Rodan & Fields again. Other days you'll be on your feet non-stop, running from one mandatory volunteer project to another, picking up Legos and laundry (yes, that counts), or chasing your dog. Look, I don't know your life, but I know this: Some days, you'll require more energy and calories than others.

So why torture yourself trying to keep up?

Wait—If Exercise Doesn't Work for Weight Loss, Why Does Everyone (and my mother) Say it Does?

Good question. Okay, so the reason you hear this advice at your doctor's office, in magazines, on Facebook, or inside any one of the million *Get Fit and Watch the Pounds Melt Away* weight loss books isn't because everyone is a pathological liar, or that they're so misinformed they need a lobotomy. It's because that approach contains an element of truth—it works the first or second time you try it.

It may be how you lost weight in college or after your first pregnancy. The problem with your past successful adventures in weight loss? It won't work again. Your body adapts to the calorie deficit.

Here's why.

Your metabolism wants your body to survive. It doesn't give a friggity frack about anything else. It doesn't care that you have a high school reunion coming up or that you just planned a Hawaiian vacation, so you need a #beachbody ASAP. Your metabolism is responsible for storing fat. It isn't because she's an evil witch; it's because she doesn't want you to die of starvation during, say, a famine.

Why Dramatic Diets and Hours of Cardio Won't Help You Lose Weight or What Your Science Teacher should have Covered under Evolution

In case you didn't know, your body is more brilliant than anything Steve Jobs created—even a MacBook Pro. It has customized, built-in programming to keep you alive without giving it a second thought.

Think about it. When was the last time you had to remind your lungs to breathe or your heart to beat? Never, right? It just knows.

Your body's response to massive calorie deficits from diet and exercise is another built-in program for your survival. Its goal is to keep your stored fat safe so you'll have it when you need it. It's your body's rainy-day fund for fat, a better-safe-than-sorry approach that keeps you alive on autopilot.

When you cut calories, and you force yourself to exercise, this built-in survival network kicks in.

Your Brain on a Restrictive Calorie + Exercise Diet

Since I'm a little insane in the membrane, I imagine this auto-survive mechanism playing out like a sci-fi movie in the brain.

You: Cut calories to 1500 per day.

Your Body: Uh, oh. Something is up; she is not getting enough food. Cue the off-the-chain hunger signals. That'll force her to eat so we can keep our fat storage safe.

You: Added a hardcore spin class to your daily routine

Your Body: Danger! Intense calorie burning is a direct threat to our fat stores and survival! Send in the big guns! Make her so hungry she feels sick. We must make up for all calorie deficits.

Okay, so I'll never be Steven Spielberg, but you get the point. Your body is designed to counteract every calorie cut, whether it is from the calories you put in or the ones you burn on the treadmill.

In other words, it's not you; it's evolution. You don't have an appetite control problem like the folks at Dexatrim would have you believe, and there's nothing wrong with your willpower, *thank you very much.*

Think about it, how many times have you hit the gym—hard—only to come home STARVING? You tell yourself you have earned it with literal sweat and maybe a few tears, but if you're trying to lose weight, you'd be better off skipping the gym.

Your weight loss problems are due to misinformation, not some deep emotional disconnect, psychological issues, or laziness.

Now that you know the truth, that 95% of extreme diets fail miserably, you can free yourself of that shame and effort and get down to business doing what works (Steele 2019).

Counting calories is a time suck and a distraction that keeps you from paying attention to your food quality—more specifically, where your calories are coming from.

Do not, I repeat, do not fall for low-fat food gimmicks. Remember, when they took out the fat, they replaced it with sugar, which does not make you feel full like fats and proteins. Sugar makes you crave more sugar. That is why you always feel like you're starving on a low-fat diet.

Then Why Does Everybody Say Calories Matter?

Calorie counting became a thing in the U.S. during World War I (that's 1914-1918 for those keeping up with the timeline) because of global food shortages. The American government needed a way to get us to cut back on food intake. So, they published the Scientific Diet, which supported their needs. The whole thing revolved around calorie counting as a means of losing weight. But it was complicated.

Enter Dr. Lulu.

You can also thank (or curse) Dr. Lulu Hunt Peters for your soul-sucking calorie counting nightmare. If the Scientific Diet lit the calorie counting flame, Lulu started the damn fire when she published *Diet & Health: With Key to the Calories* (Peters 1918).

See, Lulu wanted to sell books and weight loss advice to middle-aged American women, and that's what she did. Her book was the first of its kind to reframe the way we think about food. Thanks to this chick, food was no longer something we viewed as nourishment. It was a number. A piece of bread was no longer a piece of bread, it was 100 calories. In other words, she simplified the concept of calories and turned the food into numbers.

Of course, more calorie-restrictive diets followed suit. (That tends to happen when millions of books sell.)

You may remember the Weight Watchers commercials from the 1980s, featuring women beaming with joy over the fact that, thanks to Weight Watchers, you can have desserts! (They left out that those low-fat cheesecakes were full of sugar.)

Or maybe you or someone who lived close enough for you to smell tried Satan's weight loss plan, The Cabbage Soup diet? They may have different names, but the message to women was loud and clear: eat fewer calories and lose weight.

The good news is we know these low-calorie diets are short-term bullshit. You may lose a few pounds, but you won't keep it off because you will feel like crap. You'll yo-yo diet. You will put your body through hell, going from starving to binging—and if you have any energy left to exercise, it won't matter. Let me repeat that. Exercising will not help you because your body is working against you every step of the way.

No disrespect to exercise; there is no doubt you need it for a million reasons, but not for weight loss. It's not a reliable long-term strategy.

A Few (More) Good Reasons to Stay Out of the Gym

Remember my brain on the calorie deficit example from earlier? Well, in case you skimmed over it, here's a reminder. When your body detects any calorie deficit, it automatically sends hunger signals because it senses you are in danger of jeopardizing your fat stores. This explains why you get hungry after a workout. This hunger, combined with the self-sabotaging voice that tells you that you deserve a Snickers, often translates into canceling out all of your efforts at the gym.

Now that you know the truth about calorie restrictive diets, and exercising for weight loss, your gut instinct may be to mourn for all those years you beat yourself up over perceived failures. You may feel compelled to call your gym and tell them to stick your membership where the sun doesn't shine. That's a natural reaction, and I love your passion. Instead of wasting your energy lamenting the past, let's take that enthusiasm and apply it to learning the truth. In the next chapter, I'll break down how and why Rebel Keto works.

Just the Facts, Ma'am – Takeaways

- Counting calories to lose weight is not an effective weight loss strategy.
- Calories in versus calories out diet plans fail you because they do not take the quality of your food into account.
- Exercising is an essential practice for overall health and well-being, but it is not recommended as a tool to lose weight.

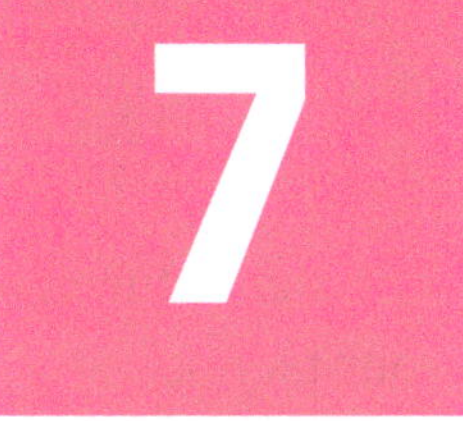

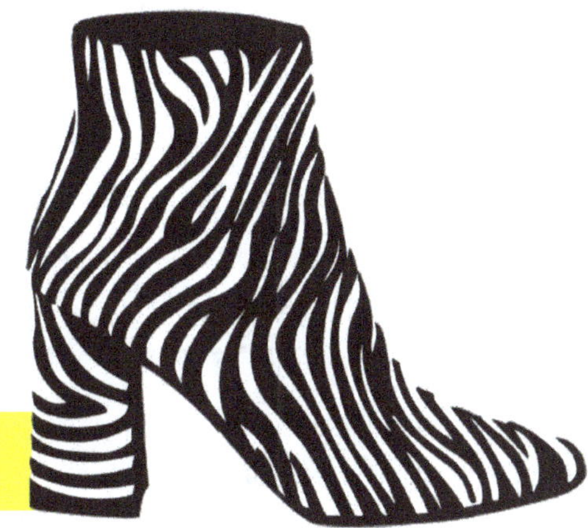

7 Why Rebel Keto And How Keto Works

Despite what you may have heard, the keto diet is not new, and it isn't a trendy diet. It's been around since 1921, when Dr. Russell Wilder developed it at the Mayo Clinic for children with epilepsy, not obesity (Wilder 1921).

The ketogenic diet's popularity didn't take off until January of 2013 when a press release for an article in *Science* claimed the keto diet could:

"… Slow the aging process and may one day allow scientists to better treat or prevent age-related disease, including heart disease, Alzheimer's, and many forms of cancer" (Tadahiro Shimazu 2013).

This is accurate A.F. The Standard American diet that's full of sugar isn't just bad for your health and weight, it also damages your skin, which causes you to look like you qualify for a senior discount way before your time. As for cardiovascular disease, Alzheimer's, and cancer? Well, the ketogenic diet may be one of the most well-researched eating plans on the planet. Numerous (and legitimate) studies have indicated that a ketogenic diet reduces cardiovascular disease (diabetes, heart disease, stroke) (Jornayvaz 2017), and some suggest it's beneficial for certain types of cancer (Tadahiro Shimazu 2013). Ketogenic diets are also known to reduce the frequency of migraines and help increase energy levels. (I can vouch for both.)

Sports Cars and Crap Gas or What's (Self) Love Got to Do with It?

You don't have to get a Ph.D. in Ketogenic Science for keto to work for you but having a general understanding of how ketosis works will help motivate you. And it turns out, it is all about self-love. Let me explain.

Let's pretend that you just got a new car, and because we are in an imaginary land, let's make it fabulously expensive—say, a Porsche. You're in love with this car. It makes you feel confident, sexy, and strong.

Inside the owner's guide, which you read like a Danielle Steel novel, you note that your new Porsche requires service every 5,000 miles, so you dutifully make a note in your planner.

Then, as you're searching for how to sync your phone because, hello, you need to pump up the jam, you notice the dashboard warning guide.

There it is in BOLD CAPS.

FAILURE TO USE PREMIUM FUEL MAY CAUSE SEVERE DAMAGE TO THE ENGINE AND VOID WARRANTY.

You then make another note in your planner—this time in red ink. 93 Octane Only!!! You underline it three times for full effect.

Now, are you going to roll the dice at the gas station the next time you need a fill-up? Opt for 87 octane because it's cheaper and readily available? Accidentally screw up by using diesel?

Hell to the no. You've been warned not to. This is one rule you decide to follow because the possibility of damage outweighs any short-term savings you may benefit from by going the cheap route.

Well, you know what else deserves high-octane fuel? Your body. No matter how expensive that dream car is, it pales in comparison to the priceless, irreplaceable vehicle that is you.

If your body came with an owner's guide like your car, that manual would tell you that its preferred fuel for optimal performance is fat, not sugar. In other words, fats are the body's preferred 93 octane, whereas carbohydrates and sugar are the cheap gas.

But to understand why your body performs better burning fat, you first need to understand your body when it's operating as a sugar burner. A sugar-burner burns carbohydrates for fuel.

When you eat carbs like bread, potatoes, candy, and rice, your body breaks them down into a sugar called glucose, which gets converted into energy.

Now, this sounds like an ideal scenario until you consider that your body has no reason to turn to its fat stores for fuel. Why should it when you're supplying it with a steady stream of carbs all day?

The fact is that running on a diet filled with sugars prevents your body from accessing stored fat for energy because it's relying on glucose. This means your body cannot oxidize fat, so you end up saving more.

To make matters worse, when you are a sugar-burner, your body can't use the fat you eat for fuel, which means instead of burning fat for energy, it stores it for a rainy day.

Another biggie is that sugar fuel is short-term. The energy you get from junk food, pasta, and bread does not last long. In other words, you are guaranteed to become hungry a few hours after eating.

That's why you are always hungry (or *hangry*). You know, hangry, the irritable state that occurs when hungry meets angry?

Yeah, well, that's the blood sugar roller coaster.

You eat more carbs and sugar and hop back on the roller coaster. You're cranky; you're irritated; you're hangry. It's a vicious cycle, and it's the reason so many people struggle with weight.

Keto = Burning Fat for Fuel

On the other hand, when you're following the keto diet and using fat for fuel, your body *can* access stored fat for energy. Your blood sugar levels stabilize, which means the days of the blood sugar roller coaster are behind you. Your energy levels improve because the healthy fats you're eating provide you with a steady stream of sustained energy. You feel full, your cravings are gone, and you no longer rely on sugar highs or suffer from sugar lows.

Nutritional Ketosis

We'll talk about how following a keto diet means cutting carbs in this chapter, but there's more to a ketogenic lifestyle than a gigantic NO list. I think it's time to talk about the bigger plan, the star of the show. And that, my friends, is ketosis. You won't get there by just cutting carbs out of your diet.

Ketosis: A safe, natural metabolic state in which the *body uses fat for fuel* instead of carbohydrates. *

* Not to be confused with diabetic ketoacidosis (DKA)—which is a life-threatening condition for people with out-of-control diabetes.

But before we talk about the path to ketosis, let's look at what our destination is all about.

Ketosis brings mental clarity, increased energy, and weight loss. A scientist or a diet guru didn't invent ketosis. It is evolution's solution to starvation. It's what our bodies naturally do to keep us alive in famine times. Fortunately, you don't have to starve to get there.

Ketone bodies, or ketones, are a natural source of energy. They're made in the liver as a by-product of the breakdown of fat. This process is known as fat oxidation.

Your body and your brain use these ketone bodies for fuel—high octane gas that primes your engine for high-performance benefits.

Let's circle back to our imaginary dream car running on premium 93 octane fuel.

My dad owned an auto parts store, and he loved cars—working on them, fixing them up, and driving them fast.

While I didn't share my dad's passion for vehicles (particularly Mustangs), I loved being his sidekick at all the car shows. One of the perks of owning a mom-and-pop parts store in the '80s was getting free tickets to all the cool car events. You know, the ones where they'd roll out the red carpet and premiere the world's most crazy expensive luxury cars. If you remembered to ask the right people, they'd let you sit in the driver's seat, and that was my jam.

Even though I still haven't made it to driving a European sports car, I like to imagine my body as an elegant, uber-luxe, six-figure dream mobile.

And you know what I wouldn't put in the tank?

Crap gas.

No, my vehicle runs smoother and performs better on high octane fuel. That's what ketones are, the most excellent fuel for your body and your brain.

Once you're running on ketones, your body has what it needs to perform at optimal performance. You've switched from sugar-burner to fat-burner, your blood sugar stabilizes, and fat burning increases.

It's a fact that ketones are a very potent fuel for your brain. Medical research suggests that ketones can play a vital role in treating brain diseases and conditions from concussions to memory loss.

You will also feel more alert; your skin will glow from the inside out, and *ding! ding!* The pounds start melting away. It's like hitting the weight loss and preventive health care jackpot.

Well, Keto Sounds Amazing ... So, Why Rebel Keto?

It's no secret that the keto diet is strict. Keeping your net carb intake to 20 per day is hard. Keeping them down to 20 net while ensuring you're getting the essential nutrients is nearly impossible without a nutritionist and a full-time chef. Add in that it's not a sustainable way to live, and you've got three damn good reasons to avoid it like the plague.

Every day, I see women in my health coaching practice who'd thrive on a keto diet, but they talk themselves out of even trying it because it's too complicated and strict. They don't want to learn how to count macros or keep up with net carbs because they know they don't have time or the desire to do math at mealtime.

I don't know a woman who *does* have that kind of time.

When I started following what I thought was keto eight years ago, I didn't play by the rules. I didn't know I needed to track macros to get to ketosis, and I would've never agreed to follow a diet that required me to do math before meals. I didn't know what ketosis was, and I still lost weight. Now, I know it wasn't luck or a fluke that I lost 148 pounds on my Rebel version of keto because I have kept that weight off for seven years.

Instead of throwing a book of rules that I didn't follow at you, I'm giving you a choice. It's up to you.

Option A: Lazy-ish

I'm not about to hand you a set of stringent, nearly impossible rules to live by and criticize you for breaking them.

Who wants to live that life? Not me.

I prefer to view what most people commonly describe as the "keto diet rules" as *guidelines.*

You get to decide how you implement these guidelines. I freaking despise the word "lazy" when referring to keto because anyone who has tried to diet before knows there is not a damn thing lazy about it.

It's freaking hard to change your eating habits; it's frustrating to have to read labels when you only have ten minutes to spare at the grocery store.

The connotations around the L-word straight up piss me off.

But the facts are the facts. *Lazy* has worked its apathetic way into the keto diet vocabulary, and I can't change that.

Doing lazy keto means tracking your carb intake only—typically keeping the amount to around 20 per day. This appeals to mass quantities of folks overwhelmed by keeping up with the other macronutrients like fats and proteins.

And I get it because that is how I did keto for the first six months. If someone had told me I would have to keep up with every bite of food when I started, I would have quit.

The "lazy" approach worked for me. I started losing weight fast; I started feeling better and more secure and confident. I was motivated, and that kept me going, and I continued learning as I went.

Look, this is your body we are talking about here, not a number on the scale, and not that size six dress you saw on PopSugar. Your body is your vehicle for life, and it is the only one you will ever have.

Whatever motivates you, whatever path you want to take that enables you to succeed, take it.

Whatever path you choose, there is no judgment here. I'm not the Keto Police.

Option B: Hardcore Tracking

You may decide that counting macronutrients (protein, fats, and carbs) for every meal will help you learn as you go and stick to it. You can feel confident that going all-in will get your body into ketosis—the ultimate fat-fueled metabolic state. I'll walk you through what you need to do to get there, step by step.

But first … set yourself up with a Macro Tracker.

You can find one at rebelketo.com/the-vault. Or use My Fitness Pal. It isn't hard to set yourself up on either tracking system, and you'll be able to log in your foods to see what percentage of fat, protein, and carbs each food or meal contains. Going this route may seem like a significant pain, but it keeps you accountable, on track, and most importantly, it helps you learn what's keto-friendly as you go.

Before you dive into counting macros and net carbs, I encourage you to learn as much as you can about the keto diet. No matter what you may have heard, there is no one-size-fits-all approach to living a ketogenic lifestyle.

Sure, there are foods on the *no* list and a few basic principles to master, but how you implement these rules is totally up to you.

Here's the thing: Both ways work for weight loss. You may or may not reach nutritional ketosis with the lazy route. As I said, I'm not here to judge you. I'm here to walk you through your options.

Know that success lies in finding the right balance for you. Either way, remember that changing your eating style is a considerable challenge. You'll make mistakes, you'll fall off the keto wagon, and there will be days you want to say screw it; life is too short to live without cookies. Be prepared for those moments. Embrace failure, and do not beat yourself up when you slip. Keep going.

You Don't Need Another Diet

What we are doing with Rebel Keto is similar to the standard keto diet in that we are cutting out most carbohydrates. Still, since we refuse to stereotype an entire food category, we're not eliminating all carbs forever.

We are not adhering to the conventional wisdom that you have to do just one diet or that you have to diet at all. You know what? I'm not too fond of the word *diet*. It's a four-letter word, just like *hell*, *shit*, and *damn*, because to hell with a damn diet. No one wants to do it. You hear the word, and you think, "Oh hell, here we go again."

Rebel Keto is not a short-term quick fix. It's an outline for a healthy, sustainable lifestyle that prolongs a quality life, helps you lose weight, helps you get off medication, helps you feel better, and works because it's based on the truth. It's honest-to-God truth and the right way to freaking eat. You deserve that.

Rebel Keto—The Best of Both Worlds

I spent the last four years researching all the latest diets available to torture yourself with. When you get past the marketing, all the shiny logos and promises that these media teams develop to sell you on these diets, they all have one thing in common: eliminating the worst carbohydrates you can eat—processed carbs and sugar.

So, it makes sense to me to take the best from the diets that work and put them into one mega-plan. Not a program that requires you to count calories, net carbs, points, or protein forever. That's not how I lost 100 pounds, and it's not how we roll on Rebel Keto.

I've taken everything I learned as a health coach and years of research and personal experience to incorporate the best aspects of keto and other dietary theories into one super plan.

We're Not Gonna Take It Anymore

Like every good teen angst song, Twisted Sister's anthem about not taking anyone's crap will fire you up and, if you're in an '80s state of mind, motivate you to rage against the Standard American Diet.

Go ahead and get stoked about the food you're not taking anymore.

Processed Carbs

We're cutting out the worst carbs: the packaged processed foods, the junk food. It's junk. Get it out of your life and your pantry.

Next, sugar. That's out, too. Especially the drinks that are half high-fructose corn syrup. That crap goes straight to your liver, where it's metabolized and stored as fat.

Sugar

Yes, technically, sugar falls into the carb category, but since many women don't automatically think of it as a carb, we're calling it out. Since it's driving an obesity epidemic, it's bad enough to call out on its own.

Counting Calories

Say *buh-bye* to counting calories.

Counting calories takes the focus off making healthy choices. If I gave you a choice between 100 calories of broccoli or the same calories of fries, you'd probably choose the fries, right? But the fries aren't going to provide nourishment, as you know. See how dangerous it is to oversimplify foods into numbers?

We're dropping the calorie counting like it's hot and giving you the resources to make choices based on your body, not a calorie count.

Obsessively Counting Macros & Net Carbs

You do not have to do keto math for every meal to reap the keto diet's health benefits or lose weight.

WTF is a Macro? And What are Net Carbs?

Chances are you've seen a macro breakdown in a recipe or heard people talk about net carbs. You may be confused, or you could be a macro-math ninja, and in that case, go ahead and skip this part. You're already a badass.

If you're going the all-in tracking every macro route, finding the right balance of carbs, fats, and proteins for you is important, and warning: It does involve a little math.

Macros 101

For those of you who are still here, "macro" is just shorthand for macronutrients, which are broken down into three categories: fat, protein, and carbohydrates.

Here are the standard percentages of macronutrients on a keto diet needed to reach ketosis.

- 5% carbohydrates,
- 25% protein
- 70% fat

Finding Your Macro Number

Unfortunately, there is no magic net carb number for everyone. Multiple factors are used to determine your ideal and oh-so-individualized macronutrient number.

- Gender: Male or Female. Our bodies are different, and so are the number of carbs we eat.
- Activity Level: Are you a marathon runner, or do you barely make it to your mailbox? Your fitness also plays into your net carbs.
- Current Weight and Goal Weight: If you have a considerable amount of weight to lose, your number will be different than if you intend to maintain your current weight.
- Health and Health Conditions: If you have Type 2 diabetes or metabolic syndrome, this will impact the number of carbs recommended, often making it lower.

Head to rebelketo.com/the-vault to get your number. It's as easy as typing in your gender, height, weight, activity level, and body fat % (there's an estimation option), adding your goals and boom! You've got your individualized macro numbers so you can plan your meals.

What if I don't want to Track All of the Macros? How many Carbs Should I Eat?

This is a question I get all the time, and the answer is always the same: It depends on the individual.

See, there are a few variables that you have to consider: age, weight, goals, and health conditions. For example, kids need more carbohydrates than adults. A marathon runner will need more carbs than someone who has Type 2 diabetes.

There isn't a hard and fast definition of a low-carb diet carb allowance, but many folks go with 25-55 net carbs per day. Keep in mind that this is a general rule of thumb that applies to adults.

If you're trying to lose weight, counting carbs may help you stay organized and successful, but you do not have to track anything if you don't want to. As far as kids go, I wouldn't count carbs unless I had been instructed to do so by a physician or nutritionist.

Start with fifty carbs per day and adjust the number as you go.

You will eventually find the right balance for your body over time.

Calculating Net Carbs

One thing you need to know when starting the keto diet is how to calculate net carbs. And I've got good news. It is easy math.

Since fiber does not affect blood sugar levels or ketosis, we subtract it from the total carb amount (listed on nutrition labels or fitness trackers) to determine net carbs.

Total Carbs—Dietary Fiber = Net Carbs

Ex: Total Carbs 6g

Dietary Fiber 2g

Net Carbs = 4 g

Simply The Best

Think of Rebel Keto as the modern woman's diet mixtape.

You'll replace sugar with heart-healthy fats that keep you full and nourished. You'll fill your plate with lots of leafy greens and vegetables, lean protein from fish and poultry, and you won't have to say *no* to fruit. Or all carbohydrates.

Just the Facts, Ma'am – Takeaways

- The keto diet is not a trend—it has been around since 1921 when Dr. Russell Wilder developed it at the Mayo Clinic for children with epilepsy.
- Ketogenic diets are backed by science—there's a ton of scientific research supporting the health benefits of low-carb diets.
- A keto diet shifts your body from sugar burner to fat burner.
- Ketosis is a natural metabolic state in which the *body uses fat for fuel* instead of carbohydrates.
- If doing math at mealtime is your jam, set yourself up online with a macro counter
- If you'd prefer not to opt out of complicated macro math, you're good to go, as long as you know how to calculate net carbs.
- Net carbs are found by subtracting dietary fiber from the total carbohydrate amount listed on nutrition labels and recipes.

8

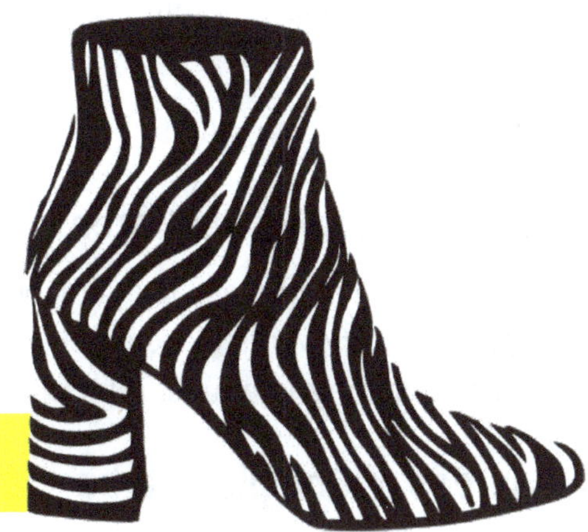

Carbs And Sugar - I Hate Myself For Loving You

Joan Jett may have been belting out one of the best (and most badass) breakup songs of all time about hating herself for loving a lowdown, cheating man who didn't love her back. Still, she could have just as easily been singing about the unhealthy relationship most of us have with carbohydrates, a.k.a. carbs.

Carbohydrates are a lot like women—they're misunderstood, complex, refined, stereotyped, and confusing A.F.

But the truth is, you don't have to be Trapper John, MD, to learn what you need to know about carbs.

If you've ever been frustrated by carb confusion, experienced PTSD-style terrifying flashbacks to eighth-grade science class, and said, "eff this shiz, I'm out," you're about to be saved by the bell with my condensed Carb Class 101.

Breaking Down the Carb Stereotype

Here's the deal. The reason diets work is that they eliminate carbs. They group them all into one "bad for you" group, which makes it freaking hard to stick to in the long run. Putting all carbs on a No List works for a short amount of time. You go all-in on a diet, cut back on junk food, processed foods, sugar, carbs, and lose weight.

Then, you go back to reality, back to your old eating habits, and the weight creeps back on.

My theory? Nothing goes on a No List. Even if it means suffering through some science stuff, getting a grip on the different types of carbs helps you lose weight and maintain your weight loss long term.

So, grab a hat and get ready to hold onto it. Carb Class 101 is in session.

Refined vs. Complex Carbs

Complex carbs take longer for your body to digest and break down. This slows digestion and absorption and prevents extreme changes in your blood sugar levels. Complex carbs provide nutrients, including vitamins, minerals, and fiber.

Sources of Complex Carbs

- *Beans*: kidney, black, garbanzo, white, pinto,
- *Starchy vegetables*: squash, pumpkin, sweet potatoes
- *Non-starchy vegetables*: asparagus, broccoli, zucchini
- *Whole grains*: quinoa, brown rice, whole wheat

2 Types of Refined Carbs

Sugar—Refined and processed sugars—including all-natural sugars.

Refined Grains—Stripped of all fibers, vitamins, and minerals, these grains are digested quickly with a high glycemic index (which means they cause rapid spikes in blood sugar and insulin levels).

Refined carbohydrates, also known as simple or processed carbs, increase your risk for obesity, chronic inflammation, and Type 2 diabetes.

Refined carbohydrates break down to sugar quickly, and they don't bring a lot of nutrients to the table, but they will give you a quick burst of energy (or a sugar high).

Sources of Refined Carbohydrates

- White flour
- White bread
- Pastries
- Soda
- Cereal
- Processed foods

- Sugars
  - Glucose
  - Sugar (sucrose)
  - Dairy (lactose)
  - Malt sugar (maltose)
  - Fruit and honey (fructose)

I look at carbs differently from your typical "keto" mindset because everyone responds to carbs differently. The only way to know is to keep up with how your body responds to each food.

That's why, even though Type 2 diabetes diagnoses are through the roof, we do not have one treatment or diet for diabetes. That's why most diets start by eliminating all carbohydrates in the beginning. Then, they suggest adding them back in one by one, so you can see how your body reacts.

I'm leaving it up to you. If you want to go all-in and eliminate all carbs, that's cool. If you want to start with cutting the unhealthiest carbs, that works too.

You'll see results by cutting out the processed, fake food carbs without doing anything else differently. And you'll allow your body time to get used to a new way of eating without having to worry about the keto flu!

Processed Fake Food Carbohydrates That Go on Everyone's NO List

Some things are just off-limits for good.

- Bagels
- Cakes, cookies, doughnuts, muffins, pastries, and other sweet baked goods
- Cereals
- Crackers
- Hamburger buns
- Hot dog buns
- Pancakes and waffles
- Pasta
- Pizza dough
- Rice snacks
- Soft sandwich bread
- White rice

Swap This For That

Not quite sure how to go about removing all the worst carbs from your diet? Start with these easy substitutions (recipes included in Chapter 15). Over time, you won't even think about your old standbys anymore.

(RK indicates Rebel Keto recipe, S indicates something you can easily find in the store. Although if the swap refers to something rebellious with a name from the '80s you can probably assume it's something you'll find here!)

Breakfast

- Cereal: Hall & Oates Grain-Free Granola Bagels or Everything But The Carbs Bagels (**RK**)
- Biscuits: The Drop Biscuits Sir Mix a Lot Would Approve Of (**RK**)
- Hash Browns: Cauliflower hash browns (**S**)
- English Muffin: When I See You Smile 90 Second Bad English Muffins (**RK**)
- Muffins: Sweet Dreams Cinnamon Muffins (**RK**)
- Oatmeal: Sowing the Chia Seeds of Love Pudding (**RK**)
- Pancakes: Just Call Me Angel of The Morning Almond Flour Pancakes (**RK**)
- Waffles: Stir Crazy Better Than Eggo Waffles (**RK**)

Snacks

- Chips: It Takes Two Ingredient Cheese Crisps (**RK**), 3 Ingredient Keto Crackers (**RK**), pork rinds (**S**), zucchini chips (**S**)
- Crackers: Almond flour crackers (**S**)
- Flavored yogurt: Sugar-free Greek yogurt (**S**)
- Nachos: It Takes Two Ingredients to Make Easy Cheese Crisps (**RK**), One-Ingredient Parmesan Cheese "Chips" (**RK**) Cheese Crisps (**S**)
- Peanut Butter: Sugar-free nut butter (**S**)

Breads

- Croutons: It Takes Two Ingredients to Make Easy Cheese Crisps (**RK**), One-Ingredient Parmesan Cheese "Chips" (**RK**) Cheese Crisps (**S**)
- Bread: Keto bread, lettuce wrap (**S**), 5-Minute Parmesan Garlic Chaffle Bread (**RK**)
- Breadsticks: Cauliflower Cheesy Bread (**S**)
- Buns: Cloud bread (**RK**), chaffle or portobello mushroom (**S**)
- Pizza crust: Fathead dough crust (**RK**), cauliflower pizza crust (**S**)
- Sandwich Bread: Keto bread (**S**)
- Taco shells: Cheddar cheese taco shells (**S**)
- Tortillas: Almond flour tortillas (**S**)

Pasta / Rice / Potatoes

- French fries: Zucchini fries **(S)**
- Lasagna: Eggplant lasagna **(S)**
- Mashed Potatoes: Mashed cauliflower **(S)**
- Pasta: Zoodles **(S)**, Zoodles with Pesto **(RK)**
- Rice: I'm All Out Of Carbs Cauliflower Rice **(RK)**
- Spaghetti: Zucchini or Spaghetti squash zoodles, Shirataki noodles **(S)**

Baking

- Breadcrumbs: Pork rinds, Almond flour **(S)**
- Chocolate Chips: Sugar Free chocolate chips **(S)**
- Margarine: Butter, Coconut oil, ghee **(S)**
- Sugar: Monk fruit, erythritol, stevia (S)
- Powdered sugar: Powdered Monk Fruit, erythritol (S)
- Vegetable Oil: Olive or avocado oil (S)
- Wheat flour: Almond or coconut flour (S)

Sauces and Dressings

- BBQ Sauce: Sugar-free BBQ sauce (S)
- Ketchup: Sugar-free ketchup **(S)**
- Maple syrup: Sugar-free maple syrup **(S)**

Drinks

- Coffee creamer: Heavy cream (S)
- Fruit Juice: Sparkling water (S)
- Lemonade: Water with lemon **(S)**
- Milk: Almond milk, coconut milk, heavy cream (S)
- Soda: Infused or sparkling water (S)

Alcohol

- Beer: Ultra-light beer **(S)**
- Sweet wine: Dry wine **(S)**

Liberate yourself from the toxic relationship you have with carbs, and your body will reward you with weight loss, good health, and a sense of control over your appetite like you've never had before.

Just The Facts, Ma'am – Takeaways

- Refined grains and sugar are the worst types of carbohydrates.
- Processed foods are universally unhealthy and causing the most health issues, including weight-gain.
- There are low-carb versions of your favorite foods that make it easier to cut carbs without feeling deprived.

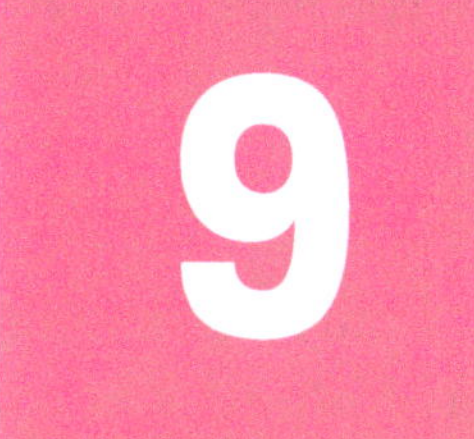

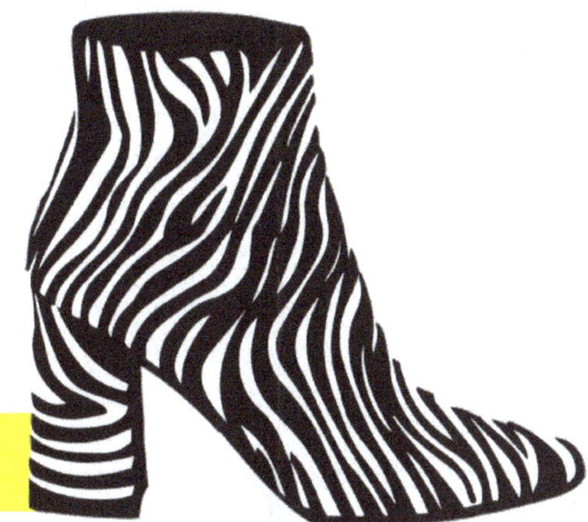

9 How Steven Tyler Will Inspire You To Take A Second Look At Sugar Labels

Okay, do you know the backstory behind "Dude Looks Like A Lady"? Because you should. Originally the Aerosmith tune was "Cruisin' for a Lady," which would have been totally lame. Thank God Aerosmith's Steven Tyler confused Motley Crue's Vince Neil for a poster-worthy hot blonde babe. The story goes, he was going to ask "her" out, but then she turned around to reveal that she was a "he." One of Tyler's buddies remarked, "That dude looks like a lady!" Song history was made.

The moral of this story? Don't assume a damned thing, and don't jump to conclusions based on appearances. Just as Vince Neil's look resembled a lady—with his metal band teased-out blonde hair—sugar comes in many disguises.

The sugar industry has seventy ways to disguise sugar on food and box labels that are easy to misunderstand. That means scanning the word *sugar* won't cut it.

This chapter will show you how to spot shady sugar techniques and give you my best tips for quitting it without losing your mind.

Cracking the Code on Sugar: What Labels Really Mean

It sucks, I know, but you have to take a closer look at the labels. You don't have to whip out a magnifying glass or spend thirty minutes trying to sound out ten-syllable words.

I've gone down that road. It wasn't too terribly long ago that I spent four hours in Walmart frantically Googling every ingredient on a Fiber One bar. People stared at me like I had six heads. My kids hated me after that shopping experience, and honestly, I didn't love being that nerdy chick at the grocery store.

Look, you do not have to memorize the Glycemic Index to figure this out. All you need to know are a few basic tricks of the sugar trade.

Natural

Natural sounds like it's healthy. It sounds clean. And let's be real, saying, "I only use natural ingredients" makes you look like you have your shit together. But guess what? *Natural* does not mean something is healthy.

Take agave, for example. Pronounced /uh-GAH-vay'/, it's labeled as healthy and natural. Look for it in energy bars, drinks, and teas. At first glance, it looks cool, and it ranks low on the Glycemic Index, so you think, "Okay, agave is the one." But not so fast. The reason it's low is that it is full of fructose, the literal worst thing for your body. But because it's natural, they can smack HEALTHY on the label and get away with it.

You may be wondering what the official rule for what is determined to be "natural." I know I did, so I hopped over to the FDA's website and found that even though the public has shown concern about labeling, there is still no formal definition of *natural*. Here's how they explain it:

"Although the FDA has not engaged in rulemaking to establish a formal definition for the term "natural," we do have a longstanding policy concerning the use of "natural" in human food labeling. The FDA has considered the term "natural" to mean that nothing artificial or synthetic (including all color additives regardless of source) has been included in, or has been added to, a food that would not normally be expected to be in that food. However, this policy was not intended to address food production methods, such as the use of pesticides, nor did it explicitly address food processing or manufacturing methods, such as thermal technologies, pasteurization, or irradiation. The FDA also did not consider whether the term "natural" should describe any nutritional or other health benefit" (U.S. Food & Drug Administration 2018).

In 2020, the FDA rolled out an update to food labels. This makes them a little easier to see with a couple of new categories like serving size and added sugar, but that doesn't cover other types of sugar content claims, such as "no added sugar" IN BOLD TEXT on the packaging.

You've got to remember that they are trying to sell you the product, not help you lose weight or lower your blood sugar. So, let's review what these claims really mean.

No Added Sugar / Without Added Sugar / No Sugar Added

What You May Think It Means: No. Sugar. Added. (Duh, right?)

What It Means: No sugar was added *during processing* or *packaging*. Naturally occurring sugars are not part of the equation, so manufacturers can label ice cream as "no sugar added" even when it has carb-carrying, blood sugar-impacting natural sugar from lactose.

Reduced Sugar / Less Sugar / Low in Sugar / Lower Sugar

What You May Think It Means: Low sugar or healthier for you.

What It Means: This version contains 25% less sugar than the original version—which could have been the equivalent of a gingerbread house.

Unsweetened

What You May Think It Means: This is unsweetened, which must mean no sugar.

What It Means: No sugars, artificial sweeteners, or sugar alcohols were *added*—another loophole for natural sugar.

Sugar-Free / Free of Sugar / Sugarless / No Sugar / Zero Sugar

What You May Think It Means: Sugar. Free.

What It Means: Sugar free doesn't mean zero sugar; it means there are less than .5 grams of sugar per serving (which adds up.)

Bottom Line: Don't fall into the trap of thinking a sugar content claim means it's better for you.

Wait—That Has Sugar In It?

Sugar isn't all cupcakes, candy, and sprinkles. There is sugar in (almost) everything. Just because you're not using sugar in your coffee or avoiding sweets does not mean you're sugar-free! Take a look at how much sugar is hiding out in your foods.

And Now, Let Me Draw Your Attention To The Worst Type of Sugar

Chances are you don't spend too much time thinking about fructose. It doesn't typically come up in casual conversations. Lots of people know of it, but few understand it. So, I'm going to break it down now, so you don't have a breakdown later when you've hit a weight loss stall or are experiencing a sugar crash that makes you feel like a depressed lunatic.

Fructose is a simple sugar that makes up 50% of table sugar. You can find it in sweeteners like high-fructose corn syrup and agave syrup.

Here's the thing about fructose. It does not trigger an insulin response. Since no insulin is triggered, your body can't tell you when it's full. Meaning you have no OFF switch for this crap.

And here's another significant fact: Unlike other types of sugar, fructose is metabolized by the liver and stored as fat.

Fructose also suppresses leptin, the hormone that tells you when you're full. Fructose doesn't suppress ghrelin, which is the hormone responsible for hunger. In other words, fructose is a beast that tricks your body into thinking it is out-of-control hungry 24/7.

Fat vs. Fructose—Why You Can't Stop

Think about it. When you grab a handful of almonds or eat a few pieces of cheese, you get full. You stay full, and you don't go on an almond binge. Compare that to drinking a super-sized drink loaded with fructose. Your body has no *off* switch for this shizzle, which explains why you can drink half a gallon of soda and want more.

Fats take longer to digest, meaning a smaller portion will keep you feeling full for longer. Eating healthy fats doesn't make you fat; it makes you full. This is why heart-healthy diets suggest you eat plenty of nuts, olive oil, and fish.

Continuing to follow low-fat logic will keep you feeling starved and dissatisfied. It will also prevent you from losing weight.

SOURCES OF HEALTHY FAT

FOOD	AMOUNT	FAT CONTENT
Almonds	10 Nuts	6 Grams
Avocado	1 Whole	30 Grams
Coconut Oil	1 TBSP	14 Grams
Eggs	1 Egg	5 Grams
Ghee	1 TBSP	15 Grams
Olive Oil	1 TBSP	14 Grams
Pecans	20 Nuts	10 Grams

Sneaky Sugar

Look for the word "sugar," which seems obvious, but hey, when the label is in teeny-tiny print, and the box is SCREAMING AT YOU IN ALL CAPS, that it's a HEALTHY choice, these things can go unnoticed.

Here are a few ways to make spotting sneaky sugars easier.

Sneaky Sugar Tip 1: Be On The Lookout for "-ose."

- Fructose
- Lactose
- Dextrose
- Sucrose
- Maltose
- Glucose

Sneaky Sugar Tip 2: Be On The Lookout for Syrup

- Corn Syrup
- Maple Syrup
- Malt Syrup
- Yacon Syrup

Sneaky Sugar Tip 3: Be On The Lookout for These Sugars

- Raw Sugar
- Confectioners sugar
- Cane sugar
- Brown Sugar

Top 6 Sources of Added Sugar

- Barbeque Sauce
- Salad Dressing
- Smoothies
- Ketchup
- Spaghetti Sauce
- Protein Bars

Right about now, you may be thinking, "This is it. This is where it ends because there's no way I have time to whip out my magnifying glass at the grocery store." I feel that. So, in the spirit of shortcuts, I'm giving you a few tips to make it easier.

6 Tips To Quit Sugar

Quitting sugar is a real bitch, so it is more important than ever to keep your eye on the prize. This means knowing your big reason *why.*

Why are you reading a book about a diet when you could be binge-watching *Scandal*? What's your goal? Keep it in mind when you're making decisions. You'll need all the motivation you can get.

Everybody has their moments. Quitting sugar is not easy, but it is worth it. Here are a few tips that I used to help me beat a lifelong sugar addiction that included not one, but four candy bars a night. If I did it, you can too.

1. Eat regularly to prevent extreme cravings later in the day. If you don't eat on the regular, your body's blood sugar levels will drop. You'll feel exhausted and hangry. Yes, hangry. It's when extreme hunger meets anger and frustration and almost always ends with bad choices. Do not starve yourself.
2. Cut out processed and packaged foods. Stick to the perimeter of the grocery store. That's where all of the healthy foods are. The canned, boxed, and bagged foods are all in the center of the store, and they are all loaded with sugars and preservatives to increase their shelf life and flavor—especially if they're low fat.
3. Add healthy fats and protein to every meal and snack to keep you full. Think nut butter, avocados, smoothies, and chia pudding. Eat eggs for breakfast, snack on almonds, and eat lots of green veggies and protein for dinner.
4. Get moving. Exercising will boost your endorphins and mood, making it less likely that you will need to rely on the sugar boost (exercise will also help you make healthier choices.)
5. Get rid of temptation. Stop sleeping with the enemy, Julia Roberts. Flex your new food detective skills and toss all the sugar-laden foods and snacks in your house.
6. Check yourself before you wreck yourself. Are you eating because of hunger or emotion? Are you eating because you're bored, or has midnight chocolate been part of your routine for so long you operate on autopilot every night and grab a Reese's?

In Case Of A Sugar Detour

Let's be real. At some point, you will cave and take a deep dive into a bowl of ice cream. It happens to the best of us. So, when that fateful day comes, instead of beating yourself up about failing or feeling guilty about eating "forbidden" foods and saying, "You know what? Since I ate a cupcake, I'm going big and chasing it with a dozen more," here's what I want you to do.

First, *do not beat yourself up!* If I find out you have smack-talked yourself even once, I will hunt you down and recite no less than one-hundred positive affirmations. This will be embarrassing for both of us, so please don't test me.

Write a note to yourself about how much sugar you ate and what prompted you to eat it:

> *Dear Diary, I caved and ate a box of Oreos today because Dan from accounting mansplained to me how my menstrual cycle worked. I hate him so much.*

Check Yourself: Why did you go for the cookies? Was it emotional? Stress? A craving? Or were you at an office party, and Maureen pressured you into it?

Be honest with yourself here.

Then pay attention to how your body feels both mentally and physically for the next few days.

How's your mood? Are you more anxious and irritable? Can you focus? What about your skin? Did you break out? Are you bloated? Do you have explosive diarrhea? Do you still hate Dan?

Checking in and noticing the correlation of your physical symptoms related to your dessert detour will keep you from making future poor decisions.

Once you figure out that every time you eat sugar, your face breaks out and your stomach blows up like a balloon, you'll be more likely just to say *no* the next time temptation or Aunt Linda comes calling.

And you'll be one step closer to breaking the sugar habit and getting control of your body.

Sugar Replacements

Some keto purists will tell you that any sugar substitutes are *no bueno,* and you'll be better off without them. And you know what? In some cases, that may be true.

If you have a hardcore sugar monkey on your back, any sweetener, even if it has zero impact on your blood sugar levels, can increase your cravings. When that happens, you could end up eating more, which leads to weight loss stalls or gains.

Also true—going 100% all-in with a no-sugar or sugar swaps policy could result in a desperate midnight chocolate binge or a deep dive into a pint or three of Cherry Garcia. So, I'm not going to recommend you go that route and set yourself up for failure and dessert, shaming yourself out of success.

There will be times when you need something sweet, and when that happens, you have options—liquid sweeteners, granular, and powdered sugar subs. Some are better than others. See, all these sugar replacements have pros and cons. Pull up a chair, and I'll fill you in on the details.

Pour Some Sugar (Swaps) On Me

When you're looking for sugar replacements, here's what I want you to keep in mind.

First, you want to use a sweetener with very few carbs and calories, with a proven safety record backed up by legit research. We aren't lab rats, we're women, and we are going to be savvy about what goes into our bodies, *capiche*?

I want you to look for something that has a zero effect on your blood sugar levels (remember, we're staying off the roller coaster!) or a positive one. You sure don't want a sweetener that negatively affects your blood pressure, cholesterol, or triglycerides.

Stevia

Let's start with *stevia*, the OG of sugar swaps used for centuries with a proven track record. In other words, this stuff is legit. stevia comes from the leaf of the stevia plant, and it does not raise your blood sugar.

There's also research that supports the theory that stevia has a positive impact on biomarkers, lowering blood pressure (albeit slightly), decreasing blood sugar and insulin levels in diabetics, and fighting inflammation.

You can get stevia in drops—which by the way, are perfect to put in your purse in case of emergency—and it comes in granulated and powdered forms.

But here's the thing about stevia: It's 300 times stronger than sugar, which is either good or bad depending on how you look at it. On the one hand, a little goes a long way, so that bottle of stevia you purchased ought to last you a while. On the other hand, it's easy to over-stevia a recipe and screw it all up.

My advice? Start with the lowest amount the recipe calls for and add a little as you go. You can also mix stevia with other low-carb sweeteners like erythritol to get the I can't believe it's not real sugar taste.

Another big selling point for stevia is the liquid comes in flavors (chocolate, vanilla, berry), which is especially handy when making a dessert or a keto cocktail. If you find yourself in a low-carb baking situation, check ***rebelketo.com/the-vault*** for my recommendation for a stevia erythritol confectioners blend that works like a champion.

Sugar Swap Tip: Swap 1 teaspoon (4 grams) powdered stevia for every cup (200 grams) of sugar.

Monk Fruit

If you're into Traditional Chinese Medicine, you may know monk fruit as Luo Han Guo, or you may have mentally checked out after reading "Traditional Chinese Medicine."

Monk fruit is another OG natural sweetener 200 times as potent as the white table variety with a 0 GI score. As far as calories and carbs? Nothing to worry about here; we're talking zero calories and zero carbs.

The only downside to using monk fruit is that it tends to have a bit of an aftertaste. You can blend it with other low-carb sugar swaps to minimize this effect.

Sugar Swap Tip: Swap monk fruit cup for cup when replacing sugar in recipes.

Allulose

Next up, allulose. At first glance, allulose looks like a dream come true. It has no impact according to the Glycemic Index, no carbs, and very few calories. A few studies suggest that allulose helps lower blood sugar levels, increase insulin sensitivity, boost fat loss, and decrease fat storage in the liver. The only problem is these studies were done on rats, and as I've mentioned, and you may have noticed, we're not rodents.

According to the FDA, allulose is "generally recognized as safe" even though the jury is still out on the long-term effects it may have on gut health (Tate & Lyle., ToxStrategies, Inc. 2019).

My recommendation is to take the wait-and-see approach. I've never used allulose, and I've never missed it. But if you feel like you HAVE to give it a try, your best bet is to start with a cookie or muffin recipe. The word on the street is that allulose contributes to the moisture level of baked goods.

Sugar Swap Tip: allulose is 70% as sweet as sugar, but you can swap it equally cup for cup with Sugar.

Sugar Alcohols

Don't let the name fool you; these sugar alcohols will not get you drunk or intoxicated. The name sugar alcohols refer to a low-key chain of chemical compounds (that I will not bore you with) and not the intoxicating alcohol molecule, ethanol.

Like sugar, these sweeteners get the party started on the sweet receptors on your tongue. And yes, they have a few more calories and carbs than the natural keto sweeteners, but much less than table sugar. They're also less sweet than sugar, and some people experience a bit of a cooling aftertaste, but that has not been my experience.

If I had to pick a favorite, I'd go with erythritol. It does not affect blood sugar or insulin, it doesn't cause stomach upset, and it is a safe choice.

Xylitol is toxic to dogs. If you have snuggly, furry family members (which I do), you might want to avoid it like the plague (which I also do). Sure, it has little effect on blood sugar, but it will cause stomach upset if you overeat it.

Erythritol

100% erythritol is a safe choice with zero calories, a 0 GI score, and next to no carbs. It also doesn't raise blood sugar or insulin levels. The only issue I've had with it is that sometimes it causes a bit of a cooling sensation on the tongue (and that takes some getting used to). When you combine erythritol with another low-carb sweetener like monk fruit or stevia, the cooling effect is less noticeable.

Sugar Swap Tip: Swap erythritol cup for cup when replacing sugar in recipes.

Swerve

Swerve is a blend of erythritol, citrus flavors, and oligosaccharides—which are technically carbs, but since your body doesn't digest these enzymes, they do not impact blood sugar.

Swerve has a 0 GI score and zero calories. Unlike many sugar swaps, Swerve can be caramelized like regular sugar, and it measures cup for cup in baking recipes.

Sugar Swap Tip: Replace regular sugar cup for cup with Swerve.

Xylitol

As I mentioned, Xylitol is not the one for you if you have pets. It's hardcore toxic for dogs (U.S. Food & Drug Administration 2021). But, if you're currently sans pets and looking for an option that's as sweet as sugar with a positive impact on dental health, give it a try.

Xylitol can be found in a lot of chewing gums because it helps to prevent cavities. It's considered safe (for humans) with a 13 GI score.

Sugar Swap Tip: Swap Xylitol cup for cup when replacing sugar in recipes.

Truvia

Truvia is a combination of erythritol, Rebaudioside A (a compound from the stevia plant), and unspecified "natural flavors." It does not impact blood sugar or insulin levels and is calorie-free with few side effects.

Sugar Swap Tip: For every 1 cup of sugar, swap with ⅓ cup + 1 ½ tablespoons of Truvia.

Slow your roll when it comes to using artificial sweeteners. Even the ones that are low glycemic and low calorie can spike blood sugar, mess with your hormones, trigger cravings, and interrupt ketosis.

And these two deserve a big Mr. Yuk warning sticker.

As in, stay far, far away from aspartame and sucralose. These are the bad guys your mother warned you about.

Aspartame

So, aspartame may have a GI ranking of 0, but it's associated with some pretty severe health issues, and there are better options available that are safer. Skip it.

Sucralose

Sucralose is an artificial sweetener that has zero carbs and calories because it's not metabolized. The most popular version of this sweetener is Splenda, which comes in more than one form. Avoid the powdered bulk versions—they have a GI score of 80, which means spikes in blood sugar.

The pure liquid form of sucralose has a GI score of 0. Your best bet is to skip sucralose and use stevia or monk fruit extract instead.

Just the Facts, Ma'am – Takeaways

- Pay attention to food labels and understand what they (really) mean.
- Natural doesn't mean healthy. The FDA's definition is too vague to put your trust in.
- No Added Sugar / Without Added Sugar / Or No Sugar Added / Reduced Sugar / Unsweetened / Sugar-Free does not mean without sugar. Always double-check the nutrition label.
- Be on the lookout for sneaky sugar in places you least expect, like ketchup, salad dressings, BBQ sauce, spaghetti sauce, yogurt, and protein bars.
- Sugar is addictive, but it is possible to quit without a 12-step program: eat healthy fats regularly to stay full and curb cravings, stay away from processed and packaged foods, exercise to prevent mood swings, and give yourself grace in case of a detour.
- Experiment with low-carb sugar swaps like stevia, monk fruit, and erythritol until you find the one you prefer.

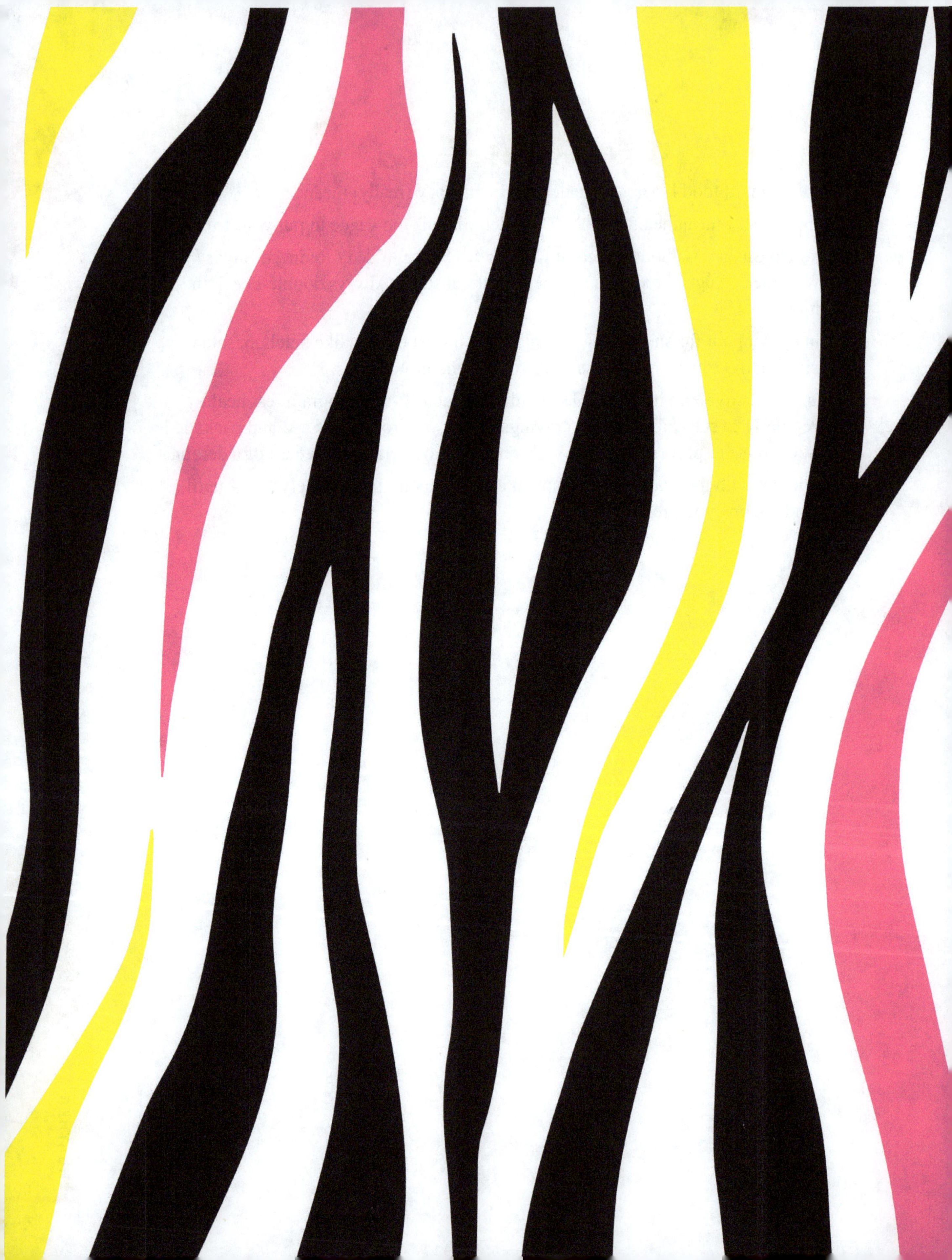

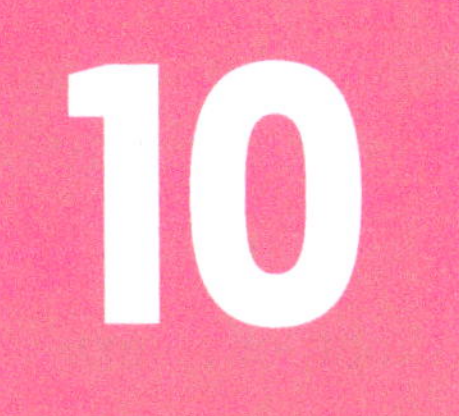

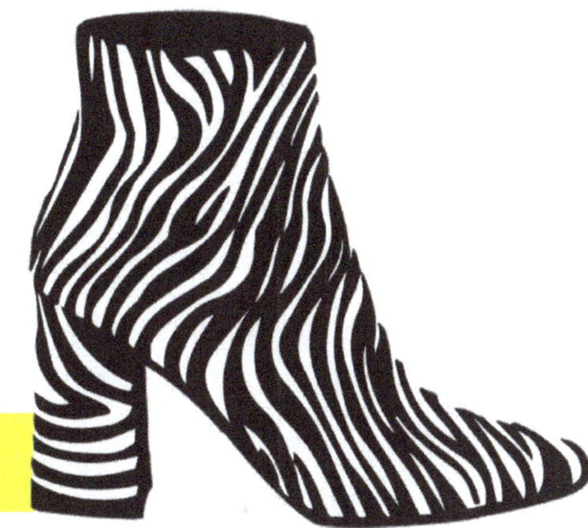

The 411 On Fat

(Or The Good, The Bad, And The Ugly Truth)

Instead of thinking about body image, look at fat for what it is: a nutrient just like protein and carbohydrates. Yes, fat is a nutrient, and no, it's not all bad.

Eating fat does not make you fat. Your body needs fat for energy, to absorb vitamins, and to protect your heart and brain. I know you've been told for decades that eating fat will raise cholesterol and make you gain weight, but that's not the case with all fats. See, just like carbohydrates, all fats are not equal. Does this mean you may have to learn a little bit about the differences? Yes, but trust me, this lesson is worth your time.

Before I put up the official "School's In Session" sign, I want to tell you what John and Sherry Singletary taught me about fat. John and Sherry were one of those, well, hate to say it but, fat couples. I swear their weights stayed within ten pounds of each other my entire life. They both struggled with weight as kids, and they were addicted to Diet Coke and Weight Watchers. Then something peculiar happened around 1988. They lost a combined amount of over 250 pounds.

I remember not recognizing them after the weight loss—and I guess they had trouble knowing each other too because they both ended up having affairs and getting a divorce (but that's not what's important here). How they lost weight is what's important. It's a story they collectively told my parents, and I overheard because, naturally, I spied on adults.

"It's the damnedest thing," John explained, "I eat steak, bacon, and eggs and I lose weight."

John reminded me of Cousin Eddie from *National Lampoon's Vacation*, except less handsome and twice as stupid. But I considered Sherry an intelligent human. I didn't understand relationships or fats back then, and I didn't need to. I was nine. I'd find out the full scoop on their adventures in weight loss from my BFF Amanda, who reported John and Sherry were on a low carb, high-fat diet.

I recall thinking they'd both end up dead of heart attacks within months because the way they lost weight was so freaking crazy. They were on the eggs and bacon diet—pretty much 100% saturated fats, 24 hours a day, seven days a week.

Don't worry; I'm not going to tell you a horror story about how they stroked out, or a survival story about how they turned their marriage around. John and Sherry are still alive, well, and divorced, again.

I will tell you that I was only half wrong about their lifestyle choice—the diet part, not the divorce. Eating fat is a good thing but eating too much saturated fat isn't.

This is where I part ways with a lot of other keto enthusiasts. They'll throw fat into a stereotype faster than you can say Weird Al Yankovic.

They'll tell you fat is filling and that all the fat that was replaced with sugar in the eighties is why we have an obesity epidemic.

But that's only partially true. See, fat is a lot like an article your husband reads on Facebook and starts quoting like the gospel because it MUST be TRUE. It was online!

Um, nope.

See, when it comes to fat, you must check the source. We went wrong in the '80s when we treated all fats like saturated fats—probably because most dietary fats fall into this category. Diets high in saturated fats are associated with obesity and cardiovascular disease. So, the John and Sherry diet isn't likely to work out. It's also why many dieticians and nutritionists recommend avoiding a keto diet. They are afraid folks will saturate it up. Which, for the record, I am saying that's what not to do!

What I recommend you do instead is get to know the heart-healthy fats. Eating a steady stream of these is what helped me lower my weight and boost my HDL, or good cholesterol, while lowering my LDL, or bad cholesterol, without a prescription.

For the record, I'm talking about polyunsaturated and monounsaturated, or PUFA and MUFA, fats.

Polyunsaturated fats are found in fatty fish, like salmon, herring, and mackerel. These are good sources of omega-3 fatty acids, which help reduce inflammation.

You'll find MUFAs in plant-based foods like almonds, hazelnuts, and avocados. These fats are, also, associated with heart health.

Do saturated fats have a place at the Rebel Keto table? Sure they do. I'm not saying to back off all the burgers and bacon. Not at all. Nothing is off-limits 100% of the time; just don't make saturated fats your kitchen's staple ingredients.

Healthy Fats

Cutting carbs and replacing sugar with healthy fats is your secret weapon to curb cravings. Aim for 30 grams of fat in every meal. You may be thinking that it sounds impossible to do, but it's pretty easy, especially if you love avocados as much as I do. But being an avocado aficionado is not required. Check out the table below for sources of healthy fats.

SOURCES OF HEALTHY FAT

FOOD	AMOUNT	FAT CONTENT
Almonds	10 Nuts	6 Grams
Avocado	1 Whole	30 Grams
Coconut Oil	1 TBSP	14 Grams
Eggs	1 Egg	5 Grams
Ghee	1 TBSP	15 Grams
Olive Oil	1 TBSP	14 Grams
Pecans	20 Nuts	10 Grams

Nuts and Seeds

Nuts and seeds are fabulous sources of fat, protein, and antioxidants that you can enjoy as stand-alone snacks, as a topping for salads and soups, and added to smoothies.

I'm going all-in graph psycho here because even though we're not counting calories, a little goes a long way in this department. Keep your portion sizes in check!

NUTS & SEEDS

NUT	SERV.	CAL.	PROTEIN	FAT	FIBER	TOTAL CARBS	NET CARBS
Almonds	23	161	5.9g	13.8	3.1	6.1	2.7
Brazil Nuts	6	184	4g	18.6	2.1	3.4	1.3
Cashews	18	155	5.1g	12.3	0.9	9.2	8.3
Chia Seeds	2 3/4 TBSP	137	4.4g	8.6	10.6	12.3	1.7
Flax	4 TBSP	150	5.1g	11.8	7.6	8.1	0.4
Hazelnuts	21	176	4.2g	17	2.7	4.7	2
Hemp Seeds	1 2/3 TBSP	161	9.2g	12.3	12.3	3.3	1.3
Macadamia	11	203	2.2g	21.5	2.4	3.9	1.5
Peanuts	28	159	7.2g	13.8	2.4	4.5	2.1
Pecans	9	193	2.6g	20.2	2.7	3.9	1.2
Pine Nuts	165	188	3.8g	19.1	2.9	3.7	2.7
Pistachios	49	156	5.8g	12.4	2.9	7.8	4.9
Poppy Seeds	1 TBSP	54	1.7g	4.3	1	2.3	1.3
Pump. Seeds	3 1/2 TBSP	151	7g	13	1.7	5	3.3
Sesame Seeds	3 TBSP	160	5g	13.9	3.3	6.6	3.3

The Incredible Edible Egg

I cannot be the only one who remembers this campaign on behalf of nature's miracle food. Eggs, with the yolk included, are one of the healthiest foods on the planet. One egg contains 6 grams of protein and 5 grams of fat that will keep you feeling full for hours.

Get the best quality eggs that you can afford—Organic, pasture-raised eggs are the best option, but I'm not going to take you to keto court if you can't afford it.

- 1 whole egg = 7 grams protein
- 1 egg white = 3 grams protein

Protein

Never underestimate the power of protein! Proteins are essential nutrients for your skin, bones, muscles, hair, and nails. Eating high protein foods will help you lose weight, build muscle, and stay full between meals. Whether you decide to get your protein from plant-based sources or animal foods, opt for local, sustainable options.

Lean meats and animal foods like eggs offer a variety of healthful nutrients, including Vitamin B12, iron, zinc, Vitamin D, and Omega-3 fatty acids.

Best Sources of Protein—Seafood

Fish is known for being rich with omega-3 fatty acids, which can protect against cardiovascular disease.

SOURCES OF PROTEIN (SEAFOOD)

FOOD	PROTEIN
Snapper (1oz)	7 g
Swordfish (1oz)	7 g
Sardines (1oz)	7 g
Tilapia (1oz)	7 g
Salmon (1oz)	6 g
Halibut (1oz)	6 g
Mackerel (1oz)	5 g
Mahi-Mahi (1oz)	5 g
Shrimp (1oz)	7 g
Mussels (1oz)	7 g
Scallops (1oz)	6 g
Lobster (1oz)	5 g
Crab (1oz)	5 g

Poultry

Poultry, like chicken and turkey, is also an excellent protein source that doesn't contain too many saturated fats.

Red Meat

Red meats are good sources of iron, Vitamin B12, zinc, and protein, all of which are essential nutrients. But you have to weigh that against the risks. According to the American Institute for Cancer Research, red meat could promote certain cancers such as colorectal cancer (American Institute for Cancer Research 2021). So limit red meats like beef, pork, and lamb to the occasional zone rather than a daily staple.

SOURCES OF PROTEIN

POULTRY	PROTEIN
Chicken (1oz)	7 g
Duck (1oz)	5 g
Turkey (1oz)	5 g

RED MEAT	PROTEIN
Pork (1oz)	8 g
Beef (1oz)	7 g
Lamb (1oz)	7 g

PLANT-BASED	PROTEIN
Asparagus (1 Cup)	2.9 g
Avocado (1/2)	2 g
Cooked Broccoli (1/2 Cup)	2 g
Brussels Sprouts (1/2 Cup)	2 g
Cooked Spinach (1/2 Cup)	3 g

Plant-Based Protein Options—Vegetables

Your mom was right about eating your veggies! Eating nutrient-dense, non-starchy veggies will support your gut health and your gut microbiome. Aim to eat four to six cups of vegetables per day. Try to buy organic when you can—check the latest version of The Dirty Dozen and The Clean Fifteen to help you make a choice. And always rinse your vegetables when you get home from the supermarket.

Carbs based on 100 grams (½ cup) serving size unless otherwise noted.

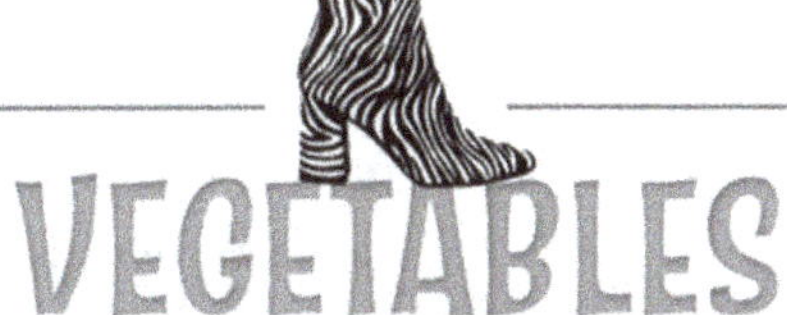

FOOD (1/2c)	CARBS	FIBER	NET CARBS
Artichokes	5.38	1.5	3.88
Arugula	3.65	1.6	2.05
Asparagus	3.88	2.1	1.78
Bell Peppers	6	2.1	3.9
Bibb Lettuce	1.5	1	0.5
Butter Lettuce	1.5	1	0.5
Bok Choy	2.18	1	1.18
Broccolo	6.64	2.6	4.04
Broccoli Rabe	3	2	1
Brussels Sprouts	8.95	3.8	5.15
Cabbage (White)	3.37	2.3	3.07
Cabbage (Green)	6.1	3.1	3
Cauliflower	4.97	2	2.97
Carrots	9.58	2.8	6.78
Celery	2.97	1.6	1.37
Collard Greens	4.81	2.7	2.11
Cucumber	3.63	0.5	3.13
Chard	3.74	1.6	2.14
Eggplant	5.58	3	2.88
Fennel	7.3	3.1	4.2
Garlic	1	1	0.9
Green Beans	6.97	6.97	4.27
Jalapeno Peppers	6.5	6.5	3.7
Kale	8.75	3.6	5.15
Kelp	3.8	0.5	3.3
Lettuce	1.63	0.5	0.93
Mustard Greens	4.67	4.67	1.47
Mushrooms	3.26	1	2.26
Okra	7.45	3.2	4.25
Olives, Black (10 small)	2	1	1
Olives, Green (10 small)	1.1	1	0.1
Onion	9.34	1.7	7.64
Pepperoncini Peppers	3.7	0.9	0.5
Pickles, Dill	2.41	1	1.41
Poblano Pepper (1)	4	3	1
Pumpkin	7	1	6
Radishes	3.4	1.6	1.8
Romain Lettuce	3.3	2.1	1.2
Rutabaga	8.62	2.3	6.32
Scallions	1.1	0.4	0.7
Spaghetti Squash	7	1.5	5.5
Spinach	3.63	2.2	1.43
Swiss Chard	3.74	1.6	2.14
Turnips	6.4	1.8	4.6
Watercress	1.29	0.5	0.79
Zucchini	13.9	1.2	2.7

Dairy to Enjoy on Keto

Raw and organic dairy products are preferred if you can swing it. Grass-fed butter, cheese, and cream are more nutritious and contain more Omega-3 fatty acids than the others. (Aubrey 2013)

- Butter
- Blue cheese
- Camembert
- Cottage cheese (full fat)
- Cream cheese (full fat)
- Greek yogurt (full fat)
- Gouda
- Half and half
- Mascarpone
- Muenster
- Ricotta cheese
- Sour cream (full fat)
- Hard and soft full fat cheeses
- Brie
- Cheddar
- Cream (heavy whipping cream)
- Feta
- Goat cheese
- Gruyere
- Heavy whipping cream
- Mozzarella
- Parmesan
- Swiss

Fruits

Limiting fruits is another place people take issue with the keto diet. They may say that a diet without fruit can't be right for you or that they couldn't live without fruit. Here's the deal. If eating fruit is going to be your deal-breaker, then let yourself have the damn fruit, in moderation. The reason fruit is limited to a recommended two servings per day is that high-fructose fruit spikes your blood sugar.

Stick to low carb fruits like berries, lemons, and limes

- Blackberries
- Grapefruit
- Lemon
- Raspberries
- Blueberries
- Kiwi
- Lime
- Strawberries

Nut Butters

Nut butter is a creamy, delicious life saver that you can use in fat bombs or eat straight up. But be warned: you'll need to flex your label reading skills when selecting the best sugar-free brand. Nut butter is creamy and full of healthy fats, and comes in several varieties: peanut butter, hazelnut spreads, almond butter, and macadamia, to name a few

- Almond butter
- Pistachio nut butter
- Sunflower seed nut butter
- Hazelnut nut butter
- Peanut butter

Here are a few guidelines to follow when hunting for your new favorite low carb nut butter.

Go for the simple ingredients, as in, two or three ingredients that you can pronounce and are familiar with. Keto-friendly nut and salt combinations are the best.

Ingredients like MCT, coconut oil, and raw nuts are other fabulous choices. Avoid nut butter with partially hydrogenated oils and high PUFA oils.

If the label lists ingredients like cane sugar, sugar, maple syrup, dates, or honey, that means added sugars. Skip these.

Herbs & Spices

Seasonings can be a little tricky on the keto diet. Some spices contain carbs, so be careful and keep an eye on what you're using to add flavor to your food.

The healthiest way to go about selecting seasonings so that you won't be adding extra carbs or lose your mind trying to track them is to avoid processed foods. Seasoning packets are convenient, but they have additives, preservatives, and yep, you guessed it, sugars. The best bet is to opt-out of the packages. (I've included recipes for all the must-haves in the recipe section.)

- Allspice (ground)
- Basil
- Bay leaves
- Black pepper
- Cardamom
- Cayenne pepper
- Celery seed
- Chili powder
- Cilantro
- Cinnamon
- Cloves (ground)
- Cream of tartar
- Cumin
- Curry powder
- Dill
- Fennel seed
- Garlic powder
- Garlic (minced)
- Ginger (ground)
- Italian seasoning
- Marjoram
- Mustard (ground)
- Mint
- Nutmeg
- Onion powder
- Oregano
- Paprika
- Parsley
- Peppercorns
- Red pepper (crushed)
- Rosemary
- Sage
- Salt
- Pink Himalayan salt
- Kosher salt
- Sea salt
- Thyme
- Turmeric
- Sugar-free taco seasoning

*Pink Himalayan sea salt, kosher salt and sea salt are always better than table salt, which is often combined with powdered dextrose.

Condiments

- Aioli
- Blue cheese dressing
- Chimichurri sauce
- Coconut oil
- Guacamole
- Hot sauce/Tabasco
- Horseradish
- Lemon juice
- Lime juice
- Mayonnaise
- Mustard
- Olive oil
- Pesto
- Salsa
- Soy sauce
- Thousand Island dressing
- Tomato paste
- Vinegar
- Vinaigrette

Flours and Baking Must-Haves

- Almond flour
- Almond meal
- Baking powder
- Baking soda
- Cocoa powder (unsweetened)
- Coconut flour
- Flaxseed meal
- Gelatine
- Glucomannan
- Hazelnut powder
- Macadamia nut flour
- MCT powder
- Peanut flour
- Protein powder (whey, collagen)
- Psyllium husk powder
- Sunflower seed meal
- Sugar-free baking chocolate
- Sugar-free chocolate chips
- Vanilla extract
- Xanthan gum

Sugar Alternatives

In case you missed the grand tour of the big three categories of sugar substitutes, go back to Chapter 9: Pour Some Sugar Swaps on Me.

- Stevia
- Erythritol
- Allulose
- Chicory root
- Monk fruit

Drinks

In a perfect world, you'd be drinking water so much that going to the ladies' room annoys you, but I get that one cannot survive and stay sane with water 24/7.

- Water
- Tea
- Bone broth
- Coconut milk (unsweetened)
- Coffee
- Almond milk (unsweetened)
- Chicken broth

Zero-Carb Zone

If you're overwhelmed with macro-nutrient data, and damn, you're hungry, welcome to the zero-carb zone. All these foods, fats, oils, and what have you all come with a big fat 0 in the net carb section.

Zero-Carb Fats and Oils

- Avocado oil
- Coconut oil
- Grass-fed butter
- MCT oil
- Animal fats (lard)
- Extra virgin olive oil
- Ghee

Zero-Carb Proteins

- Beef
- Duck
- Hen
- Turkey
- Quail
- Venison
- Lamb
- Chicken
- Goose
- Pork
- Veal
- Exotic meats

Zero-Carb (Processed) Meats

Go easy on the processed meats. They're okay once in a while, but if your diet consists of nothing but hot dogs and bacon, you need to circle back to the veggie list, um-kay? Also, check the label for added sugars!

- Bacon
- Corned beef
- Ham
- Jerky
- Smoked meat
- Canned meat
- Deli meats/lunch meat
- Hot dogs
- Sausage

Zero-Carb Seafood

Here's the zero-carb selection from the sea. In a perfect world, you'll choose wild-caught salmon and sardines. They're the healthy choice with the most Omega-3s and the lowest mercury.

- Bass
- Cod
- Grouper
- Haddock
- Sardine
- Swordfish
- Tuna
- Catfish
- Flounder
- Halibut
- Salmon
- Sole
- Trout

Zero-Carb Sweeteners

Remember that choosing the right sweetener depends not only on net carbs, but also on how it impacts any health condition you may need to consider. For instance, if you have diabetes, pay attention to where it ranks on the GI (Glycemic Index.) The following sweeteners fall into the zero-carb zone as long as they don't have additives or fillers.

- Erythritol
- Stevia (liquid and granular)
- Blends of stevia, monk fruit, and erythritol
- Monk fruit
- Swerve

Zero-Carb Herbs & Spices

- Basil
- Chives
- Mustard
- Rosemary
- Thyme
- Black pepper
- Dill
- Oregano
- Salt

Zero-Carb Drinks

You're free to drink up selections with 0 net carbs as long as you don't add anything to them!

- Club soda
- Seltzer water
- Tea
- Coffee
- Sparkling water
- Water

You Can't Touch This—Foods to Avoid on Rebel Keto

You know I hate a *don't* list, because I feel like the minute someone tells you that you cannot have something, you want it more than ever. I wish I could wave a magic wand and give you the results you want with no restrictions, but since that isn't possible, the least I can do is provide you with damn good reasons to avoid these foods.

Avoid These Ingredients with Sugar

Remember, in Chapter 9, how we talked about the shady sugar aliases? You may want to revisit that—and avoid the following ingredients. Some are pretty easy to spot—hello, white sugar—while others, like pretty much anything ending in -ose, are on the sneakier side.

- White sugar
- Brown sugar
- Coconut sugar
- Dextrose
- Glucose
- Maple syrup
- Agave
- Corn syrup
- Fructose
- Lactose
- Honey

Starchy Vegetables

It may be hard to wrap your head around a veggie being on any diet's don't list. When it comes to vegetables that grow underground, like potatoes and sweet potatoes, the rule of thumb is to avoid these higher-carb vegetables. But this doesn't mean you'll have to live without sweet potatoes forever. After a few months of getting adjusted to keto, you can slowly add these back into your life.

STARCHY VEGETABLES

FOOD	CARBS	FIBER	SUGAR	PROTEIN
1 Medium Potato	37 g	4.7	1.7	4.3
1 Ear Sweet Yellow Corn	19 g	2	6.4	3.3
1/2 Cup Greeen Peas	11 g	3.6	3.5	4.1
1 Medium Sweet Potato	26 g	3.9	5.4	2
1 Cup Yams	42 g	6.2	0.7	2.3
1 Cup Yuca	78 g	3.7	3.5	2.8

Grains

As in, all grains—wheat, rice, oat, rye, spelt, barley, buckwheat, quinoa, and corn. (Yep, corn is a grain, not a veggie.)

Keep in mind that bread, pasta, crackers, cookies, and pizza crusts typically contain these ingredients, so don't forget to double-check the label or the ingredient list!

Avoid Legumes

Also known as beans and peas, legumes are another high-carb food you'll want to avoid for the first few months. If you find yourself missing them and want to try adding them back, feel free, but add them back in moderation. As long as you're aware of where your carbs are coming from, you'll be in control.

The nutrient information for the legumes below is based on a one-cup serving.

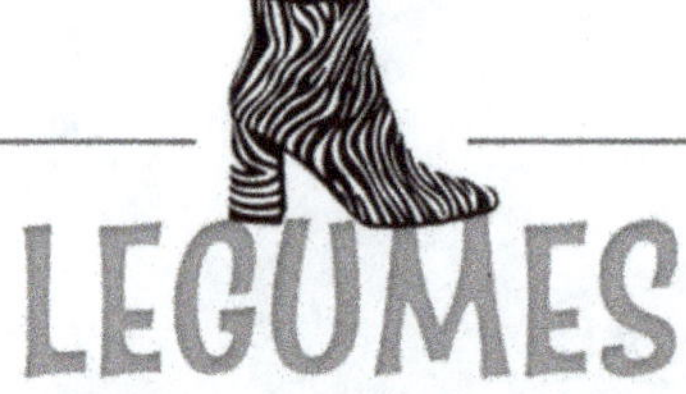

LEGUMES

FOOD	CARBS	FIBER	SUGAR	PROTEIN
Baked Beans	55	14	7.78	14
Black Beans	40	16.6	0.6	14
Black-Eyed Peas	32	8	6	6
Cannellini Beans	38	10	2	16
Chickpeas	35	9.6	6	10.7
Fava Beans	22	9	12	10
Great Northern Beans	88	52	4	32
Kidney Beans	40	13.4	0.6	15.6
Lima Beans	31.4	70.6	2.4	10.6
Pinto Beans	45	15	0	15
Soybeans	56	17	14	68
Navy Beans	47	19	0.7	15

Fruits to Avoid

We're going to take a hard pass on most fruits—also known as nature's candy. I know, I know. You thought fruit was healthy. And you weren't all wrong. Compared to other sugar sources, fruit does have more fiber, vitamins, and nutrients, but that doesn't make it suitable for your waistline. Giving sugar from high GI fruits a free pass because it's "natural" or has a few vitamins is like giving your kids a free pass to attend a keg party as long as they chase every beer with a vitamin.

- Apple
- Apricot
- Banana
- Cantaloupe
- Cherries
- Cranberries (fresh)
- Cranberries (dry)
- Dates
- Fig
- Grapefruit
- Grapes
- Guava
- Honeydew
- Kiwi
- Mango
- Orange
- Papaya
- Peach
- Pear
- Pineapple
- Plum
- Watermelon

Dairy to Avoid

While lower-carb full-fat cheeses and heavy cream are Kool & the Gang, dairy sources like cow's milk should be avoided. Since we're saying no to sugar, here are a few of the worst offenders in the dairy department.

- Milk sourced from cows (both full fat and low-fat versions—heavy cream is okay)
- Condensed milk
- Rice milk
- Soy milk
- Low-fat cheeses
- Creamed cottage cheese
- Yogurt (fat- free and low fat)
- Ice cream

Oils to Avoid

- Canola oil
- Corn oil
- Cottonseed oil
- Crisco
- Grapeseed oil
- Margarine
- Safflower oil
- Soybean oil
- Vegetable oil
- Vegetable shortening

Processed Foods to Avoid

Look, I love convenience just as much as the next girl, but if it comes in a box, it's not healthy. And it's not only the carbs and sugars we are avoiding here. (Although we are skipping those, too.)

Think about it: Why do you think the shelf life is so long on cereal? Natural, whole-food comes with a deadline—there are only so many days that zucchini can ride it out in your refrigerator drawer before it begins to turn into mystery mush. But your average box of cereal? Oh, it has staying power. Up to two years. That's because the food companies have added preservatives and chemicals to enhance their longevity while decreasing yours.

Baked Goods

- Cakes
- Muffins
- Bread
- Chips
- Pancakes
- Snack bars
- Cookies
- Pastries
- Cereal
- Crackers
- Pretzels
- Ice cream

Starchy Flours and Thickeners to Avoid

- Arrowroot
- Corn starch
- Inulin
- Powdered cellulose
- Tapioca
- Cornmeal
- Chickpea flour or Gram
- Modified starch
- Sago

Drinks to Avoid

- Fruit and vegetable juice
- Flavored coffees
- Ginger ale
- Lemonade
- Smoothies (check labels)
- Sweet tea
- Vitamin Water
- Energy drinks (unless sugar-free)
- Frappuccino
- Hot chocolate
- Soda
- Sports drinks
- Tonic water (unless sugar-free)

Alcoholic Drinks to Avoid

Not all beer is to fear, and not all wine is fine. And your best bet on mixed drinks and cocktails is to pass, especially on the pre-mixed gallons of margaritas and pina coladas. But that doesn't mean you will have to steer clear of all your rowdy friends forever. Check out Chapter 13 for all the details on drinking.

- Beer (check labels)
- Dessert wines
- Mixed drinks (check ingredients)
- Sangria
- Wine coolers
- Cocktails (margaritas, pina coladas)
- Moscato
- Ports
- Sherry

Condiments to Avoid

- Barbeque sauce
- Jelly/jam
- Ketchup
- Maple syrup
- Nutella
- Teriyaki sauce
- Light and fat-free or low-fat salad dressings

Just the Facts, Ma'am – Takeaways

- Eat healthy fats with every meal.
- Chose quality, lean protein.
- Enjoy 4-6 cups of non-starchy vegetables per day.
- Limit high-fructose fruits to two servings per day.
- Aim for no more than 50 net carbs per day.

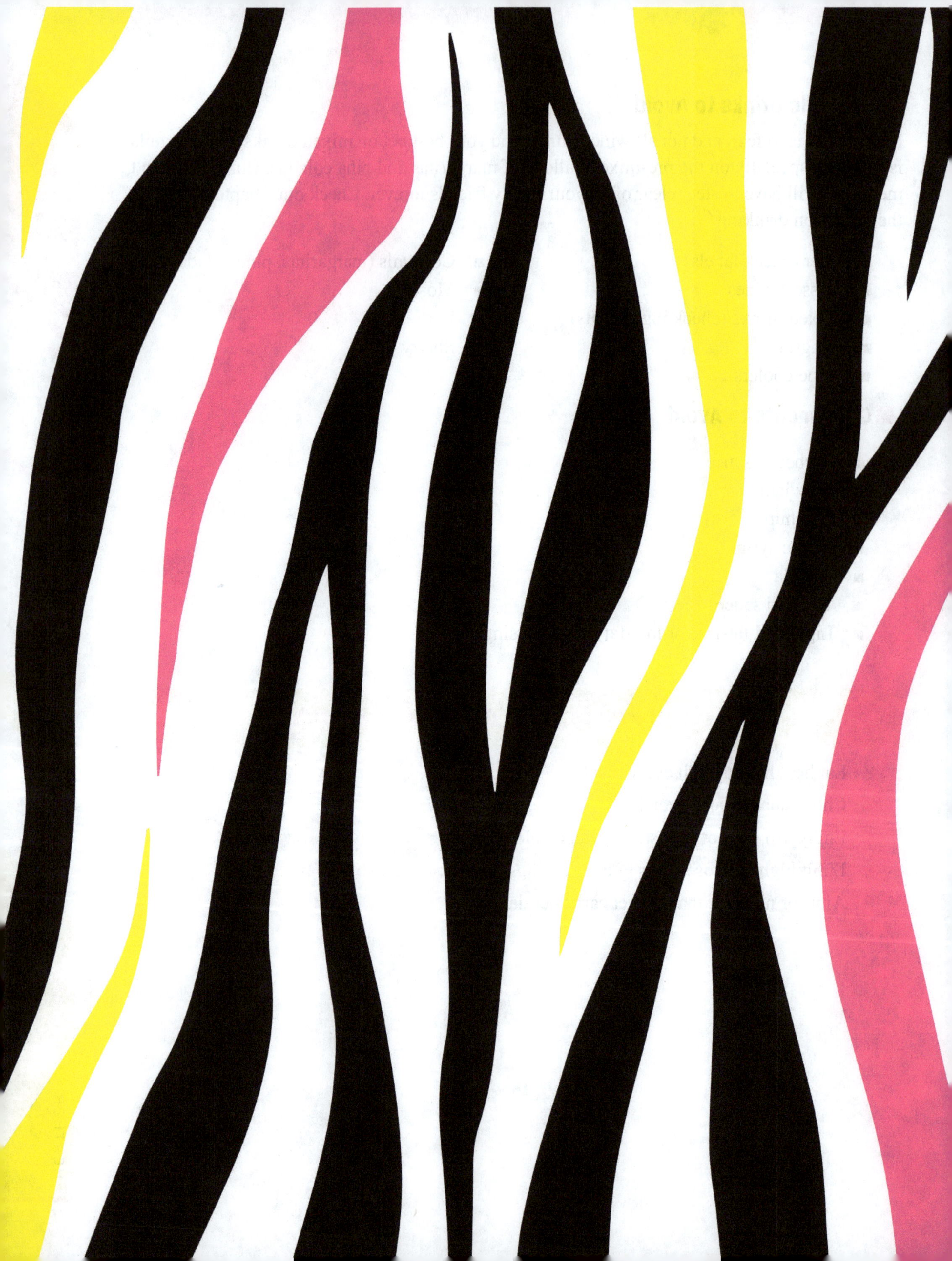

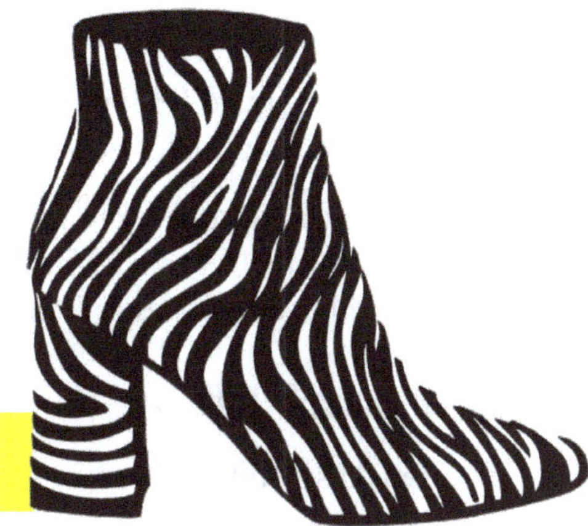

Overcome Self-Sabotage

Moment of truth time, y'all. If you've struggled with losing weight and keeping it off, chances are your battle isn't only with food, it's with yourself. More specifically, with the self-sabotaging thoughts that keep you from achieving your goals. In this chapter, I'll show you how to hit the delete button on that voice in your head telling you to give up or that you can't do it.

What Is Self-Sabotage?

> *"Self-sabotage is when we say we want something and then go about making sure it doesn't happen."*
>
> —Alyce Cornyn-Selby

When your rational, logical mind (the one that tells you to eat healthy foods and exercise) is not on the same page as your subconscious mind (the one telling you to eat pie, dammit), you've got yourself some inner sabotage going down.

To be fair, your subconscious mind isn't an evil witch, and you're not nuts. Your brain is doing what it is supposed to do. It thinks it's protecting you by stopping you from experiencing pain, fear, and failure.

Whenever you think of trying something new, like starting a new diet, or switching careers because at 45 you've realized accounting is no longer your jam, it automatically kicks in with a million reasons you can't do "the thing." You're not crazy, and you're not the only one who has this built-in bee-otch.

Once you learn how to identify these negative Nancys and talk back to them (in your head, not out loud because that would get weird), you'll be on your way to being unstoppable. Once you learn how to reframe your brain's negative thought patterns, you will be in control. You'll resist tempting foods, even if you're staring at a triple hot fudge brownie with whipped cream on top.

By the way, I've struggled with my inner critic for, oh, I don't know, all my life? And if you're reading this, I'm willing to bet you've experienced your fair share, too.

When I was trying to lose weight, my brain gave me all kinds of excuses to quit. I like to call them my Greatest Hits list. You know, like a screwed up go-to playlist of sad, self-defeating songs that would never be featured on The Rick Dees Weekly Top 40.

Evil Self Smack Talk

- What makes you think you can lose weight when you've failed 1,000 times?
- You don't deserve to lose weight.
- OMG, my thighs look like cottage cheese.
- Where can I buy a tent to wear this summer?
- What's the point? You're just going to give up again.
- I don't have the willpower to stick to a diet.
- I look just like Fat Bastard in this outfit.
- I can't risk offending Aunt Linda by not eating her famous sour cream Bundt cake—that would be rude.
- I've already cheated on my diet today, so I might as well eat this gallon of ice cream and Google "drastic plastic surgery makeovers" because, clearly, that's my only option.

You may not notice it, but you always have thoughts before making a choice. Now, these thoughts can be positive and encouraging, but nine times out of ten, they're on the negative end of the spectrum for women who have issues with weight and food. It's been my experience that we all have one or more of these saboteurs.

Saboteur 1—The Permission Giver

I'm starting with the easiest to recognize one first, The Permission Giver. She manipulates you by using partial bits of truth mixed with familiar excuses and why it's really "okay" just this once. Her greatest hits include:

- I know I shouldn't eat this, but it's okay, it's been a tough day.
- I know this piece of pecan pie is not good for me, but it's okay because it's Thanksgiving.
- Oh, my gah, pizza? I can't resist a double pepperoni Brooklyn style pie!
- I'm sad. I deserve to eat cookies.

- I'm depressed. I need a lasagna. An entire frozen lasagna.
- It's my birthday so carbs don't count!
- If I eat at night after everyone goes to bed, it doesn't count.
- If I eat it on vacation, it doesn't count.
- I know I shouldn't eat this but screw it. One cheat meal won't hurt.
- I'll start tomorrow.
- Life is short; one Oreo won't kill me.

Or my personal favorite, which seems to appear when she's desperate:

- I know I don't need to eat this leftover apple pie, but it will go to waste if I don't.

Yeah, the one that convinces you to eat to avoid waste is one of the worst. But look, it's all good because once you start to recognize these thoughts, you'll be able to stop the saboteur. Here's how to put her in her place.

- Yeah, I shouldn't eat that, and I'm not going to because I know every decision I make counts as a stepping stone toward my goal.
- That pecan pie is out of the question. Why would I celebrate being thankful by punishing myself with a slice of food that I'll feel guilty about later?
- Stay the hell away from me, Satan's layer cookie! I know eating just one of you is impossible, and I'm not falling for it.
- I think I'll give this pie to my neighbor. That way, it won't go to waste, and I'll be doing something kind for someone instead of mentally kicking my ass later for eating it.

Saboteur 2—The Wicked Witch Who Lays on The Guilt

Warning: The Wicked Witch is mean spirited. Straight up evil. She appears whenever you have fallen off the diet wagon or when you hit a weight loss stall. Some of The Wicked Witch's favorite go-tos are:

- You're so weak. See, I told you, you couldn't stick to a diet.
- Since you ate that candy bar, you might as well eat ten more. Cheater.
- Oh, so you didn't lose weight this week? After no carbs? This sucks. This diet doesn't work. Quit.

I told you she was mean. Now, here's how to put her in check.

- So, what if I ate a cookie? I'm human. I make mistakes, but I learn from them, and I don't use them as excuses to make more.
- Okay, so I didn't lose weight this week, but you know what? I stuck to the plan, and I feel better than ever! I know I am making progress.

Saboteur 3—The Perfectionist

In one way or another, we all struggle with The Perfectionist as women. But when you're trying to be perfect on a diet? Well, that's a special kind of soul-sucking self-sabotage.

Out of all the lies I used to tell myself and believe as Gospel, I *wasn't* a perfectionist is my favorite. I knew perfection wasn't real; I didn't expect my kids, husband, or anyone else to be perfect; I just had incredibly high standards for myself. I wasn't struggling with perfection. I was just trying to do my best. Nothing wrong with that, right? No, as long as you're cool with having anxiety attacks every five minutes, you feel paralyzed by fear, and you beat yourself up every time you make a mistake.

The Perfectionist saboteur believes in an all or nothing approach to every-freaking-thing, including dieting. Sometimes she convinces you that YOU are capable of speeding things along by skipping out on meals, doing more exercise than Richard Simmons and Jane Fonda combined, and suffering in the name of losing weight.

Here are some of her tactics.

- She will tell you to throw in the towel after one mistake.
- She will tell you to start on Monday.
- She may tell you to starve yourself.
- She may be telling you right now that before you can start this diet that you must first learn everything there is to know about carbohydrates, memorize all the recipes, remodel your kitchen because how can you cook in an oven that isn't spotless? And become an overnight meal prepping freezer meal maker by 6 PM. tonight.

Do not fall for the lies of The Perfectionist. She's a big Debbie Downer who will bring you down every time. You'll be weaker, with less resolve, less confidence, and oh, way less energy because she keeps you on the go all the time—both physically and emotionally.

The Perfectionist will keep you from giving yourself credit when you deserve it. She is never impressed. There's always something more to do. Her greatest hits list usually starts with a big ol' *but.* And not a fun Sir-Mix-A-Lot-style butt. A self-deprecating *but.*

You successfully quit eating your beloved French fries and haven't had a potato in weeks. You lost twenty-five pounds this month. That's a milestone that The Perfectionist will celebrate by reminding you that you still aren't at your goal weight, and summer is just around the corner.

You started keto with your best friend Jenny, who isn't nearly as dedicated as you, yet she's down ten pounds more than you are. Sure, you've got more energy than ever, and yes, you've lost weight, but something inside of you will not allow you to stop thinking of Jenny's success as your failure.

If this is starting to sound familiar, good. Now that you notice the thoughts, you can address them. And you can overcome this negative way of thinking without months or years of therapy. You're welcome.

Just the Facts, Ma'am – Takeaways

- Your brain tries to protect you whenever you try something new by talking you out of it, to prevent pain.
- Recognize your self-defeating thoughts.
- Identify your saboteur. Put her in her place.
- And give yourself grace. Nobody—I repeat—*nobody* is perfect.

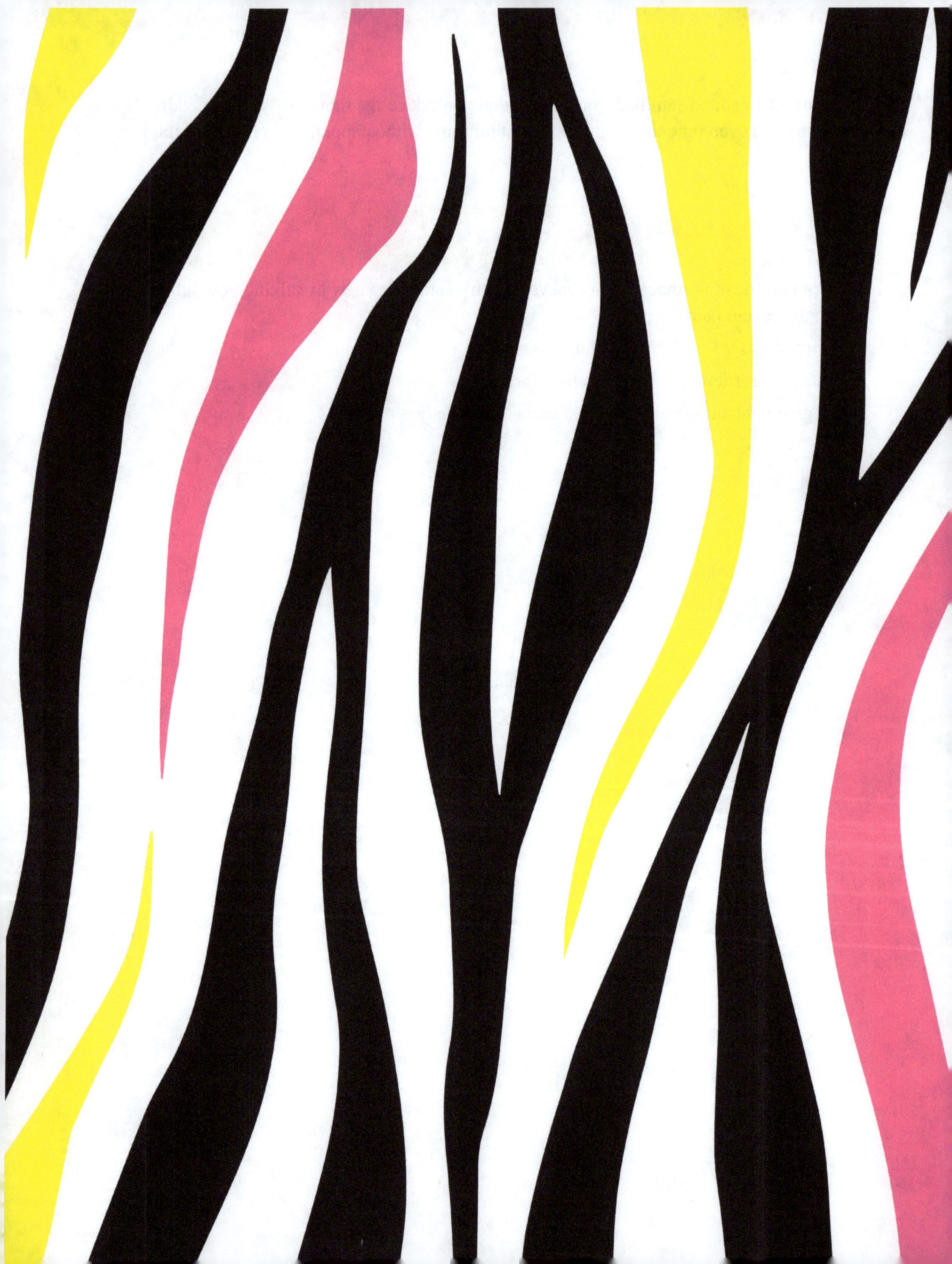

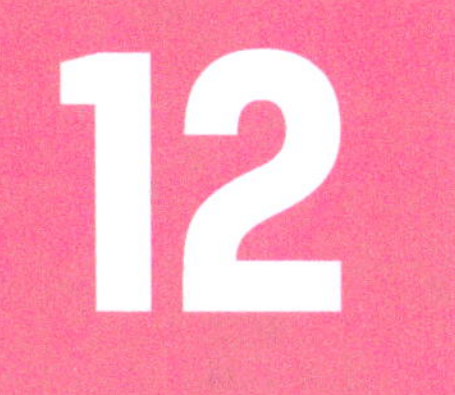

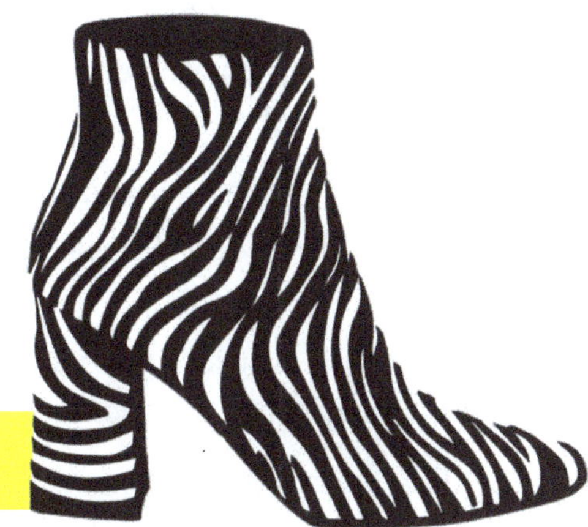

12 Meal Prep And Planning On A Budget

Do you know those diet books that tell you that the key to losing weight is spending hours on Saturdays making freezer meals? Yeah, well, this isn't one of those books.

I'm a firm believer in enjoying your lazy Saturdays and Sundays, and if preparing meals ahead sounds like a special kind of hell to you, then hello, soul sister! Let's swap friendship bracelets.

The truth is, a little can go a long way when it comes to hairspray and meal prep. In this chapter, I'm going to make it easy for you. My meal prep routine involves cooking and prepping so you can spend less time and effort in the kitchen. You'll get more done and get the hell out of there so you can enjoy running a marathon, KonMari-ing your closet, or not doing one damned thing (which is one of my personal favorites).

In this chapter, we're going to cover all you need to know about making meals in advance. I'll cover why you should consider meal prep even if the thought makes you nauseous. I'll show you how to get your butt in gear if you hate the idea of make-ahead meals and what you can and cannot freeze. I'll tell you what you seriously do need on hand to become a keto meal prep queen and the recipes that will save your sanity.

As with all things in life, when it comes to meal prep and keto, ladies, you have a few choices. You can 100% go all-in and cook your weight in freezer meals once a month. You may find that you enjoy the gratification of taking care of so much business and become a marathon meal prepper for life. You may also find this old-school technique burns you out or makes you tired just thinking about it. The good news is you can succeed either way.

Before you decide which category you fall into, you may want to consider all the benefits the magic of meal prep offers.

Making meals ahead means you always have something on hand to eat, which means you are less likely to go off the rails on a crazy Domino's pizza train on a night where you have zero time to cook.

Meal prepping will also save you money. If you prepare your meals using ingredients you buy on sale, you'll find your money, and your cauliflower, goes a lot further.

Another, dare I say "fabulous" in the same sentence as "meal planning" benefit? Having meals planned may save you the drama of the dreaded "what's for dinner" decision every night.

You may be surprised at how much a teeny tiny bit of prep work can have your back.

Full disclosure: It took a long time for me to become anywhere close to qualifying as a "meal prep person." I hate the grocery store. I'm not always the best planner, and, since we're sharing today, I don't love cooking.

I also do not enjoy last-minute hangry situations that almost always end in making awful choices (also known as pizza) and figuring out what to make for dinner every night.

If you're already a "prepper," then you'll be happy to know there are tons of keto-friendly ingredients that you can batch cook and freeze. Feel free to skip to the recipes for the freezing section below.

And if you're straight-up new to the idea? Well, girlfriend, I have a few tricks up my apron that will help take the suckage out of both planning and prepping just for you!

Make-Ahead Freezer Meals Tips for Beginners

Know thyself and thy freezer.

- You may think you'll remember that killer chili you carefully froze last Wednesday, but we both know deep down that it will become mystery meat if you do not label it. In other words, get into the habit of labelling everything you freeze with the name of the recipe, date you froze it/use-by date, reheating instructions, and any other special tips (like adding cream cheese or shredded cheddar to top it).
- Here's a fact: you can freeze almost every keto ingredient safely—except for cream cheese. That means other cheeses and eggs (cooked eggs—not raw) are fair for freezer meals. As for that soup with the cream cheese you want to keep on hand? You can still freeze it—without the cream cheese—and add it in after you reheat it.

- Timing is everything. Veggies usually last up to six months in the freezer. Ground beef, chicken, and seafood last up to three months. The same goes for casseroles, soups, and stews.
- Finally, make sure there's room in the freezer and fridge. You don't have to do a complete clear out, but you do want to avoid an unfortunate "I have no space" scenario when you unload the groceries!

Batch Cooking Time Savers

If you're not feeling the full-on freezer meal vibe or don't have the time, know that is okay. You'll be amazed at what you can accomplish in an hour, without a ton of effort.

Double or triple-up on the ground beef or turkey you're cooking for dinner and then freeze it to use later in casseroles, soups, or salads. Doubling up on an ingredient you are planning to cook anyway will only take you a few extra minutes, and it will save you tons of time down the road. It's also a fabulous way to get the most out of those large family value packs, especially when they are on sale.

Roast all the veggies for your upcoming meals and portion them out in airtight containers. Use these for salads, side dishes, or soups. Cook chicken, make a roast, and batch cook bacon and eggs.

A few of my favorite batch cooking time savers are:

Chicken: You can pre-roast a chicken on meal prep day and use it for making soups, salads, and sandwiches later in the week. Head over to **rebelketo.com/the-vault** to see how I use the Instant Pot to prep a whole chicken—Rotisserie Style! Shredded chicken crockpot recipes are another favorite.

Veggies: Roast cauliflower, zucchini, and broccoli together—they have similar cook times.

Bacon: Batch cook bacon to keep on hand in the fridge or freezer for recipes—if you can keep it! Mine has a way of disappearing into my mouth.

Eggs: I swear having hard-boiled eggs on hand has shaved a million minutes off hundreds of recipes from breakfast to lunch. And they make a super convenient snack, especially when covered with salt and pepper.

Fat bombs: I love fat bombs. You love fat bombs. We both hate waiting for them to set in the freezer. So, make them ahead in batches!

How Long Will It Last in The Freezer?

Here's a handy chart to help you know how long stuff will stay safe and tasty.

(Information is from https://www.fda.gov/media/74435/download and is current as of date of publication. Please check website for any updates.)

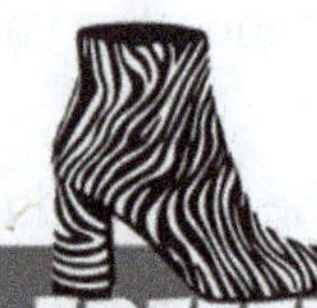

REFRIGERATOR & FREEZER STORAGE CHART

These short but safe time limits will help keep refrigerated food 40° F (4° C) from spoiling or becoming dangerous. Since product dates aren't a guide for safe use of a product, consult this chart and follow these tips.

- Purchase the product before "sell-by" or expiration dates.
- Follow handling recommendations on product.
- Keep meat and poultry in its package until just before using.
- If freezing meat and poultry in its original package longer than 2 months, overwrap these packages with airtight heavy-duty foil, plastic wrap, or freezer paper; or place the package inside a plastic bag.

Because freezing 0° F (-18° C) keeps food safe indefinitely, the following recommended storage times are for quality only.

PRODUCT	REFRIGERATOR	FREEZER
EGGS		
Fresh, in shell	3 - 5 weeks	Don't freeze
Raw yolks, whites	2 - 4 days	1 year
Hard cooked	1 week	Don't freeze
Liquid pasteurized eggs or egg substitutes, opened	3 days	Don't freeze
unopened	10 days	1 year
TV DINNERS, FROZEN CASSEROLES		
Keep frozen until ready to heat		3 - 4 months
DELI & VACUUM-PACKED PRODUCTS		
Store-prepared (or homemade) egg, chicken, tuna, ham, macaroni salads	3 - 5 days	Don't freeze
Pre-stuffed pork & lamb chops, chicken breasts stuffed w/dressing	1 day	Don't freeze
Store-cooked convenience meals	3 - 4 days	Don't freeze
Commercial brand vacuum-packed dinners with USDA seal, unopened	2 weeks	Don't freeze
RAW HAMBURGER, GROUND & STEW MEAT		
Hamburger & stew meats	1 - 2 days	3 - 4 months
Ground turkey, veal, pork, lamb	1 - 2 days	3 - 4 months
HAM, CORNED BEEF		
Corned beef in pouch with pickling juices	5 - 7 days	Drained, 1 month
Ham, canned, labeled "Keep Refrigerated," unopened	6 - 9 months	Don't freeze
opened	3 - 5 days	1 - 2 months
Ham, fully cooked, whole	7 days	1 - 2 months
Ham, fully cooked, half	3 - 5 days	1 - 2 months
Ham, fully cooked, slices	3 - 4 days	1 - 2 months
HOT DOGS & LUNCH MEATS (IN FREEZER WRAP)		
Hot dogs, opened package	1 week	1 - 2 months
unopened package	2 weeks	1 - 2 months
Lunch meats, opened package	3 - 5 days	1 - 2 months
unopened package	2 weeks	1 - 2 months

PRODUCT	REFRIGERATOR	FREEZER
SOUPS & STEWS		
Vegetable or meat-added & mixtures of them	3 - 4 days	2 - 3 months
BACON & SAUSAGE		
Bacon	7 days	1 month
Sausage, raw from pork, beef, chicken or turkey	1 - 2 days	1 - 2 months
Smoked breakfast links, patties	7 days	1 - 2 months
FRESH MEAT (BEEF, VEAL, LAMB, & PORK)		
Steaks	3 - 5 days	6 - 12 months
Chops	3 - 5 days	4 - 6 months
Roasts	3 - 5 days	4 - 12 months
Variety meats (tongue, kidneys, liver, heart, chitterlings)	1 - 2 days	3 - 4 months
MEAT LEFTOVERS		
Cooked meat & meat dishes	3 - 4 days	2 - 3 months
Gravy & meat broth	1 - 2 days	2 - 3 months
FRESH POULTRY		
Chicken or turkey, whole	1 - 2 days	1 year
Chicken or turkey, parts	1 - 2 days	9 months
Giblets	1 - 2 days	3 - 4 months
COOKED POULTRY, LEFTOVER		
Fried chicken	3 - 4 days	4 months
Cooked poultry dishes	3 - 4 days	4 - 6 months
Pieces, plain	3 - 4 days	4 months
Pieces covered with broth, gravy	3 - 4 days	6 months
Chicken nuggets, patties	3 - 4 days	1 - 3 months
FISH & SHELLFISH		
Lean fish	1 - 2 days	6 - 8 months
Fatty fish	1 - 2 days	2 - 3 months
Cooked fish	3 - 4 days	4 - 6 months
Smoked fish	14 days	2 months
Fresh shrimp, scallops, crawfish, squid	1 - 2 days	3 - 6 months
Canned seafood (Pantry, 5 years)	after opening 3 - 4 days	out of can 2 months

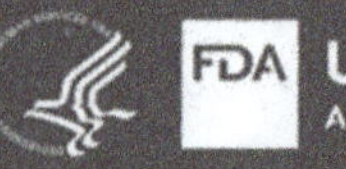

March 2018

Stuff You Need to Be A Keto Meal Prep Queen (Yes, Really)

Chances are unless you're living in a teepee in the desert, you probably have everything you need in your kitchen to make meal prep day (or minute) happen. You don't need to invest your paycheck in a food saver vacuum sealer or a custom label printer.

Sure, you may evolve into someone who seals her food, but let's hold off on the significant purchases until we know for sure, okay? In my opinion, you can get by and even get ahead with these necessary tools.

Slow Cooker/ Crock Pot

No other kitchen appliance in the history of womankind has liberated us like the crockpot. Get one in every color. Just kidding—just get one that has a lid, and you'll be in business.

Sharp Knives

Nothing cues the evil inner critic like attempting to saw through a spaghetti squash with a dull knife. Don't believe me? Grab a butter knife and use it to slice through a tough vegetable. I guarantee your negative Nancy will chime in within thirty seconds with a joy-stealing message like, "I told you you couldn't do it," or my personal favorite, "Dog the Bounty Hunter has more kitchen sense than you do, Heather. Time to quit!"

If you buy a set, make sure the one you choose includes a chef's knife.

Measuring Spoons

Did you know they make measuring spoons that fit right inside a spice jar? Yeah, well, I didn't either, but turns out that feature comes in very handy, especially if you're prone to spilling.

Stand or Hand Mixer

Going all-in on a KitchenAid stand mixer isn't necessary, unless you want one. But you do need a dependable hand mixer, especially for baking.

Food Processor

I never knew how much I was missing one of these until I made the ultimate executive decision to buy a $10 cheap model at Walmart. In other words, you don't have to buy a high-ticket version to get the job done. You will use it to chop and dice veggies, shred blocks of cheese, and mix, especially for baking with almond flour. I use mine to make sure I always have a lump-free batter for muffins and cookies.

Freezer Bags

Freezer bags are fabulous space savers for storing soups and stews. You can stack them if you freeze them on their sides. I tend to splurge on the name brand here because I don't like rolling the dice when it comes to off-label freezer bags that can and will rip, may or may not be sealed, and overall, make me feel a little too insecure about my meal prep game.

Sharpies

Permanent markers are a must-have when you are labeling. Otherwise, you up the chances of having mystery meat on your hands, and you'll get to play WTH Is This? a not-so-fun guessing game your whole family despises.

Dash Mini Waffle Maker

The perfect size to make chaffles!

Spiralizer

This one is a little on the advanced beginner side, but if you're a pasta fan and you know you'll be zoodling your heart out, it is worth the investment.

Rebel Keto on A Budget

It can be easy and aggravating to go grocery shopping and find yourself with a considerable bill and nothing to eat. (And no energy left to cook!)

But seriously, keto does not have to mean broke. The truth is, you can follow Rebel Keto and stick to a budget. I'll walk you through how to make it happen right after I tell you about the day I almost killed my teenager for going keto.

Those of you who follow my blog may be familiar with my oldest daughter's obsession to be a "skinny queen"—a term I hate, by the way, because it implies skinny is the solution (which it is not).

Anyway, since part of the mom job requires me to be supportive without fail or judgment, I told myself I was empowering Savannah by giving her my debit card to go buy "all of the keto things" to jumpstart her new plan.

I never dreamed she would fall into the keto consumer traps—buying more avocado oil than we could use in a lifetime or ¼ of the entire bill in unsweetened chocolate chips.

Turns out, I was wrong.

Imagine my surprise when she handed me my card along with a $430.00 receipt and then asked me what we were having for dinner!

What?

Had she not just been to the store?

Sure, I was stating the obvious at this point, but in the name of all things keto and holy, how does one spend over $400 and have NOTHING to eat for dinner?

Well, I'll tell you how. When that someone has no list, shops hungry, and buys ten different varieties of low-carb boxed snacks and a five pound "value" bag of nuts, the money runs out fast.

Here's how you can plan your way around a huge grocery bill and have plenty of food on hand without needing 101 ways to use pine nuts.

Plan. Then plan some more. I know, I know; you hate planning. You are a grocery store thrill seeker. You're a maverick. You like to shop on the fly and rip the tags off mattresses that demand you DO NOT REMOVE with reckless abandon. I feel that.

I also feel that you're spending way too much time and money at the grocery store! Factor in that we spend around 17% of our weekly grocery budget on impulse items (not including tabloid rags at the checkout). Every quick trip to the store adds up, y'all. So, it makes sense to make a list and stick to it as if your life depends on it.

Select recipes with ingredients that are on sale. Use a coupon app or go old school and check the Sunday paper for ads and coupons before you pick your meals for the week. Train your brain to be on the lookout for deals: When you see a major price drop on ground beef, stock up! Then go home and freeze it raw or batch cook it and freeze it. Boom! You're now budgeting and a make-ahead queen.

Keep your meals simple. Think five ingredients or less. The fewer ingredients, the cheaper the meal will be.

Then shop your cabinets for ingredients you have on hand. Start with the seasonings—there's no sense in having three or four half-full containers of garlic powder! Work your way through the cooking oils, baking essentials, and canned items and conduct an inventory of your refrigerator and freezer. Let no zucchini or spaghetti squash go unused.

Choose store brands over name brands. Look, I love a label as much as any other Sarah Jessica Parker-loving Sex and the City fan, but if I can save a few cents on canned diced tomatoes, I'm not above going the no-name canned route. Spoiler alert: They taste the same because nine times out of ten, they are the same thing.

Know that it is okay if your meat is not grass-fed, and your eggs are regular. I know, I know, I'm setting myself up for gasps from the peanut gallery, but the thing is, until the day the Keto Police start paying for food, you decide according to your bottom line. Yes, organic and grass-fed beef, poultry, fish, and vegetables are better for your health, but regular ground beef is always better than a McDonald's double cheeseburger extra value meal! Choose the highest quality food you can afford.

Money-Saver: Save money and time on chicken by buying whole cooked chickens and freezing any unused portions for later.

Skip the pricey fruits and veggies until they go on sale or are in season. You do not need to have an avocado on your person or in your shopping cart to be keto. Look, I love good guacamole, and anything with kale in it makes me happier than it should, but these ingredients are on the expensive side. Put those on the "one day I'll use" list and roll on.

Feel free to buy frozen fruits and veggies. Frozen fruits and vegetables are just as healthy as fresh—and sometimes they're better. They often have a higher level of antioxidants and vitamins because they're picked at their peak.

Money-Saver: Frozen berries, broccoli, and cauliflower are less expensive than fresh, and they last longer

Buy in Bulk

When you can, buy the value-sized containers of nuts, seeds, shredded coconut, and cooking oils (like avocado oil in bulk) at discount stores or online.

Buying chicken and turkey in bulk, will save you around $1 per pound. Stock up when you can and freeze it for up to six months until you're ready to use it.

Skip Packaged Keto Foods

Are pre-portioned sized cheese crisps convenient and low-key cute? Absolutely. But the thing about packaged keto snacks and desserts is they are pricey, and you can't eat them for dinner. Well, technically, you can, but chances are you won't be happy after, and you may be broke.

Cook at Home

Dining in will always be cheaper than going out. It doesn't matter if we're talking about drive-through, buffet style, or sitting down at a five-star restaurant. You will always come in cheaper by cooking at home. You will also be healthier. Think of cooking as the ultimate control: You're in control of every ingredient, every step of the way. No second-guessing, no getting grossed out by behind-the-scenes kitchen glimpses, no more worries about whether the employees wash their hands properly after bathroom breaks.

Just the Facts, Ma'am – Takeaways

- You don't have to spend all weekend in the kitchen to prep meals ahead.
- You can meal prep for success in less than two hours.
- You don't need a bunch of kitchen gadgets to cook at home.
- You can follow a healthy diet and stick to a budget.

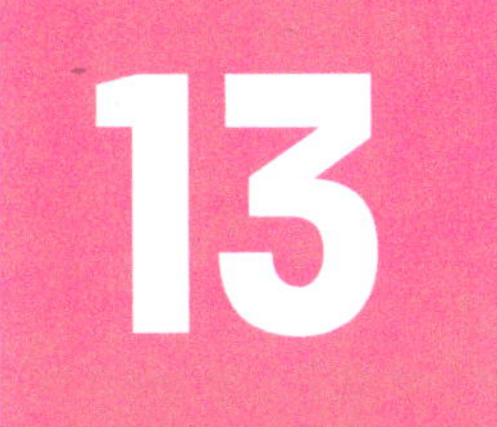

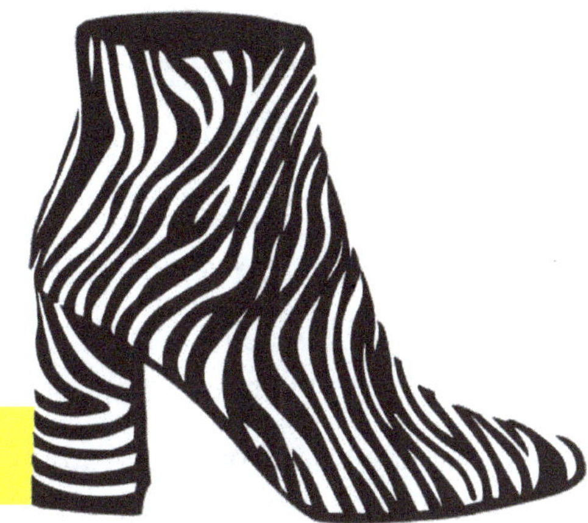

13 Cheers! Drinking on a Low-Carb Diet

You know, I try not to be 100% that keto chick 24/7. Sure, it helped me lose over one hundred pounds which gave my confidence the boost needed to completely change my life. If I led every conversation with, "Hey, guess what keto did for me!" I'd lose the five friends I still have.

When I started my website, I needed someone to help me with the technical side, which tends to stress me out more than my two teenage girls. Enter my friend Henderson from North Carolina. I found her on Etsy, and after a few "getting to know you" style conversations, my success on keto came up. She casually mentioned how she needed to lose the thirty pounds she put on with her last pregnancy.

I was no stranger to the need to lose baby weight, and over 75% of all women find themselves in this predicament after giving birth. I figured this conversation with Henderson would flow like all the other new keto convos with questions about meal planning and foods to avoid, but she shocked me with her first and only question:

"All I need to know is if I can drink wine!?!"

Henderson explained that while she was sure she wasn't an alcoholic, she did know for sure that she could follow any diet plan no matter how strict—as long as she could still enjoy her afternoon cocktail hour.

Enjoying an occasional beer or cocktail won't throw you out of ketosis as long as you follow a few guidelines.

Because of the popularity of the keto diet, it seems like new brands of wine, beer, and mixers are launched every day, which is good news for your 5 o'clock cocktail hour.

But before you party like a rockstar, there are a few things you need to know about being fat-fueled and drinking.

Your Tolerance for Alcohol Is Not What It Used to Be

Now that you've lowered the number of sugars and carbs you're consuming, you have also reduced your body's tolerance to alcohol.

Back in the day when you ate bread, pasta, and rice on the regular, you had plenty of glycogen stored up, which acted as a buffer of sorts when you took part in Happy Hour.

Now? Not so much.

On the bright side, you'll save money on Happy Hour. But there is also a significantly higher chance of you making a complete fool out of yourself and suffering a wicked hangover. Knowing your tolerance level is lowered and pacing yourself will help with both.

But first let's look at what you can and can't drink on a keto diet. Most alcohol contains 0 carbs, that means you're good to go with this list:

- Vodka
- Tequila
- Bourbon
- Rum
- Whiskey
- Gin
- Scotch
- Brandy

What you choose to mix with these spirits is where the low-carb dilemma comes in.

Mixers & Chasers to Avoid

Most mixers and chasers contain loads of sugar. These are a no-can-do.

MIXERS & CHASERS TO AVOID

FOOD	AMOUNT	CALORIES	CARBS
Simple Syrup	1 oz	50	14
Cranberry Juice	1 oz	17	4.27
Margarita Mix	4 oz	110	27
Daiquiri Mix	4 oz	190	46
Pina Colada Mix	4 oz	180	43
Whiskey Sour Mix	4 oz	260	40
Sweet & Sour	4 oz	90	23
Amaretto	1 oz	110	17
Grand Marnier	1 oz	76	6.5
Trip Sec	1 oz	103	11
Peach Schnapps	1 oz	72	6.6
Kahlua	1 oz	91	14.7
Creme de Menthe	1.5 oz	187	21

Low Carb Keto-Friendly Mixers and Chasers

Fortunately, there are plenty of sugar-free versions of your favorite mixers for you to experiment with, which means that you have options. If you thought hating your best friend's go-to LaCroix Lemon Vodka Drop meant you needed to tag out on the keto diet—you were wrong!

- Flavored stevia drops
- Sparkling water: LaCroix, Bubly
- Diet soda: Sprite Zero, Zevia, Diet Coke
- Sugar-free energy drinks: Red Bull, Monster
- Angostura Bitters
- DaVinci Sugar-Free Syrup
- Berries
- Swerve
- Club soda
- Water enhancers: Mio, Stur, Dasani Drops, Crystal Light
- Sugar-free cranberry juice
- Extracts
- Citrus Fruits

Cheers! Best Low-Carb Alcohol Drinks to Order

Just in case you're not familiar with the bar scene (and who are you if you aren't?), I'll set things up for you if you want to go where everybody knows your name.

On any given night, even Tuesdays, your typical all-American bar is crowded, loud, and full of drunk people spouting off orders to the one bartender tending the alcohol.

In other words, do not depend on your bartender to make your drink low carb. They may or may not know what the hell you are talking about, and depending on their mood, if you sound or appear a little too high maintenance, may serve you a few extra carbs.

To make life easier on you and your bartender, order one of these simple drinks.

Keto-Friendly Drinks

- Dirty martini: 0 Carbs
- Vodka & soda Water: 0 Carbs
- Gin & soda Water: < 1 Carb
- Tequila shot: 0 Carbs
- Whiskey: 0 Carbs
- Jack & Diet Coke: 0 Carbs

Quick Tip: The flavored stevia drops will fit into your purse without taking up too much room—keep them on hand in case of a low-carb cocktail emergency.

Drinks to Avoid Ordering (The Worst Offender List)

Unless you can jump over the bar and go full-on Tom Cruise and make it yourself, you'll be better off avoiding these popular drinks loaded with sugar and carbs.

- Gin & Tonic: 16 Carbs
- White Russian: 17 Carbs
- Mimosa Sherbet: 27 Carbs
- Vodka & Orange Juice: 28 Carbs
- Rum & Coke: 39 Carbs
- Pina Colada: 61 Carbs

Red, Red (and More) Keto-Friendly Wine

My friend Henderson isn't the only person who has asked me about drinking wine on keto. If you enjoy a little red or a little white, then I've got good news. A little wine is fine.

Now, this does not give you a free pass on all wines. I've picked out a few of the worst offenders. Steer clear of the following wines—they have too much sugar to qualify as keto.

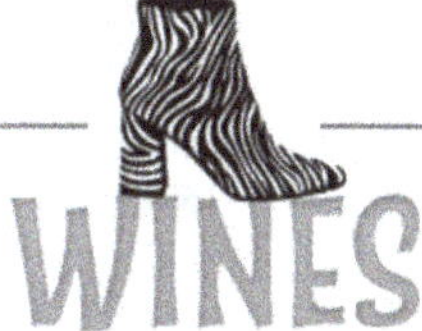

TOP CHOICES OF WHITE WINE (5 OZ)	CAL	CARBS
Chardonnay	123	3.1
Pinot Grigio	122	3.2
Sauvignon Blanc	120	2.7
Sparkling White	96	1.5
Brut Champagne	147	2.8

TOP CHOICES OF RED WINE (5 OZ)	CAL	CARBS
Pinot Noir	121	3.4
Merlot	122	3.7
Cabernet Sauvignon	122	3.8
Syrah	122	3.8
Zinfandel	130	4

Wines to Avoid

WINES TO AVOID + TOP CHOICES

WINES TO AVOID	CAL	CARBS
Dessert Wines	165	14
Sangria	89	10
Moscato	127	11
Ports	79	6
Sherry	165	14

TOP CHOICES OF BEER (12 OZ)	CAL	CARBS
Greens Trailblazer	119	0.5
Bud Select 55	55	1.9
Rolling Rock	92	2.4
Michelob Ultra	95	2.6
Miller Lite	96	3.2

Beer—The Lowdown on Your Favorite Brews

Also known as liquid bread, beer is full of gluten and carbs. Most beer contains seven carbs per 12-ounce serving/bottle/can. If you can avoid it, do. But if beer is your jam, you don't have to let the liquid bread thing scare you out of trying keto. There are low-carb options that don't taste like total garbage.

Keto-Friendly Cocktail Recipes

If you're a cocktail lover, all is not lost. I've got some cautions but some good news for you, too, and some delicious recipes. (See Drinks in the Recipe section).

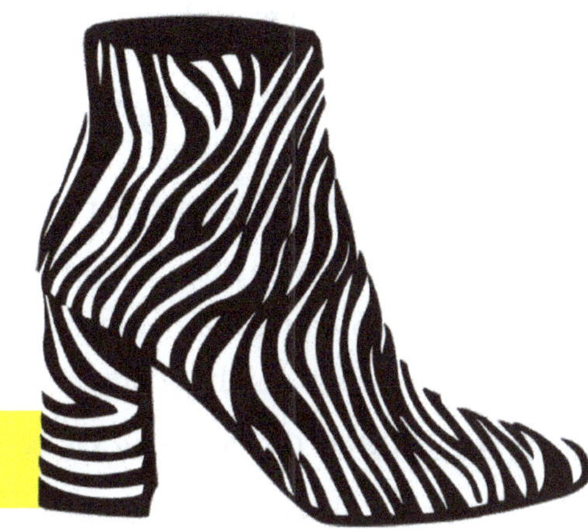

Dining Out

Unless you're on house arrest, all the keto-compliant foods you've stocked in your kitchen won't matter. Sooner or later, you'll need to get your grub on and go out to eat.

Let me warn you: This can be a slight bit overwhelming in the beginning. So, I'm going to walk you through how you can enjoy a meal with friends without desperately seeking Google's advice on macros or having to say, "I can't eat that!" once.

Focus on what you can have rather than what you can't. Nothing says I'm about to spoil everyone's night out like an "I can't eat that" declaration.

Helpful Tips to Make Dining Out Less Awkward

With a few new, simple habits, you can handle the restaurant circuit like the boss lady you are.

1. **Plan Ahead: Look Up the Menu Online**

   Last-minute menu selections stress me out. Avoid making a split-second choice by looking up the menu online before you get to the restaurant. You can always ask for nutrition information when you arrive.

   Restaurants are required by law to have nutritional information available.

2. **Be A Chatty Kathy**

   Waiters and waitresses are there to help you find something fab to eat because if you enjoy your food, you'll enjoy the experience, and they're more likely to get a good tip. Don't be afraid to talk to them! Tell him or her you're on the most fabulous eating plan (give them the name of this book) and ask for substitutions (even if they're not on the menu).

I promise you won't be the first one!

3. ***Just Say No* to the Starch**

   Take a pass on the pasta, ask the server to hold the bread, refuse the rice, and fight for your right to a potato-free plate.

   - Swap the hamburger bun with a lettuce wrap.
   - Swap loaded or mashed potatoes with steamed vegetables.
   - Skip anything breaded or fried, wraps, tortillas, chips, and croutons.

4. **Side Dishes (Or No, You Do Not Want Fries With That)**

   Most entrées come with a heaping pile of carbs on the side, but that doesn't mean you have to do without a side dish. Opt-out of the twice-baked potato and go with a side salad or steamed vegetables.

5. **Won't They Look at Me Like I Have 2 Heads? How to Ask for a Low-Carb Order Without Feeling Like an Outcast**

   You may get a couple of stares when you don't dive into the chips and dip or buttered rolls. Expect a little Judge Judy action and deal with it accordingly. Do not let a look from your server, your friends, or co-workers shame you into eating something because you're the lone holdout.

   If you aren't used to asking for what you want, this will be an adjustment for you. In the beginning, it may be challenging to try to explain your diet in thirty seconds—especially if you've just picked up this way of eating. You may risk saying, "forget it," cave into peer pressure, and go off-plan. I don't want that to happen to you.

So here are a few of my favorite ways to get the message across without seeming like a demanding diva. (Which, by the way, there is nothing wrong with being!)

The "I Have Medical Issues" Approach

You can always use a canned script like,

- "I have stomach issues."
- "Doctor's orders!"
- "I'm on a keto diet because the Standard American Diet has caused an obesity epidemic and is crippling our nation's healthcare system."

Okay, well maybe skip that last one!

The "I'll Be Honest" Approach

Honesty is always a good policy. Try these on for size.

- "I'm doing this thing where I eat healthy because, otherwise, I feel like garbage."
- "I'm trying to lose weight, so I need to keep all carbs at least 25 feet away at all times."
- "I've made a commitment to going all-in low carb."
- "I hate to be demanding here, but could you help me order XYZ?"

The Make 'Em Laugh Approach

This approach is one of my personal faves.

- "I made a bet with my friends to see who could be more high maintenance."
- "I'm participating in a research study that requires me to make life harder on every server I encounter for the next three to six years."

How to Dine Out Like A Boss

Love ethnic foods? Me, too! Here's how to navigate exotic menus.

Chinese Restaurants

You can keep it keto at a Chinese place by avoiding rice, even the brown versions. Your server should be able to substitute steamed vegetables for any rice. Some safe order ideas are chicken with mushrooms, beef with broccoli, chicken with broccoli, Szechuan prawns, and egg drop soup.

Indian Restaurants

No naan bread (sorry, not sorry). Feel free to order Tandoori chicken, kabobs, chicken and goat options, from mild (korma) to medium (tikka masala) to hot (vindaloo). Avoid curries with potatoes and carb-filled side dishes like papadums, pakoras, and samosas.

Order creamy saag (toasted cheese and spinach) instead. To add flavor to any meal, ask for ghee (clarified butter).

Italian Restaurants

Good news—a few Italian restaurants are now offering spaghetti squash as an alternative to grain-based noodles and cauliflower crusts for their pizzas that you can load up with meats and veggies and make a meal.

If you're not finding any keto-friendly options, don't worry, you won't have to go hungry. You can start with an antipasto platter—also known as an assortment of meats, cheeses, and vegetables. Or try the carpaccio, which is thinly sliced beef or fish served with vegetables.

Main dish options include meatballs (as long as they don't involve breadcrumbs), steak with a side salad, shrimp, steamed clams or mussels, or cioppino (a fish stew).

Opt-out of croutons, bread, and heavily breaded dishes like chicken and veal parmesan.

Japanese Restaurants

Ever noticed that the hibachi chef often cooks in butter? You will now! Japanese steakhouses are fabulous dine-out places for folks on the keto diet. Go all-in on chicken, shrimp, steak, scallops, or lobster—skip the rice and ask for extra vegetables (mushrooms, onions, and zucchini.)

You'll also want to opt-out of the "yum yum" sauce—it's usually too carb-y to be keto, but the brown ginger sauce is okay!

Because of the rice, sushi isn't keto, but sashimi (raw fish only) is. Dumplings, tempura, and sweet sauces are off-limits, but miso soup, edamame, and seaweed dishes are fine.

Mexican Restaurants

Skip the chips. Better yet, ask the server not even to bring them out so you won't be tempted.

Order-wise, fajitas without the tortillas are your best choice. Coming in at a close second is the taco salad—skip the beans and any hard-shell or tortilla bowl and chips used as croutons. Order extra guacamole to make it more filling and to keep up your intake of healthy fats.

The Main Course

Here are some general rules of thumb.

Do: Feel free to go all-in on steak, salmon, shrimp, grilled chicken, pork, and turkey.

Don't: Order anything fried or topped with a sauce you can't spell or say (when in doubt, ASK!)

Do: Order a burger.

Don't: Eat the bun. Ask your server to leave out the bun and get your burger in a lettuce wrap or over extra lettuce in a bowl.

Do: Order a salad. Bonus points for adding grilled chicken, salmon, filet, or shrimp.

Don't: Cover your salad with dressing until the lettuce is unrecognizable.

Do: Ask for the dressing on the side.

Don't: Eat the croutons or any other crunchy salad topping.

Just Say No to Sugary Starches

Bread: Includes breadsticks, rolls, biscuits, croutons, and breaded or fried foods.

Pasta: Includes spaghetti, fettuccini, macaroni, ravioli, etc.

Rice: No rice—including brown rice.

Potatoes: Includes mashed, baked, and French fries.

Salad Dressing: Go with olive oil or you risk getting a dressing loaded with sugar.

Dessert: Skip it.

Now, let's move onto where to go and what to order.

For the latest nutritional information make sure to check out the restaurant's websites!

Applebee's

The shrimp and parmesan sirloin and the grilled chicken breast are good go-to options. Applebee's also provides full nutrition content for everything on their menu.

Buffalo Wild Wings

The BWW nutritional guide shows you the amount of sugar, carbs, and everything else you may want to know about your food—love them for that! Try the traditional wings with medium sauce.

Olive Garden

Skip the breadsticks, the 25 grams of carbs in each one may make you want to tell the server to avoid bringing them at all. Go for the herb-grilled salmon (with 4 net carbs), the chicken margherita (with 6 net carbs), or the chicken piccata (with 9 net carbs).

Dave and Busters

The wings over at Dave and Busters have a few too many carbs, but their ancho caesar lettuce wraps have a healthy choice with 13 nets. You could also opt for the Fresh Garden salad (hold the tortilla strips) or the Parmesan Caesar salad (without the croutons).

Quizno's

Go for the regular-sized cobb salad (without the pita bread wedges).

Papa John's

Because sometimes ordering pizza is your only hope of eating dinner! Thankfully, you have options other than picking off the toppings and feeling sorry for yourself while watching people you love to scarf down a deep-dish pepperoni. Try an eight-piece order of Papa John's buffalo wings with sauce (7 carbs) or without sauce (4 carbs). Speaking of sauce, their garlic butter and bleu cheese sauce have zero carbs. Oh, and don't fall for the gluten-free crust, which has 17 carbs per slice. Need more details? Papa John's nutrition info is a click away.

Panda Express

It turns out you have several options at Panda Express, including the kung pao chicken and the string bean chicken breast. For more low-carb options, check out Panda Express's food and allergen guide. And don't forget to skip the rice!

Carrabba's Italian Grill

The Tuscan grilled filet or the pollo rosa maria are excellent options. Take a look at your other options on Carrabba's nutrition guide.

Outback Steakhouse

It's pretty easy to find something low carb at Outback Steakhouse. My only word of caution would be to skip the Bloomin' Onion™ and the potatoes on the side. Stick to steamed veggies or a side salad.

Fast Food

We know the drive-thru is not the healthiest source of a meal, but sometimes, life happens, and we have no other choice. Here are a few options for those times.

Kentucky Fried Chicken

Grilled chicken with green beans.

Subway

Order your sub without the bread—in a bowl. Also known as a "sub tub," or order a double chicken chopped salad.

Chipotle

Bowl or salad.

Chick-Fil-A

Cobb Salad with grilled chicken nuggets with coleslaw.

Wendy's

Southwest avocado chicken salad or spicy chicken salad or any burger (without the bun).

Carbs in Sauces & Condiments

Net carbs per 2 tablespoons

- Oils
- Butter 0
- Macadamia oil 0
- Salad Dressings
- Bleu cheese dressing 1.3
- Tahini dressing 4.3
- Vinaigrette 0
- Dijon mustard 0.2
- Mayonnaise 1
- Sauerkraut 0
- Sauces
- Béarnaise sauce 0.6
- Avocado oil 0
- Coconut oil 0
- Vinegar 0
- Balsamic vinegar 5
- Ranch dressing 1.8
- Thousand Island dressing 1
- Condiments
- Harissa 4
- Mustard 0.1 (watch labels for added sugar)
- Sriracha 2.2
- Aioli 0.3
- Buffalo wing sauce 0

- Chutney 2.5
- Miso 3.4
- Pesto 2.1
- Soy sauce 1.3
- Teriyaki 5.6
- Worcestershire sauce 6.6
- Guacamole 0.58
- Tomato paste 4.8 (watch labels for added sugar)
- Hollandaise sauce 0.8
- Oyster sauce 3.9
- Salsa 1.5 (watch labels for added sugar)
- Tartar sauce 3.9
- Tabasco 0.1
- Dips/Spreads
- Hummus 3

High Carb Sauces & Condiments

Net carbs per 2 tablespoons

- Cocktail sauce 6
- Honey mustard 6.9
- Maple syrup 26
- Relish 10.7
- Wasabi 16
- Barbeque sauce 14
- French dressing 5
- Ketchup 26
- Marmalade 25.7
- Steak sauce 6

Just the Facts, Ma'am – Takeaways

- Check the menu ahead of time before going out to eat.
- Don't be afraid to ask your server for details.
- Avoid bread, chips, and croutons.
- When in doubt, go for olive oil as a salad dressing.
- When desperate, a bun-less burger will work.

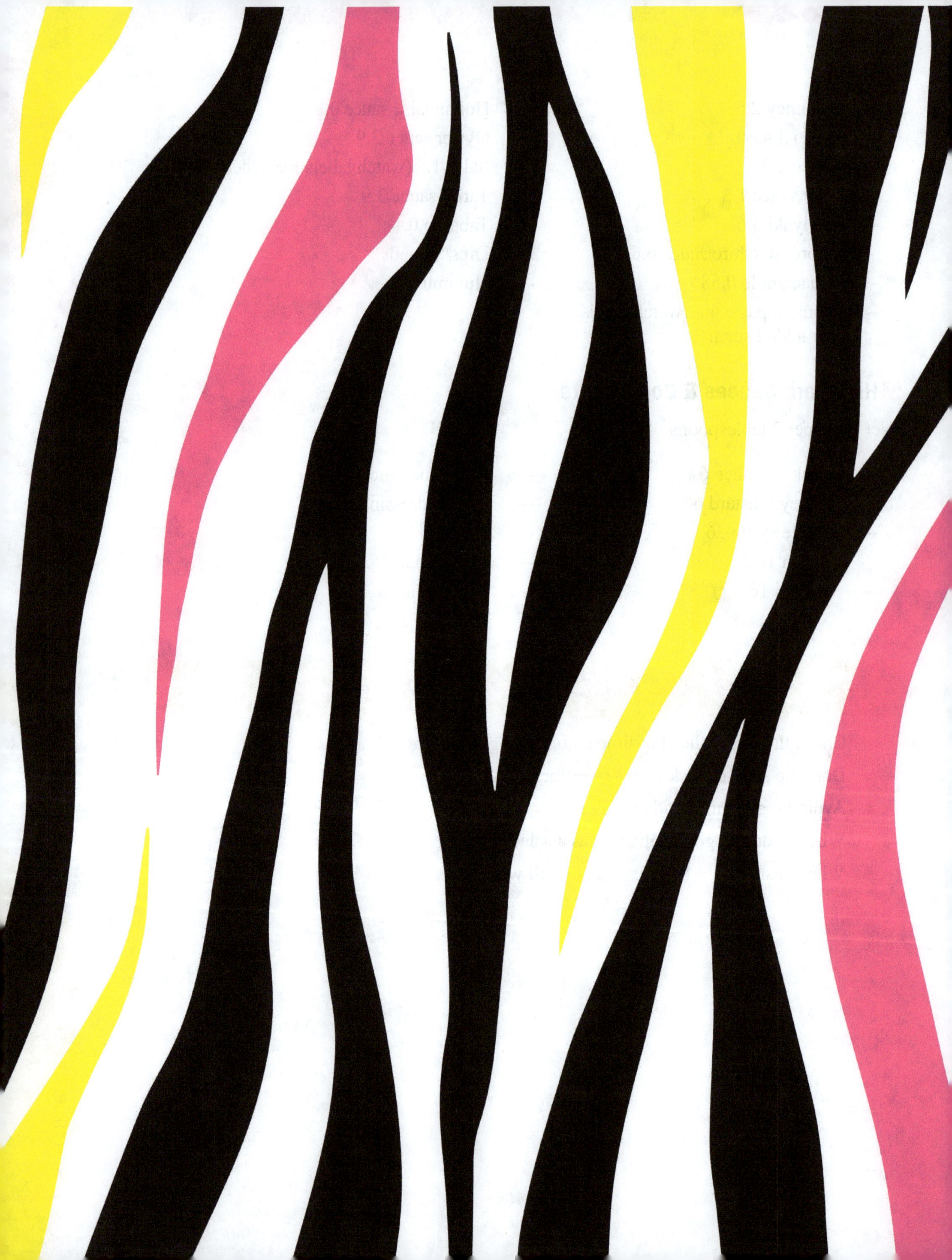

15

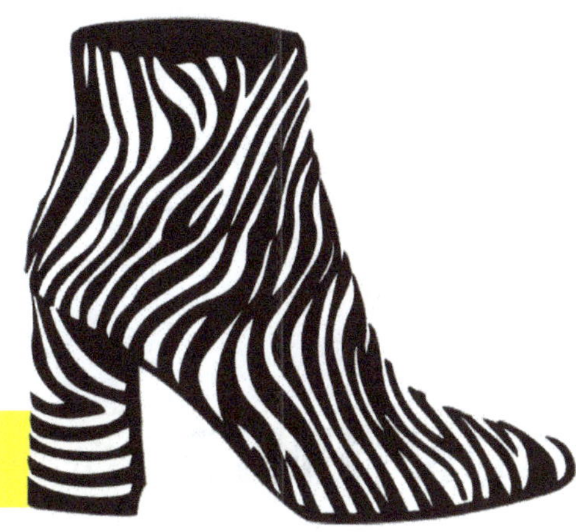

Ta Da! It's Recipe Time

Here's a handy chart to help you know what temperature to cook foods to so you know it's safe and tasty! (Information is from https://www.fda.gov/media/93628/download and is current as of date of publication. Please check website for any updates.)

SAFE MINIMUM INTERNAL TEMPERATURES
AS MEASURED WITH A FOOD THERMOMETER

FOOD TYPE	INTERNAL TEMPERATURE
Beef, Pork, Veal, and Lamb (chops, roasts, steaks)	145°F with a 3-minute rest time
Ground Meat	160°F
Ham, uncooked (fresh or smoked)	145°F with a 3-minute rest time
Ham, fully cooked (to reheat)	140°F
Poultry (ground, parts, whole, and stuffing)	165°F
Eggs	Cook until yolk & white are firm
Egg Dishes	160°F
Fin Fish	145°F or flesh is opaque & separates easily with fork
Shrimp, Lobster, and Crabs	Flesh pearly & opaque
Clams, Oysters, and Mussels	Shells open during cooking
Scallops	Flesh is milky white or opaque and firm
Leftovers and Casseroles	165°F

August 2017

FDA U.S. FOOD & DRUG ADMINISTRATION

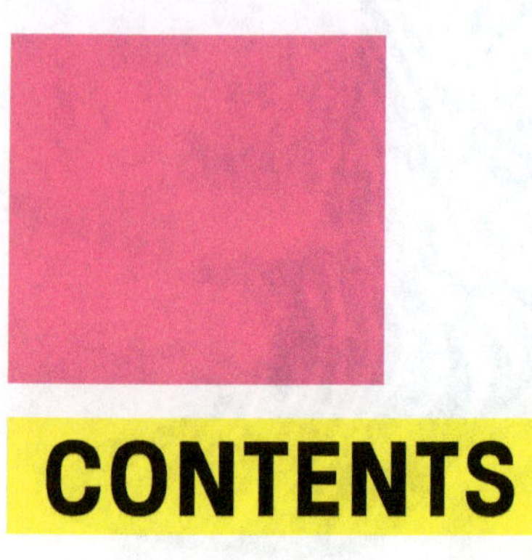

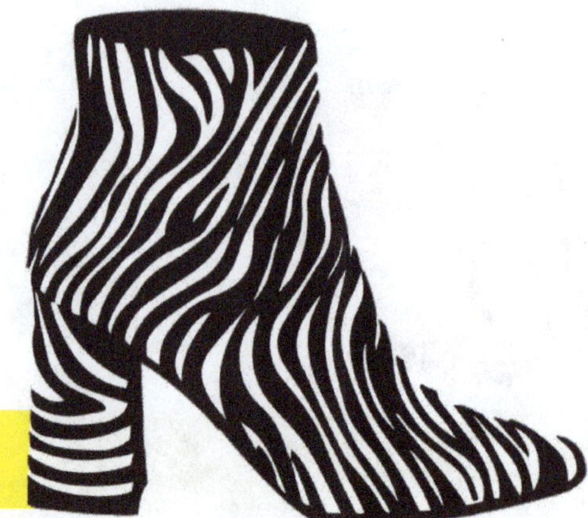

CONTENTS

Breakfast

Lunch

Dinner

Appetizers & Snacks

Bread

Sides

Sauces

Seasonings

Desserts

Drinks

Breakfast

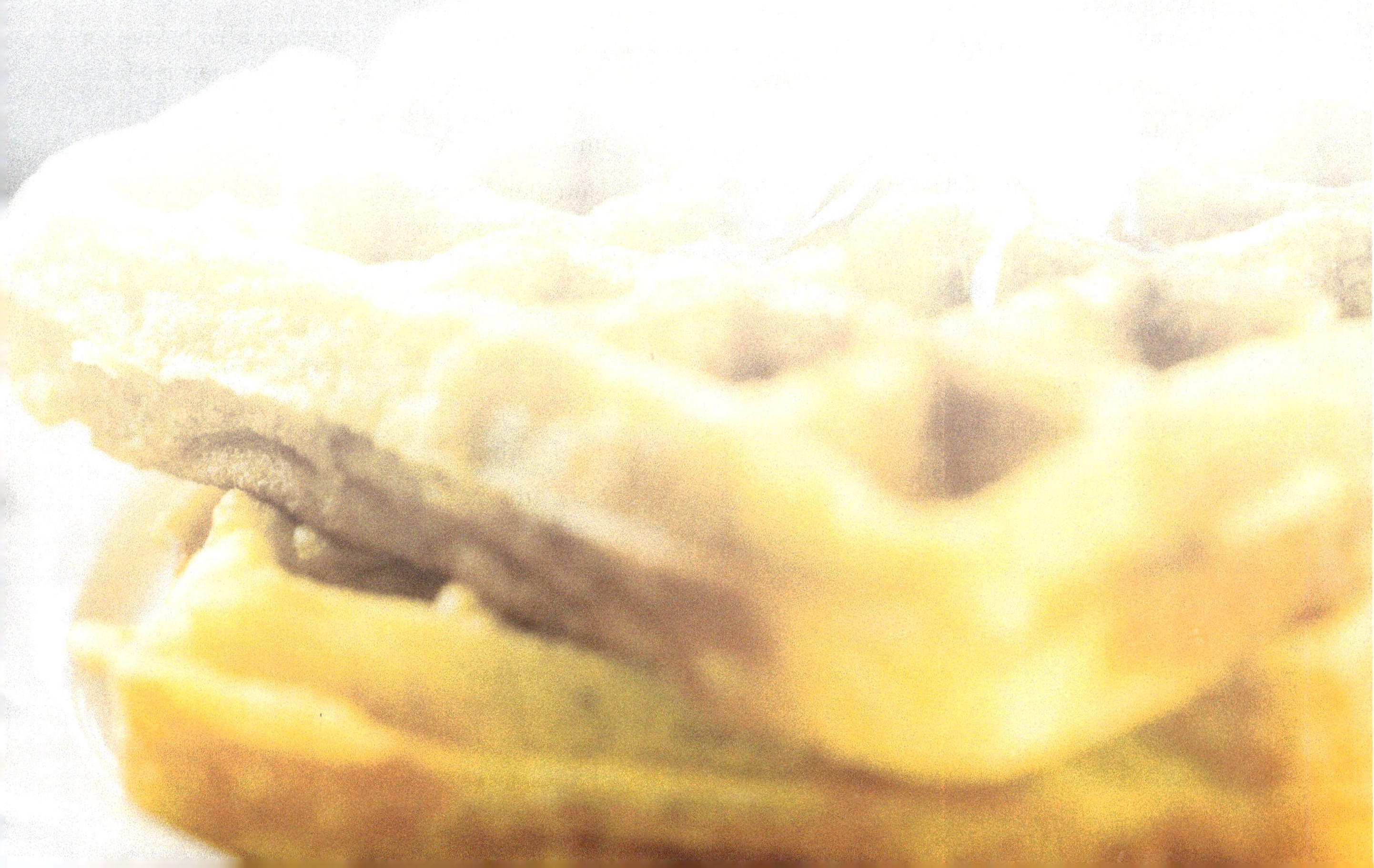

The Breakfast Club Casserole

Prep Time: 10 minutes

Cook Time: 35 minutes

Yield: 6

Saturday, March 24, 1984

Shermer High School, Shermer, IL 60062

Emilio Estevez, Ally Sheedy, Molly Ringwald, Judd Nelson, and Anthony Michael Hall, also known as an athlete, a basket case, a princess, a criminal, and a brain, prove that stereotyping and detention is pointless.

The epic soundtrack, the classic lines, and Bender's unforgettable fist pump in the last frame will forever be known as timeless.

This breakfast is like that.

A combination of sausage, eggs, and cheese with a hint of garlic and onion that pairs well with Sunday brunches, high school memories, letters to prickish school administrators, and a killer Simple Minds song.

1 tablespoon butter

4 cloves garlic, minced

⅓ cup yellow onion, chopped

1 pound breakfast sausage

8 eggs

⅓ cup heavy cream

1 teaspoon salt

½ teaspoon black pepper

1 cup cheddar cheese, shredded

Preheat the oven to 350° and grease an 8 x 8 or 9 x 9 casserole dish. (The smaller the better). In a medium-sized pan, heat the butter until melted.

Add the garlic and onions.

Sauté over medium heat for 4 minutes or until tender.

Add the breakfast sausage, break it up into smaller pieces with a spatula, and cook for about 10 minutes until browned.

Drain excess fat and spread evenly into the casserole dish. Whisk the eggs, cream, salt, and pepper.

Pour this mixture over the sausage, and top with cheese.

Bake at 350° for 30 minutes until eggs are set and the top is golden brown. Cool and serve.

Store leftovers in an airtight container in the refrigerator for up to 4 days.

To Freeze: Freeze this casserole after baking for up to 3 months covered in plastic wrap and foil. Thaw overnight in the fridge and reheat in the microwave or oven.

Nutrition Per Serving
(1 cup = 1 serving)

Calories: 395

Fat: 30.8g

Protein: 26g

Fiber: 0.2g

Total Carbs: 2.2g

Net Carbs: 2g

Just Beat It Scrambled Eggs

Prep Time: 2 minutes

Cook Time: 5 minutes

Yield: 2

The incredible edible egg meets a legendary music video that shows us if you can unite gangsters through music and dance, anything is freaking possible.

3 tablespoons unsalted butter

4 eggs

⅓ cup heavy cream

½ teaspoon salt

¼ teaspoon pepper

Melt the butter in a medium-sized pan over low heat.

Whisk the eggs, heavy cream, salt, and pepper until they're combined. Take a moment to remember the tri-fold *Thriller* album Michael Jackson released in 1982. That album was everything. It had "Beat It," "Billie Jean," "PYT," and "Human Nature"—every song was killer.

Add the eggs to the skillet and cook until the eggs are no longer runny. Serve garnished with cheese or chopped green onions.

Nutrition Per Serving
(2 eggs = 1 serving)

Calories: 330

Fat: 31.7g

Protein: 10.3g

Fiber: 0.1g

Total Carbs: 1.3g

Net Carbs: 1.2g

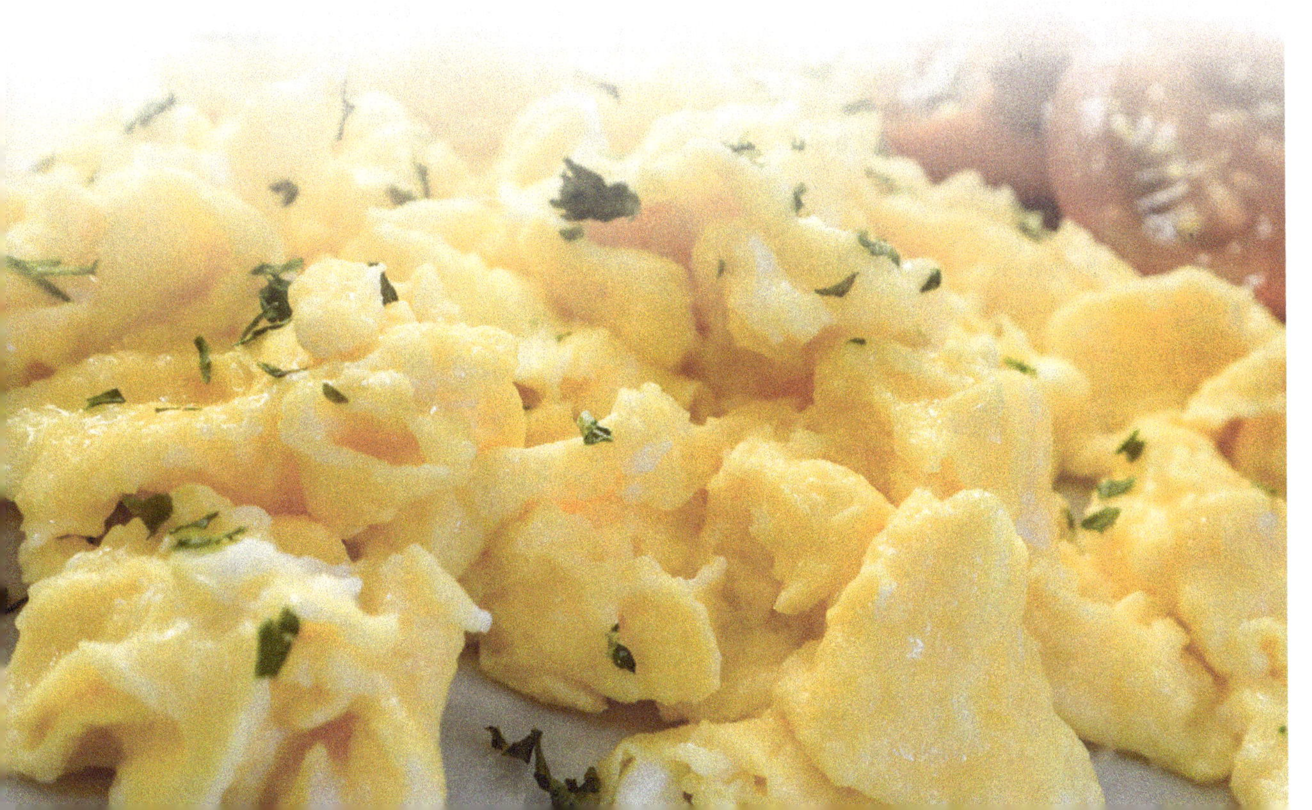

I'm So Egg-Cited Cheesy Egg & Sausage Bites

Prep Time: 15 minutes

Cook Time: 20 minutes

Yield: 32

Excitement.

The thrill of getting ready for a night on the town with the apple of your eye. The anticipation of what the night will bring when all eyes, especially his—are focused on you.

That night will come, but first, these sausage egg bites.

A breakfast that is filling, satisfying, and will deliciously help you get to your goals. Pairs well with The Pointer Sisters.

1 pound breakfast sausage or ground beef, cooked

4 ounces cream cheese

3 eggs

1 cup sharp cheddar cheese, shredded

⅓ cup coconut flour

½ teaspoon baking powder

⅛ teaspoon salt

Preheat the oven to 350° and prep a baking sheet with parchment paper.

Brown the sausage in a large pan over medium-high heat until it is no longer pink. Remove from heat.

Drain the fat, stir in cream cheese, and set aside to cool.

In a large mixing bowl, combine the eggs, cheddar cheese, coconut flour, baking powder, and salt. When the sausage and cream cheese mixture is cooled, you can add it and stir a little more.

Next, we're going to chill the batter in the refrigerator for 10 minutes. If you skip this step, you will be disappointed because you will end up with sad, flat discs instead of fluffy bites. Please don't say I didn't warn you.

Remove from the fridge, stir one more time.

Grab a mini cookie scoop (or a teaspoon), and portion out 32 servings (or however many you darn well please) onto the lined baking sheet or a silicone mat.

Bake at 350° for 18-20 minutes.

Store in an airtight container in the refrigerator for up to 5 days. Reheat wrapped in a paper towel in the microwave until warm.

To Freeze: These freeze well for up to 3 months. Let the bites cool entirely, then flash freeze them for an hour. Store in a heavy-duty freezer bag.

Nutrition Per Serving

(1 egg bite = 1 serving)

Calories: 79

Fat: 6g

Protein: 5g

Fiber: 0.5g

Total Carbs: 1.2g

Net Carbs: 0.7g

Hall & Oates – Grain Free Granola

Prep Time: 10 minutes

Cook Time: 30 minutes

Yield: 3 cups

Daryl Hall. John Oates. A staple duo in the '80s.

Hall belts outs the lyrics as the lead vocalist while Oates holds down the melodies on the guitar. It worked.

"Rich Girl," "Private Eyes," "She's Gone," and "Maneater"—a few unforgettable collaborations. Another collaboration you'll want to have on standby? This grain-free granola.

It's a snack—it's cereal—it's a two bird, one stone recipe that you'll want to put on repeat like that 45 you had in junior high.

1 cup sunflower seeds

1 cup pecans, chopped

1 cup coconut flakes, unsweetened

¼ cup blanched almond flour

¼ cup salted butter, melted

¼ cup granular erythritol

1 teaspoon vanilla

⅛ teaspoon liquid stevia

1 egg white

Preheat your oven to 325°

Line a large baking sheet (or two small sheet pans) with parchment paper. Combine the sunflower seeds, pecans, coconut, and almond flour in a large bowl. In a separate bowl, dissolve the erythritol into the butter.

Then add vanilla, liquid stevia, and egg white.

Once that's well combined, pour it over the pecan mixture and stir until all the nuts and seeds are coated.

Spread it evenly onto your baking sheets.

Bake for 20–30 minutes—with one stir break at the 10-minute mark. When it's ready, the granola will be golden brown.

Don't worry if it doesn't look perfect—it will crisp as it cools. Cool completely before serving.

Store in an airtight container at room temperature for up to 3 weeks.

Nutrition Per Serving
(¼ cup = 1 serving)

Calories: 186

Fat: 18.1g

Protein: 4g

Fiber: 2.9g

Total Carbs: 4.5g

Net Carbs: 1.6g

Sowing The Chia Seeds of Love Pudding

Prep Time: 5 minutes

Chill Time: 8 hours

Yield: 2

You reap what you sow.

Philosophers remind us that our current realities are manifested by decisions and actions we previously planted.

Some take longer than others.

A Madagascar palm takes 100 years to bloom. The giant Himalayan lily takes 5–7 years.

This chia pudding takes 8 hours. Pairs nicely with Tears for Fears.

¼ cup unsweetened almond milk

¾ cup full fat coconut milk

¼ teaspoon vanilla

4–5 drops liquid stevia

1 tablespoons chia seeds

1 tablespoon protein powder

½ cup blueberries

2 tablespoons hemp seeds

Combine almond milk, coconut milk, vanilla, and stevia in a medium bowl. Add the chia seeds and protein powder—combine well.

Refrigerate overnight to let it thicken and to give the chia seeds time to absorb the liquid. Divide into two bowls and top with blueberries and hemp seeds.

Nutrition Per Serving
(1 bowl = 1 serving)

Calories: 337

Fat: 23g

Protein: 11g

Fiber: 5g

Total Carbs: 14g

Net Carbs: 9g

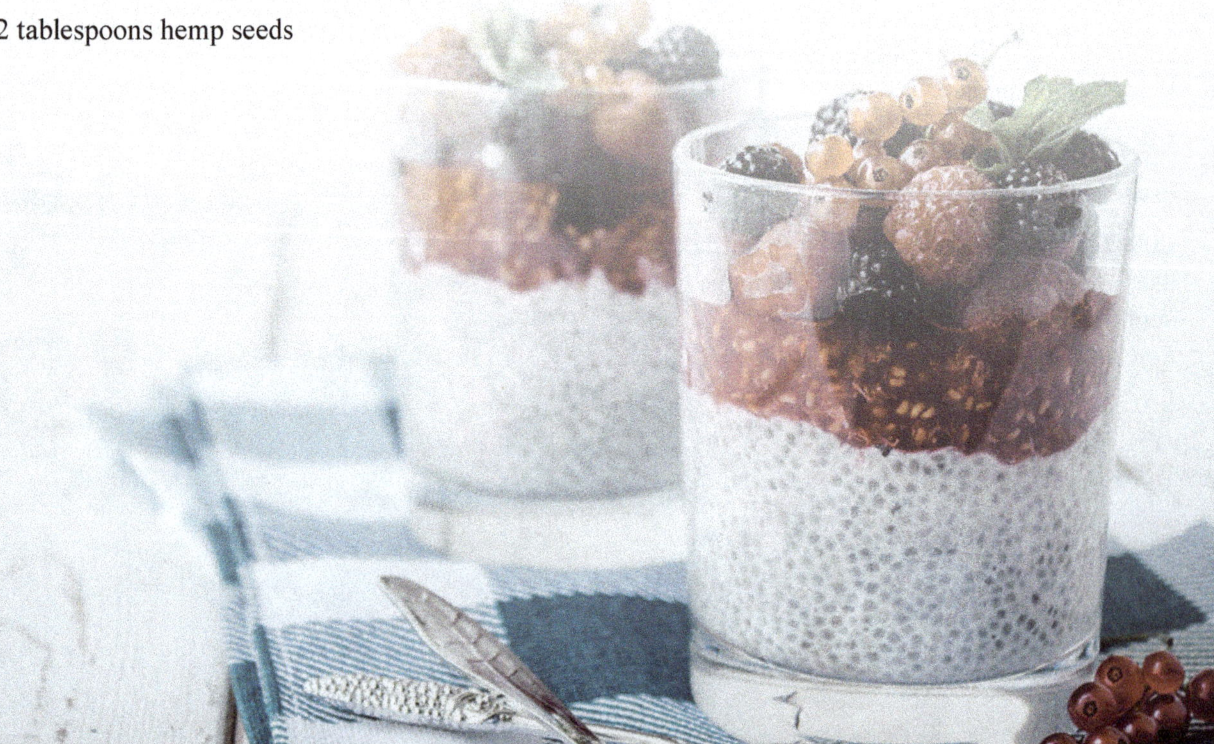

Stir Crazy Better Than Eggo Waffles

Prep Time: 10 minutes

Cook Time 20 minutes

Yield: 2

Create the easy, grab-and-go Eggo vibe with this recipe for low carb waffles that seriously taste better than the original, and they're freezer-friendly.

Pairs well with the 1980 comedy classic, *Stir Crazy* featuring Gene Wilder and Richard Pryor.

5 eggs, separated

1 tablespoons coconut flour

1 teaspoon baking powder

2 tablespoons granulated monk fruit (use less or more depending on your taste)

½ cup butter, melted

2 teaspoons vanilla

3 tablespoons heavy cream

Preheat your waffle iron and grease it with butter or cooking spray. Grab two mixing bowls and get ready to get your waffle on.

The first step is to separate the egg yolks from the whites. You'll be tempted to skip it, but don't.

Whisk the egg whites like your life depends on it—until they get bubbly and form "stiff peaks," which makes them look like a whipped cream dollop. We're going through this trouble to make the waffle texture as close to the legit version as possible. You can use a whisk, an electric mixer, or a stand mixer to make this stir-crazy action happen.

Meanwhile, in bowl #2, you're going to mix up the egg yolks, coconut flour, baking powder, and sweetener. Stir in melted butter, vanilla, and heavy cream.

Fold in the egg whites.

Add the batter to your waffle iron and cook until your waffles look so golden and perfect that you cannot take it anymore!

(For those of you who have yet to master the art of waffle-making, take a peek at the 3-minute mark to see how your waffles are looking.)

Serve with butter and sugar-free syrup—if that's your thing.

Try Lakanto Sugar-Free Maple syrup if you haven't already. In my opinion, it is the most realistic tasting of the sugar-free options available.

To Freeze: Make a double batch and freeze these suckers for up to 4 months. Just let them cool off, then freeze in Ziploc bags—separate each one with wax or parchment paper so they don't stick together. Reheat them in the oven, toaster, or microwave.

Nutrition Per Serving
(1 waffle = 1 serving)

Calories: 287

Fat: 26.5g

Protein: 7.2g

Fiber: 2g

Total Carbs: 5.3g

Net Carbs: 3.3g

Just Call Me Angel Of The Morning Almond Flour Pancakes

Prep Time: 15 minutes

Cook Time: 10 minutes

Yield: 6

A new day. Another beginning. A fresh start.

Make it count.

English pancakes are flat like crepes. In China, they use dough instead of batter, and Ancient Greeks combined wheat flour, olive oil, honey, and curdled milk.

Empowered women today use this combination of almond flour, eggs, and cream cheese. Pairs nicely with wispy bangs, high-waisted denim, and any Juice Newton LP.

2 eggs

4 ounces cream cheese

½ cup almond flour

1 teaspoon vanilla

¼ teaspoon baking powder

1 teaspoon powdered sweetener (I like So Nourished erythritol)

2 teaspoons unsalted butter or coconut oil

Salted butter (optional)

Sugar-free maple syrup (optional)

Combine eggs, cream cheese, almond flour, vanilla, baking powder, and sweetener in a food processor or blender and pulse until smooth.

In a medium-sized pan, heat butter or coconut oil over medium heat. Once the butter melts, add ¼ cup batter and flip after batter bubbles evenly throughout the pancake.

Cook another 2–3 minutes.

Transfer to a plate and repeat with the rest of the mixture. Serve plain or topped with butter and sugar-free maple syrup.

Lakanto Maple Syrup is keto-friendly (1 net carb), sugar-free, all-natural, and low glycemic.

To Freeze: Freeze individually (between sheets of parchment or wax paper) in Ziploc bags for up to 3 months. Reheat in the oven or wrapped in a paper towel in the microwave.

Nutrition Per Serving
(3 pancakes = 1 serving)

Calories: 487

Fat: 34.2g

Protein: 18g

Fiber: 0.9g

Total Carbs: 9g

Net Carbs: 4.5g

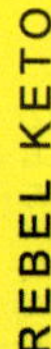

Stand By Me Spinach Sausage & Cheese Frittata

Prep Time: 15 minutes

Cook Time: 15 minutes

Yield: 6

You don't have to know that frittata means "fried" in Italian or that a frittata is pretty much an omelet with the fillings mixed with eggs in the pan instead of folded in.

But hey, knowledge is power, right? Speaking of knowledge...

In the coming-of-age film, Stand by Me, a group of 12-year-old boys learned a few life lessons the hard way—don't believe in stereotypes, support your friends, seize the moment, and never give up on your dreams.

The 12 ingredients in this frittata come together to help you do the same. Here's how to make it happen.

1 tablespoon avocado oil

1 pound ground pork

1 teaspoon dried thyme

1 teaspoon dried sage

¼ teaspoon ground nutmeg

¼ teaspoon red pepper flakes

½ onion, diced

3 garlic cloves, minced

10 ounces fresh spinach or frozen spinach (thawed & drained)

8 eggs

½ cup heavy cream

1 cup feta cheese

Heat the oil in an oven-safe pan or cast-iron skillet over medium heat.

Add the sausage, and when it starts to brown, add the thyme, sage, nutmeg, and red pepper flakes. Stir and cook for another 5 minutes until sausage is cooked.

Drain the majority of fat—but try to leave around 2–3 tablespoons worth in the pan.

Transfer the pork to a separate bowl and add the onions to the skillet. Sauté on low for 5 minutes until the onions are transparent.

Add the garlic and sauté for another minute.

Stir in the spinach and the sausage. Combine well.

In a small bowl, whisk the eggs and the heavy cream together, then pour the egg mixture over the veggies in the skillet.

Don't bother stirring.

Cook for 8 minutes until eggs are set.

Sprinkle the top with feta cheese and place it in an oven set to low broil.

Broil for 5 minutes until eggs are cooked, and cheese is golden brown. Cool before serving and enjoy.

Nutrition Per Serving
(⅙ of recipe = 1 serving)

Calories: 424

Fat: 33.7g

Protein: 26.2g

Fiber: 1g

Total Carbs: 3.5g

Net Carbs: 2.5g

The Drop Biscuits Sir-Mix-A-Lot Would Approve Of

Prep Time: 15 minutes

Cook Time: 15 minutes

Yield: 12

Nope. Your eyes aren't fooling you. You can make biscuits happen on a low carb diet. These are ready to serve in 30 minutes—and yes, in case you're wondering, they are also gluten-free.

So, they're not quite the buttermilk biscuits that inspired the sick rhyme of the '80s, but at least you'll have that song in your head all day. But seriously, these drop biscuits couldn't be easier to put together—no kneading or rolling required!

1 cup almond flour (blanched)

2 teaspoons baking powder

½ teaspoon salt

⅓ cup butter, melted

2 eggs

½ cup sour cream

Preheat the oven to 350° and line a baking sheet with parchment paper. In a large bowl, combine almond flour, baking powder, and salt.

Add melted butter, eggs, and sour cream. Stir well.

Now, grab a cookie scoop or a spoon to drop the dough onto the parchment paper. Use about two tablespoons of batter per biscuit.

Bake at 350° for 15 minutes. Serve topped with butter.

Store in the fridge in an airtight container for up to a week.

To Freeze: Freeze for up to 3 months in freezer bags or a freezer-safe container. Reheat in the oven, toaster, or microwave.

*You can substitute butter with coconut oil or ghee for dairy-free biscuits

Nutrition Per Serving

(1 biscuit = 1 serving)

Calories: 216

Fat: 19g

Protein: 7g

Fiber: 2g

Total Carbs: 5g

Net Carbs: 3g

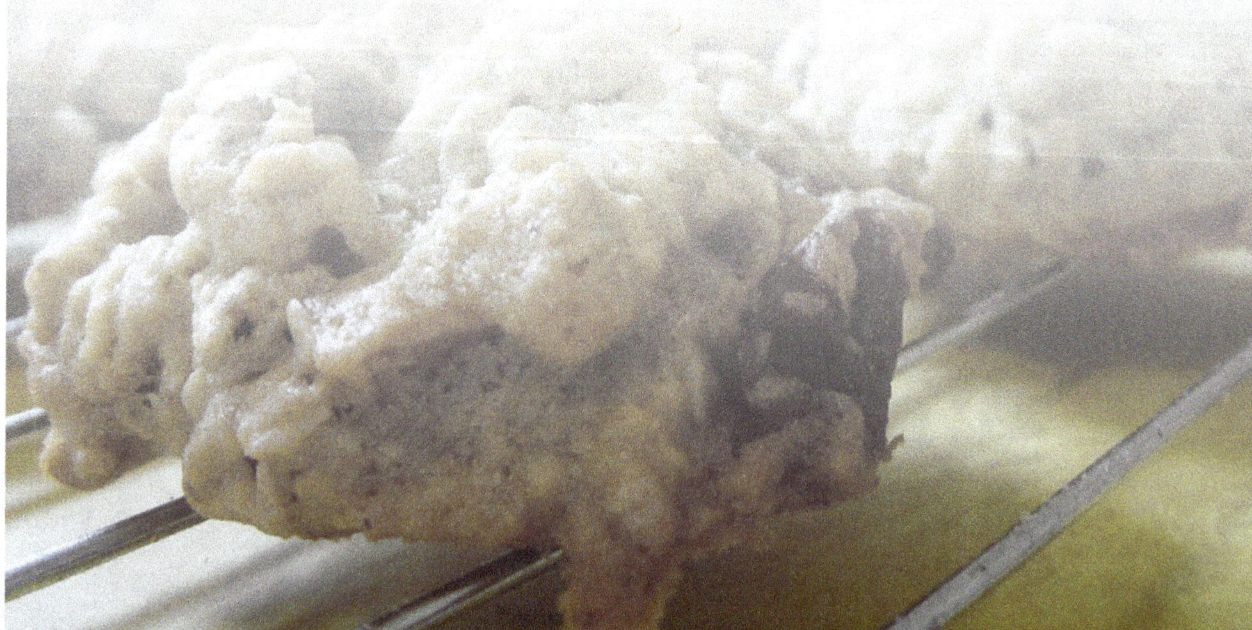

Mary Mary Make-Ahead Omelette Muffins

Prep Time: 10 minutes

Cook Time: 20 minutes

Yield: 12

Mary.

She has it together. Always on time?

Check.

Dressed for the day at 7:45 am?

Check.

P.T.A. Yoga enthusiast. Goal weight after three kids? Check. Check. Check.

Mary has it all together. What's her secret weapon? Meal prep.

She may be buggin', but she's got it going on.

Thanks to these easy egg muffins that are as versatile as ripped denim jeans. Dress 'em up or dress 'em down.

They'll be your new secret go-to breakfast weapon.

Pairs well with any Run-D.M.C. classic as well as an empowering Spirit of Mom competition.

12 eggs

1 cup ham, cooked & diced

1 cup sharp cheddar cheese, shredded

½ cup baby spinach, shredded

¼ cup mushrooms, chopped

¼ cup red bell pepper, diced

3 tablespoons onion, diced

½ teaspoon seasoned salt

¼ teaspoon garlic powder

¼ teaspoon black pepper

Swap the ham with sausage or bacon—switch up the type of cheese and vegetables to make life more exciting or to use what you have on hand.

Preheat the oven to 350°. Grease a 12-cup muffin tin. In a medium-sized bowl, beat the eggs until fluffy.

Stir in the rest of the ingredients.

Divide evenly into muffin cups—about ¾ full. (I use a ⅓ cup for each, and it works.) Bake for 20–25 minutes.

(The center of each muffin will be cooked through.) Cool and serve.

Store in an airtight container in the fridge for up to 4 days or freeze for up to 2 months.

To Freeze: Let the egg muffins cool completely before attempting to freeze. Once cool, place in a heavy-duty freezer bag or freezer-friendly container and freeze for up to 2 months.

To Reheat from thawed: Thaw overnight and reheat wrapped in a paper towel in the microwave for 20 seconds.

To Reheat from frozen: Reheat frozen muffins in the microwave wrapped in a paper towel for 1 minute.

Nutrition Per Serving

(1 muffin = 1 serving)

Calories: 141

Fat: 10g

Protein: 11g

Fiber: 1g

Total Carbs: 1g

Net Carbs: 1g

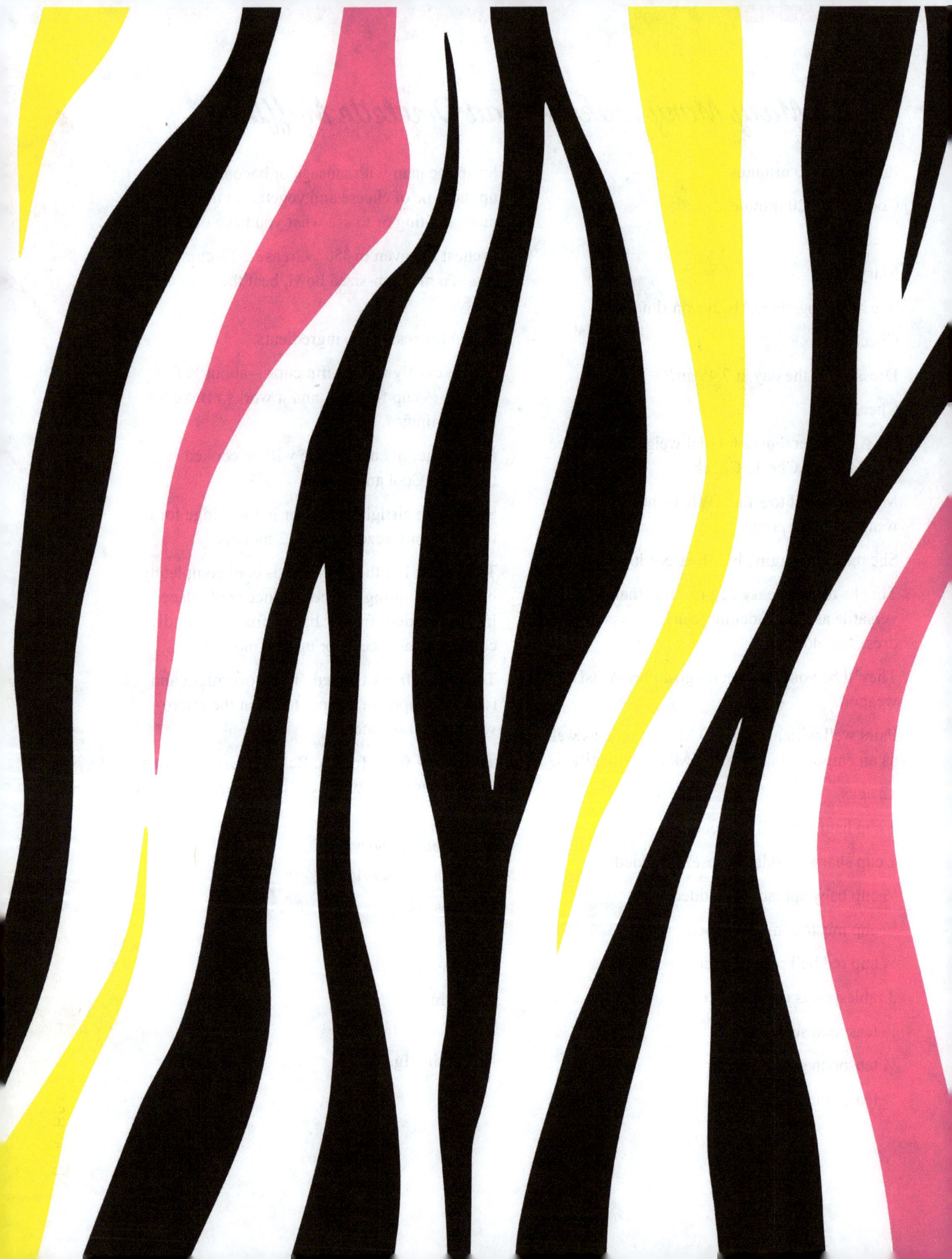

Lunch

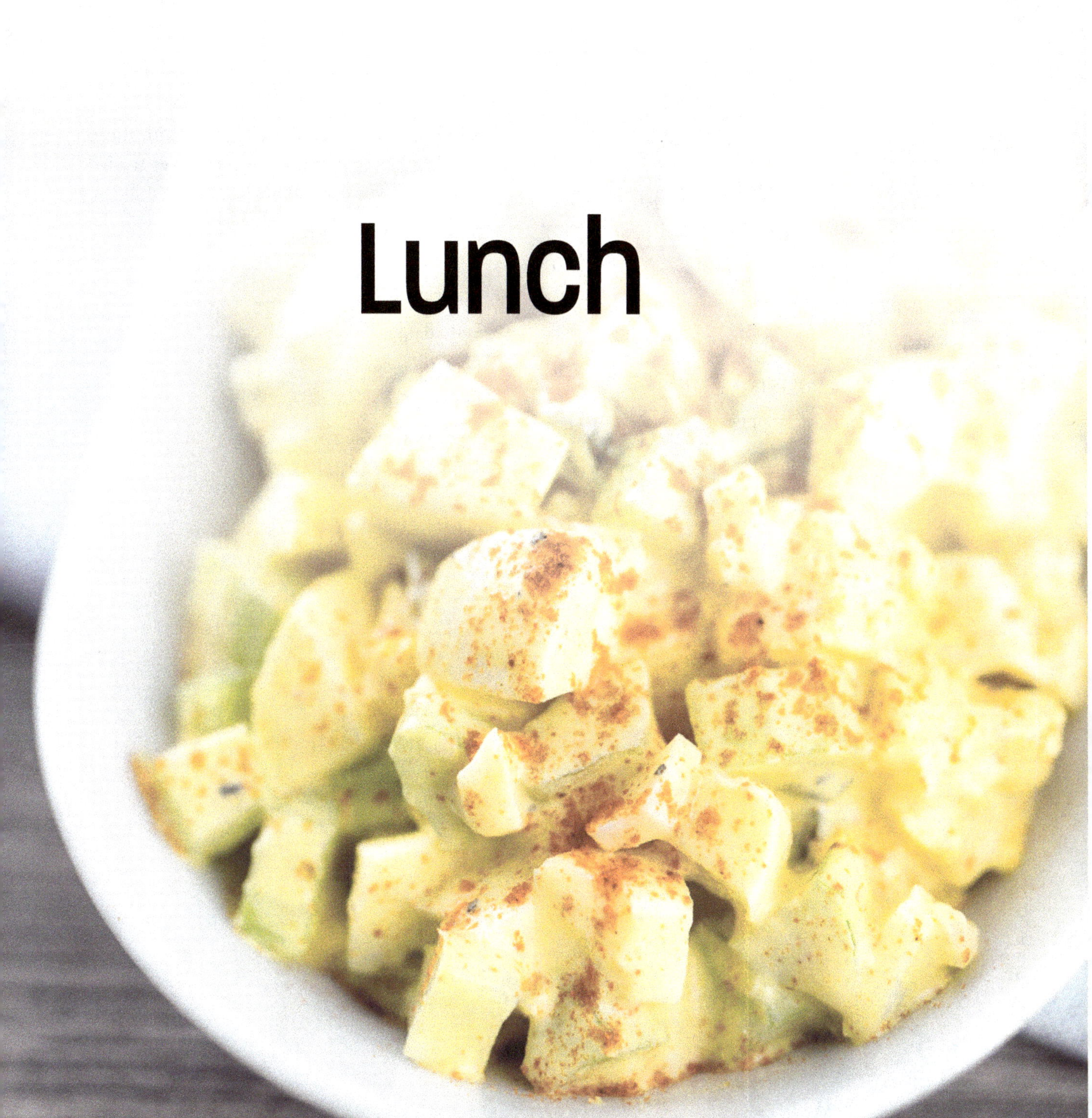

Bill & Ted's Egg Salad Adventure

Prep Time: 10 minutes

Cook Time: 0

Yield: 4

Something strange may have been afoot at the Circle K, but there's nothing weird about this Egg Salad, which is perfect for meal prep as well as any adventure that you may find yourself on. (Regardless of time-travel.)

6 hard-boiled eggs, peeled and chopped

2 stalks celery, chopped

1 tablespoon dill pickle relish

1 tablespoon onion, chopped

¼ cup mayonnaise

1 teaspoon prepared yellow mustard

¼ teaspoon sweet paprika

¼ teaspoon black pepper

⅛ teaspoon salt

Boil and peel eggs and prep vegetables.

In a medium bowl, combine all of the ingredients—chopped eggs, celery, dill pickle relish, onion, mayonnaise, mustard, paprika, pepper, and salt. Refrigerate until you're ready to serve and eat.

Store any leftovers in an airtight container in the fridge for up to 3 days.

Serving Ideas: Stuff this egg salad with sliced bell peppers or tomatoes or serve over fresh spinach leaves or romaine lettuce.

Nutrition Per Serving

(¼ recipe = 1 serving)

Calories: 218

Fat: 18.4g

Protein: 9.8g

Fiber: 0.5g

Total Carbs: 2.6g

Net Carbs: 2.1g

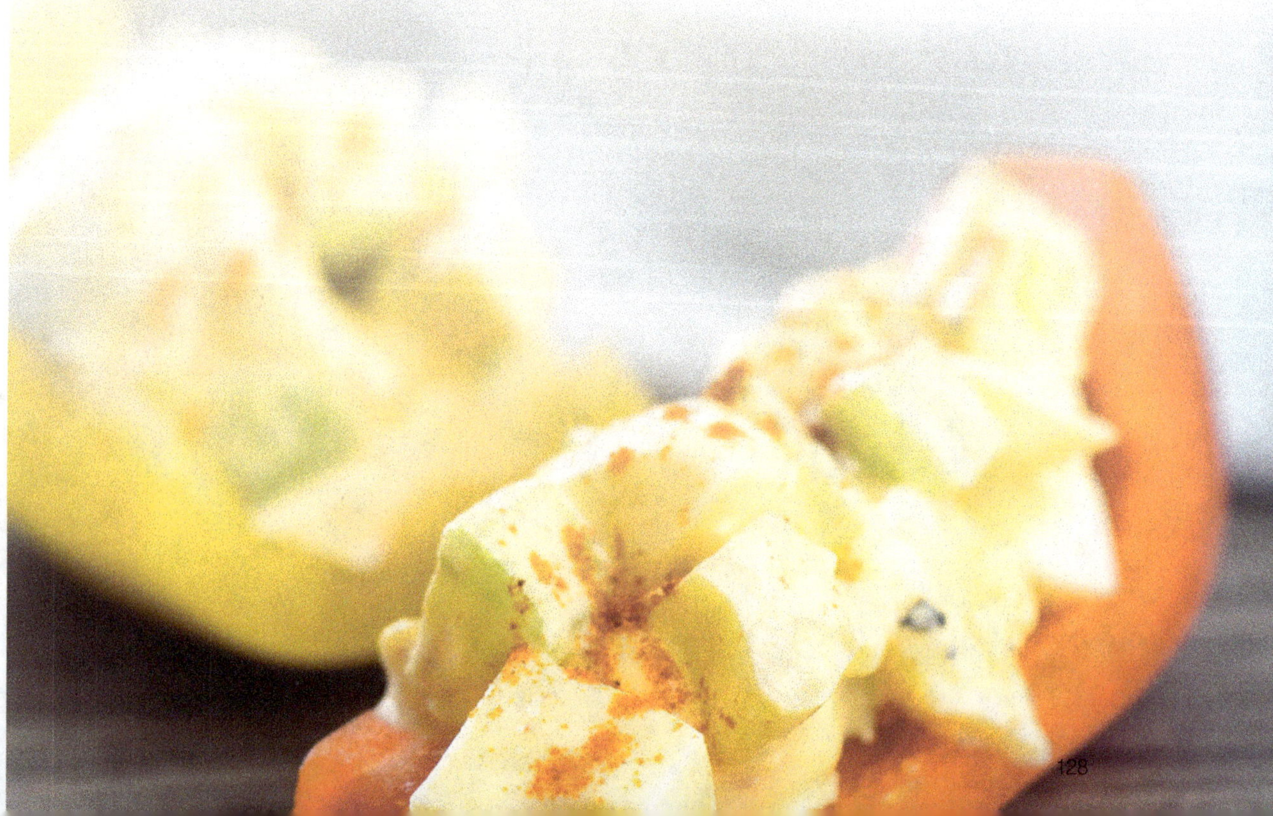

Catch You on The Flip Side Egg-Wrapped Club Sandwich

Prep Time: 10 minutes

Cook Time: 15 minutes

Yield: 4

If you grew up listening to '80s radio, then you'll recall "see you on the flip side" was code for we're about to play the B side—or the less popular, not-what-you-were-hoping-for song. It was usually a major disappointment.

These easy to customize with whatever you have handy egg wraps will not be.

If you have a skillet, a few eggs, and a few pieces of lunch meat or leftover ham, you can make an egg-wrapped club happen.

Note: You can use any skillet you want, but an 8-inch non-stick one makes perfectly sized egg wraps every time.

5 eggs

¼ teaspoon garlic powder

¼ teaspoon salt

⅛–¼ teaspoon pepper

2 teaspoons butter

2–4 teaspoons mayonnaise or mustard

8 slices turkey or ham

4 slices bacon, cooked

1 avocado, sliced

1 small tomato, sliced

1 cup lettuce

Prep a plate or a piece of wax or parchment paper to place your egg wraps on before you get carried away and start cooking.

Whisk eggs with garlic powder, salt, and pepper.

Put the butter in the skillet on low, then add just enough of the egg mixture to cover the bottom of the pan.

(About ¼ of the eggs will do—remember you're making four wraps.) Cook for around 1–2 minutes and flip.

The flip side only needs to cook for around 45 seconds, depending on how state-of-the-art your stove is.

Once you've got the first wrap under your belt and it's on the platter—you'll need to repeat this process three more times.

Once the wraps are ready, prep your roll-ups with mayonnaise or mustard, two slices of turkey, two pieces of bacon, avocado, sliced tomato, and lettuce.

Wrap or fold and serve.

Nutrition Per Serving
(1 wrap = 1 serving)

Calories: 279

Fat: 20.3g

Protein: 19.7g

Fiber: 2.7g

Total Carbs: 4.8g

Net Carbs: 2.1g

Some Kind of Wonderful Chicken Salad

Prep Time: 10 minutes

Cook Time: 10 minutes

Yield: 4

It's the classic John Hughes misfit movie. The outcast falls in love with the A-list girl. Complications arise, eventually love wins.

Here's to happy endings and Eric Stoltz getting the girl. And to easy chicken salad!

Perfect for lunch or brunch.

Pairs well with any John Hughes movie.

1 cup chicken, shredded (You can also use a store-bought rotisserie chicken)

2 hard-boiled eggs, chopped

¼ cup dill pickles, chopped

¼ cup red onion, chopped

¼ cup celery, chopped

¼ cup pecans, chopped

½ cup mayonnaise

1 teaspoon prepared mustard

1 teaspoon dill

Salt & pepper

Grab a large bowl and combine the ingredients—chicken, hard-boiled eggs, dill pickles, red onion, celery, pecans, mayonnaise, mustard, dill, salt and pepper, and chill for an hour before serving.

Serve in a lettuce wrap or a hollowed-out tomato.

Nutrition Per Serving
(1 cup = 1 serving)

Calories: 394

Fat: 32g

Protein: 21g

Fiber: 1g

Total Carbs: 3g

Net Carbs: 2g

Not Chicken of The Sea Tuna Salad

Prep Time: 15 minutes

Cook Time: 0

Yield: 6

When I was a kid, I hated tuna with a passion. I especially hated it when my grandmother would try to sell me on the idea of eating it by calling it the chicken of the sea, which always summoned images of snobby chickens swimming in the ocean turning down their beaks on the lowly tuna.

But you know what? As you get older (ahem, broke in college) and you have to get most of your protein out of a can—your opinion on tuna changes. Well, mine did anyway!

1 5-ounce can tuna packed in water

2 hard-boiled eggs, peeled and chopped

1 stalk celery, chopped

¼ cup green bell pepper, chopped

1 tablespoon white onion, chopped

2 tablespoons dill relish

½ cup mayonnaise

¼ teaspoon salt

¼ teaspoon pepper

Boil and chop eggs, and prepare the celery, green bell pepper, and onion.

Drain the tuna and add to a medium-sized bowl. Add the egg, celery, bell pepper, onion, relish, mayonnaise, salt, and pepper. Stir until combined. Refrigerate until you're ready to eat it!

Serve garnished with fresh dill if you like fresh dill.

If you're about the presentation, you can serve it in a hollowed-out tomato or a lettuce wrap. Store any leftovers in an airtight container in the refrigerator for up to three days.

Nutrition Per Serving
(½ cup = 1 serving)

Calories: 216

Fat: 16.9g

Protein: 13.5g

Fiber: 0.2g

Total Carbs: 1.6g

Net Carbs: 1.4g

Club Salad in a Mason Jar

Prep Time: 15 minutes

Cook Time: 5 minutes

Yield: 1

I'm all about the club. Give me a salad that includes bacon, and I'll be happy every time.

Feel free to switch up the proteins and the veggies, depending on what you have available. Or throw everything but the kitchen sink in, as long as you layer it properly.

The rule for mason jar salads is the dressing goes in first, otherwise, you'll end up with a jacked-up soggy salad (and nobody wants that).

Remember that, and you'll be good to go.

1 ounce turkey (2 slices deli meat), chopped

2 ounces ham (2 slices deli meat), chopped

1 hard-boiled egg, diced

2 slices crispy cooked bacon, crumbled

½ avocado, diced

1 teaspoon lemon juice

1 tablespoon blue cheese, crumbled

1½ cups romaine lettuce, chopped

2 tablespoons blue cheese dressing

Chop the veggies and your choice of protein.

Start by putting two tablespoons of blue cheese dressing in a quart-sized mason jar, followed by the chopped tomato and cucumber.

Add your choice of protein (chicken or ham & turkey), egg, and bacon. Top with crumbled blue cheese.

The last layer is the chopped romaine.

Now place the lid on the jar and put it in the fridge until you're ready to eat. Shake it up and pour into your favorite salad bowl or eat it from the jar.

Nutrition Per Serving

(1 jar salad = 1 serving)

Calories: 425

Fat: 30g

Protein: 31.4g

Fiber: 2g

Total Carbs: 7.9g

Net Carbs: 5.9g

Taco Salad

Prep Time: 15 minutes

Cook Time: 15 minutes

Yield: 4

If you need a crowd or a kid-pleaser, you cannot go wrong with this taco salad that is healthy, filling, and simple!

1 tablespoon avocado oil or olive oil

1 pound ground beef

3 tablespoons Homemade Taco Seasoning (See recipe in Seasonings) or store bought

2 cups lettuce, chopped

1 cup cherry tomatoes, sliced

1 avocado, sliced

1 cup cheddar cheese, shredded

½ cup green onions, chopped

½ cup sour cream

⅓ cup salsa

Heat oil in a pan over high heat on the stove.

Brown the ground beef until it's done—as in, no longer pink. Add in the taco seasoning and cook on low for about 5 minutes. Rinse and chop lettuce, tomatoes, green onions, and avocado.

In a large bowl, toss veggies, avocado, seasoned ground beef, cheese, and salsa. Top with sour cream and serve.

Store any leftovers in the fridge in a DO NOT TOUCH container, so you'll know it will be safe.

Nutrition Per Serving
(¼ recipe = 1 serving)

Calories: 280

Fat: 18.2g

Protein: 22.6g

Fiber: 2.8g

Total Carbs: 6.9g

Net Carbs: 4.1g

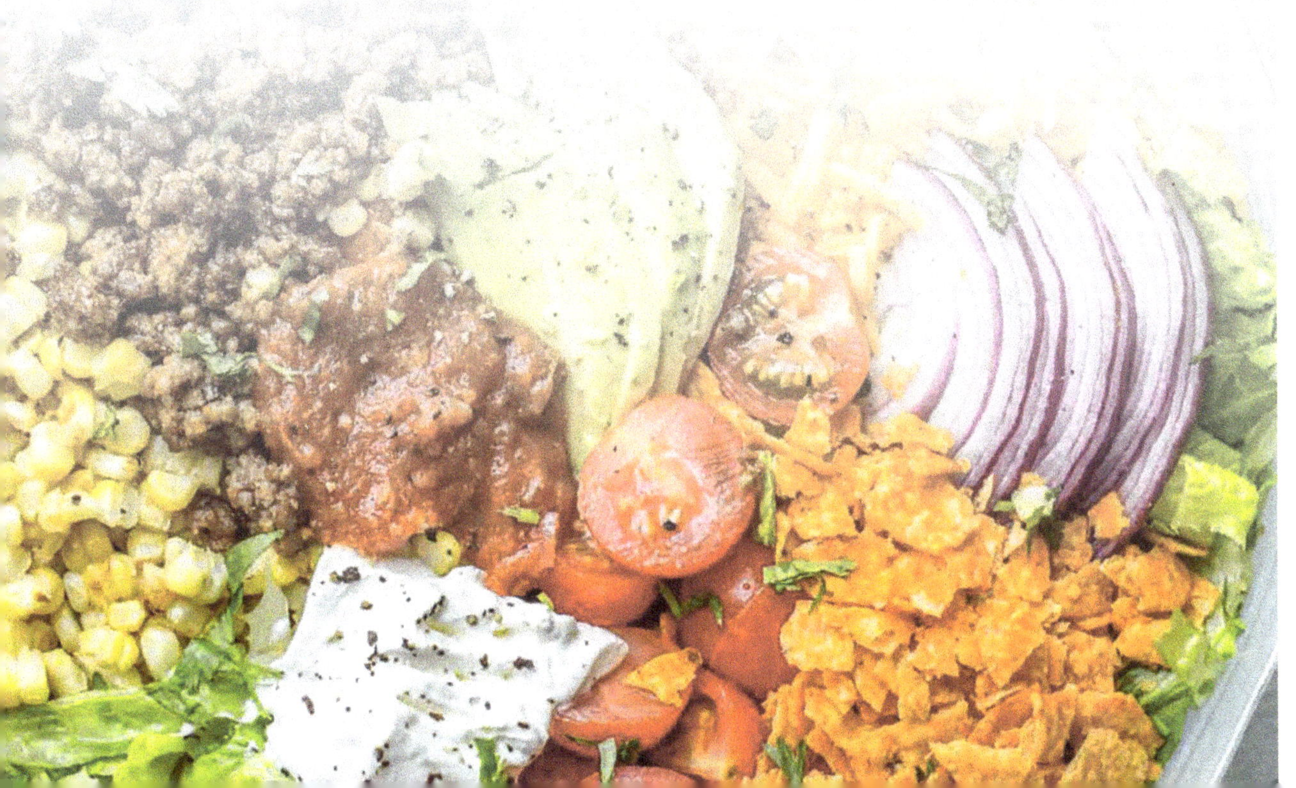

I'll Take Your Man Meatloaf Muffins

Prep Time: 10 minutes

Cook Time: 15 minutes

Yield: 12

So, I've been pretty clear about my struggle with meal prep. The idea of spending my weekend in the kitchen flash freezing and batch cooking makes me sick to my stomach. I like to stick with a few simple make-ahead recipes that I can customize in case of complete boredom. This is one of those recipes.

Bonus points if you blast Salt-n-Pepa while you make 'em.

Let's start with the "base" recipe, and I'll list substitutions on the other side.

½ medium-sized onion, diced

¼ green bell pepper, diced

1½ pounds ground beef

1 clove garlic, minced

½ teaspoon dried oregano

½ teaspoon black pepper

¼ teaspoon salt

1 egg

1 cup pork rinds

Preheat the oven to 350° and grab your favorite muffin tin-no need to grease it.

Chop the onion and bell pepper by hand or by using your food processor. (Don't pulse for too long, or it will get too mushy to use.)

In a large bowl, mix ground beef, onion, bell pepper, garlic, oregano, pepper, salt, egg, and pork rinds. (You'll have to use your hands—it's the only way.)

Then evenly distribute this mixture into 12 muffin cups. (About ⅓ cup each.) Bake for 15–20 minutes.

Variations: I promised you a few variations of this recipe, so here are a few ideas for when you need to switch things up.

Swap ground turkey for ground beef

Add ¾ cup cheddar cheese or a blended Italian or Mexican cheese.

Add spice: chili powder or crushed red pepper.

Top with grated Parmesan cheese.

Top with sugar-free ketchup

To Freeze: Let the mini meatloaves cool and then transfer them to a lined baking sheet and cover them.

Freeze for an hour until they're firm. Then put them in an airtight container and freeze for up to 3 months.

To Reheat: Thaw it in the fridge overnight. Reheat in an oven set at 350 degrees for about 10 minutes.

Nutrition Per Serving
(1 muffin = 1 serving)

Calories: 180

Fat: 8g

Protein: 24.6g

Fiber: 0.2g

Total Carbs: 0.7g

Net Carbs: 0.5g

Lettuce Go Crazy Avocado Egg Salad Wraps

Prep Time: 10 minutes

Cook Time: 10 minutes

Yield: 6

Have you ever sat down and listened to Prince's lyrics? He may have looked like an '80s pop star, but he was a deep-thinking observer with a knack for the synthesizer. His unique combination of the spoken word blended with multiple sound elements always culminated in a musical masterpiece.

While this Egg Salad Wrap may not be as brilliant as a Prince song, it does clearly combine the healthy fats of avocado with the powerful protein of egg to create a flavorful lunch that will keep you full for hours.

Hot tip: Leave the avocado pit in the salad to prevent it from turning brown!

6 hard-boiled eggs, peeled

1 avocado, peeled & diced

¼ cup red onion, chopped

1 teaspoon lemon juice

2 teaspoons fresh thyme

½ teaspoon salt

¼ teaspoon pepper

6 Butter, Green leaf or Romaine lettuce leaves

Mix the egg yolks and avocado until smooth.

Add chopped egg (whites), onion, lemon juice, thyme, salt, and pepper. Serve wrapped in lettuce.

Nutrition Per Serving
(⅙ recipe = 1 serving)

Calories: 150

Fat: 11.7g

Protein: 7.2g

Fiber: 3.2g

Total Carbs: 5g

Net Carbs: 1.8g

Cobb Salad with Last-Minute Ranch

Prep Time: 10 minutes

Cook Time: 0

Serves: 4

10 ounces Romaine lettuce, chopped

1 ounce chicken, chopped (Rotisserie is perfect)

4 hard-boiled eggs, chopped

1 slices bacon, cooked and crumbled

2 medium tomatoes, chopped

2 avocados, sliced

4 ounces blue cheese, crumbled

Combine ingredients in a bowl—romaine lettuce, chicken, eggs, bacon, tomatoes, avocados, and blue cheese.

Serve topped with your favorite low carb dressing or the last-minute Ranch recipe below!

Last Minute Ranch

6 tablespoons mayonnaise

1½ tablespoons What's Hiding in the Valley Ranch Seasoning (See recipe in Seasonings)

¼ teaspoon pepper

4 tablespoons water

Nutrition Per Serving
(¼ recipe = 1 serving)

Calories: 485

Fat: 35.4g

Protein: 27.3g

Fiber: 6.7g

Total Carbs: 11.3g

Net Carbs: 4.6g

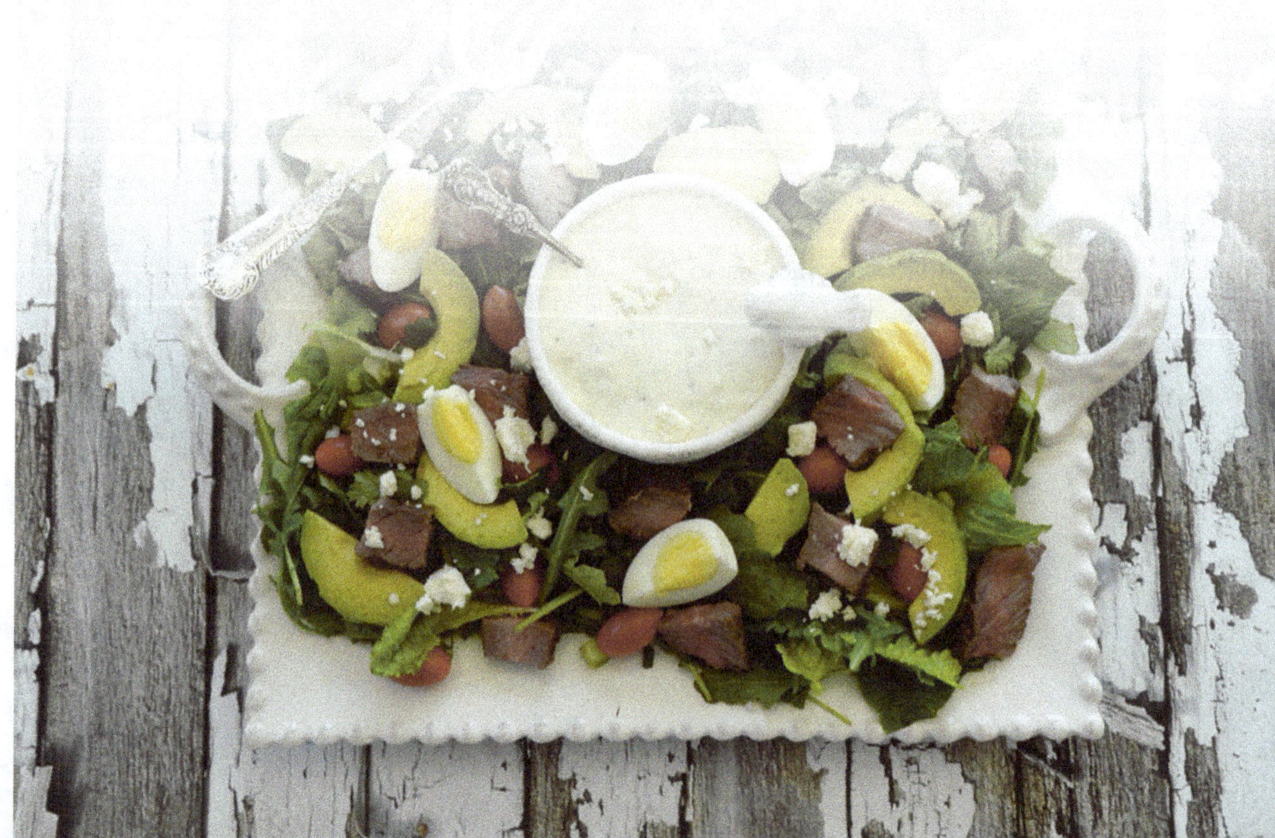

Dead Poet's Society Chicken Caesar Salad with Avocado

Prep Time: 15 minutes

Cook Time: 0

Yield: 2

I watch Dead Poet's Society at least once a year, and I always see something new and learn a lesson every time. But one is always evident: never miss an opportunity to seize the day. Make your life extraordinary—you only get one.

9 ounces romaine lettuce

6 cherry tomatoes, halved

1 avocado, cubed

6 ounces cooked chicken—chopped (you can use Rotisserie chicken)

¼ cup Parmesan cheese

¼ teaspoon black pepper

1 slice cooked bacon, crumbled (optional)

2–3 tablespoons of Carpe Diem Caesar Salad Dressing (See recipe in Seasonings)

Rinse the romaine and pat it dry with a paper towel.

Rinse and halve the cherry tomatoes and cube or slice the avocado. In a medium bowl, combine the romaine, chicken, and tomatoes.

Toss with Caesar dressing.

Top with avocado, parmesan cheese, pepper, and bacon. Enjoy every bite!

Nutrition Per Serving
(½ recipe = 1 serving)

Calories: 594

Fat: 48g

Protein: 30g

Fiber: 7g

Total Carbs: 13g

Net Carbs: 4.5g

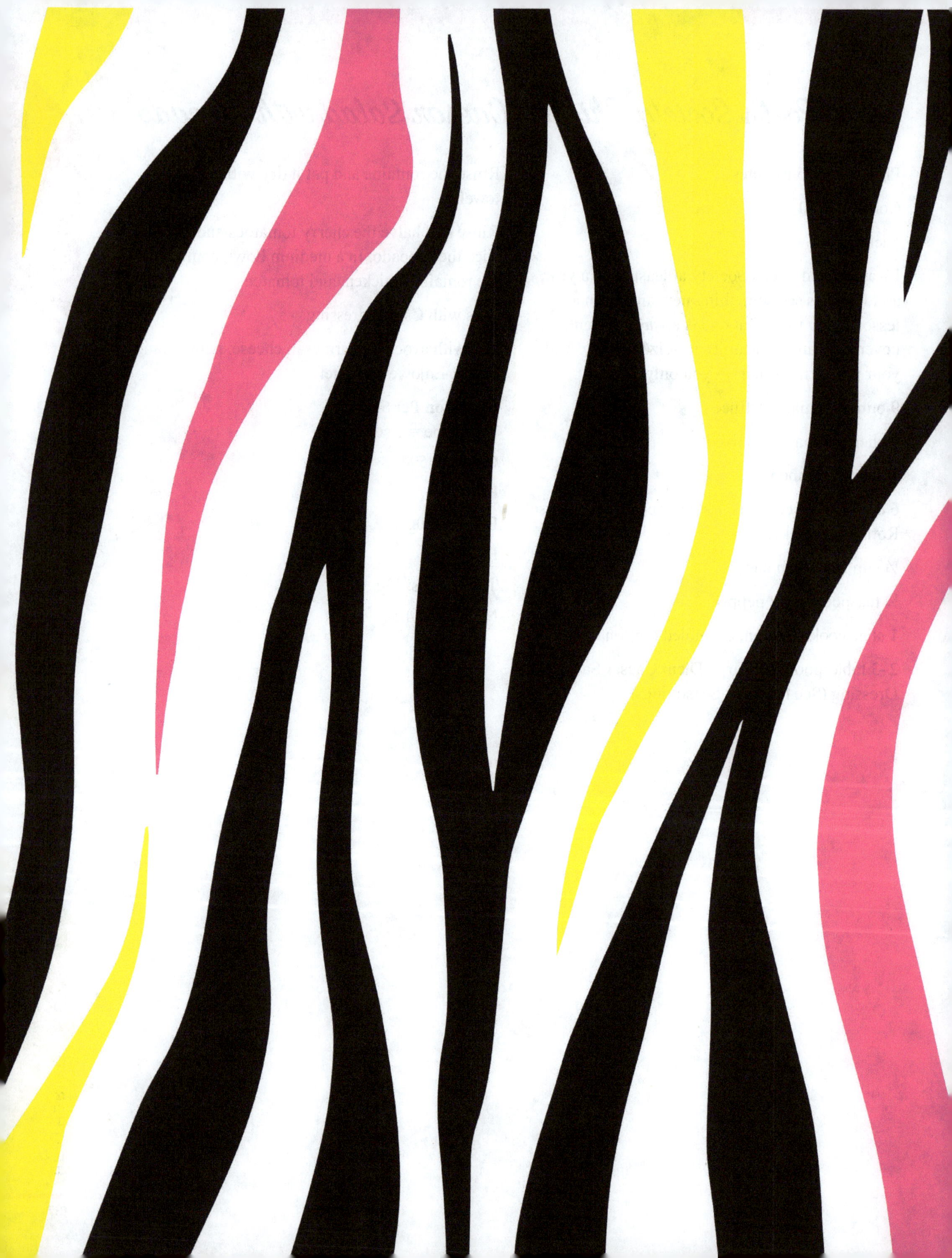

Dinner

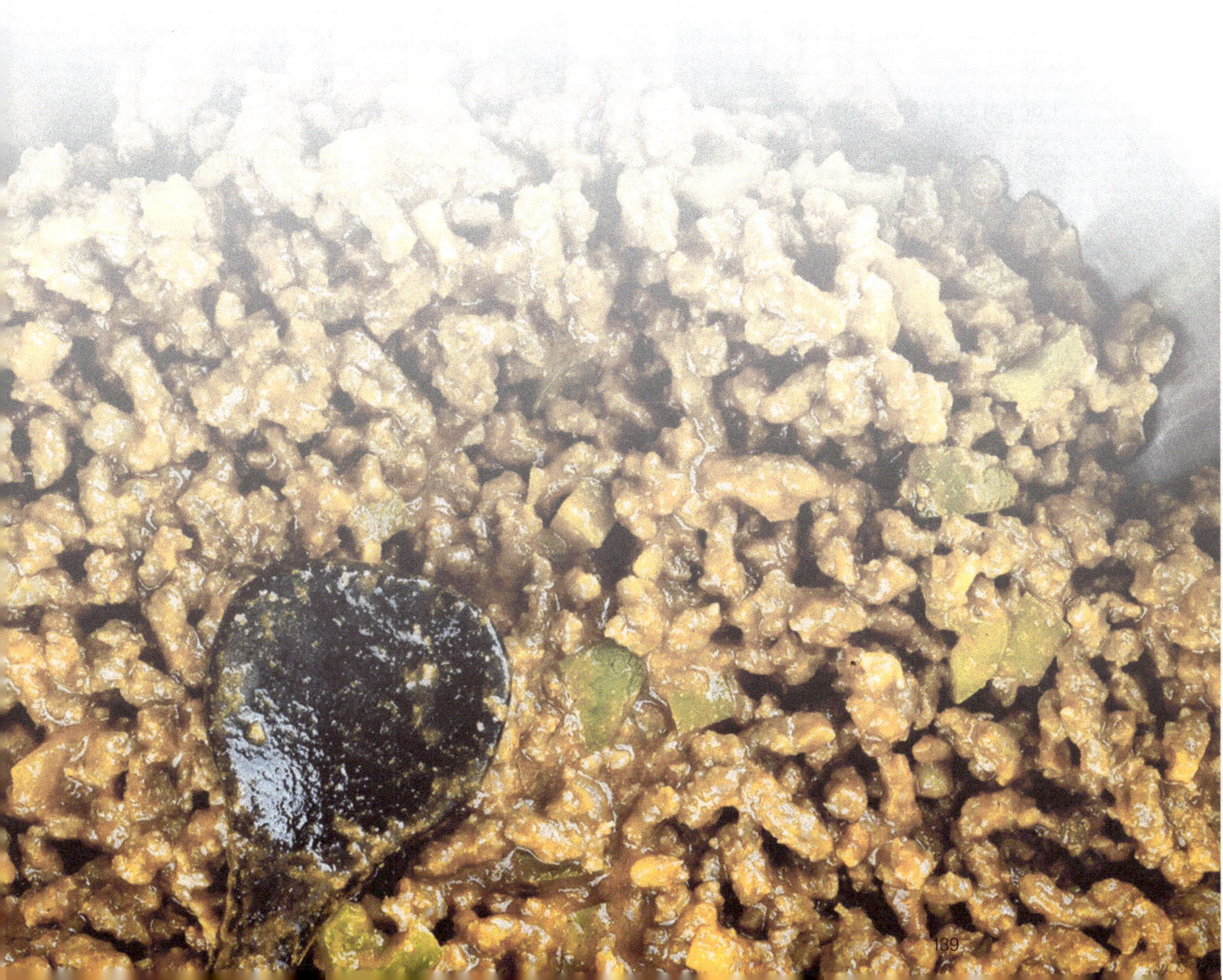

30-Minute Hold The Buns Sloppy Joes

Prep Time: 10 minutes

Cook Time: 20 minutes

Yield: 6

One meal every kid in the '80s could count on (like it or not) was Sloppy Joe night. It may have been every '80s mom's go-to dinner. Whether she went "homemade" with tomato sauce and seasonings or with the even simpler Manwich canned version, the classic Sloppy Joe was always served on a hamburger bun. And it almost always meant leftovers for dinner the following day.

Like the '80s version, this recipe for Sloppy Joes is a quick fix dinner that kids and moms love—without the bun!

1 pound ground beef (or ground turkey)

1 small onion, chopped (½ cup)

1 green bell pepper, chopped

1 clove garlic, minced (or 1 ½ teaspoons minced garlic)

1 8-ounce can tomato sauce

½ cup beef broth

2 tablespoons brown Swerve

2 tablespoons Worcestershire sauce

1 tablespoon prepared yellow mustard

1 teaspoon chili powder

¼ teaspoon salt

¼ teaspoon pepper

In a large skillet, cook the ground beef on medium-high heat until it is no longer pink. (You'll have to break the meat up into smaller pieces as you go.)

Add the onion, bell pepper, and garlic and cook another 2–3 minutes until the veggies are tender. Drain as much fat as you want to.

Stir in the tomato sauce, add in the beef broth, brown Swerve, Worcestershire sauce, yellow mustard, chili powder, salt and pepper.

Turn the heat down to low and simmer for 20 minutes, stirring occasionally.

Serving Ideas:

- Stuff into hollowed-out bell peppers.
- Serve in a lettuce cup.
- Serve over roasted spaghetti squash.
- Serve over mashed cauliflower.
- Serve over cauliflower rice.
- Serve with nothing and eat it straight outta the skillet.

Store any leftovers in an airtight container in the fridge for up to 5 days.

Nutrition Per Serving
(1 cup = 1 serving)

Calories: 347

Fat: 22.9g

Protein: 22g

Fiber: 0.8g

Total Carbs: 4.5g

Net Carbs: 3.7g

Working 9-to-5 Cheeseburger Casserole

Prep Time: 10 minutes

Cook Time: 20 minutes

Yield: 10

This casserole is legit, folks. You'll love it, your family and friends will love it. It may become your favorite thing ever.

Pairs well with the classic film, 9 to 5, starring Dolly Parton, Jane Fonda, and Lily Tomlin.

4 eggs

1 cup cheddar cheese, divided

1 cup heavy cream

1 tablespoons horseradish mustard (or yellow)

6 slices bacon, cooked and crumbled

3 pounds ground beef

1 cup onion, diced

4 garlic cloves, minced

5 teaspoons Worcestershire sauce (I suggest Lea & Perrins)

Salt & pepper to taste

3 ounces cream cheese

4 dill pickles

Shredded lettuce (if you have it)

Chopped or sliced tomatoes (if you have it)

Preheat the oven to 350°

Combine the eggs, 2 cups of cheese, heavy cream, and mustard in a medium bowl and set it aside—you're going to use this after you have cooked the ground beef.

It is going to rock your world so wait for it.

Brown the ground beef in a skillet. Once you've got it browning, add the diced onions, garlic, Lea & Perrins, salt & pepper.

Once you've got it all browned—drain as much fat as you feel comfortable with giving up – the fat does add flavor.

Final skillet step – add the cream cheese.

Now grab a casserole dish, grease it, and throw the ground beef mixture in it. Then add the eggs, cream, and bacon.

Add the other 2 cups of cheddar cheese and the pickles. Bake it at 350° for 20 minutes.

Serve over shredded lettuce or straight up without anything extra, because you cooked, damn it. Store any leftovers in an airtight container in the refrigerator for up to 4 days.

Nutrition Per Serving
(1 cup = 1 serving)

Calories: 517

Fat: 38.1g

Protein: 38.3g

Fiber: 0.3g

Total Carbs: 3.9g

Net Carbs: 3.6g

No Sides Required Stuffed Bell Peppers

Prep Time: 10 minutes

Cook Time: 30 minutes

Yield: 6

Stuffed peppers were a staple at my house when I was a kid. My mom loved stuffed peppers because there wasn't a ton of work involved. She hated cooking with a passion—a trait she passed on to me. Another feature my mom loved to point out was that since the ground beef and rice were delivered inside vegetable side dishes were unnecessary. Love that.

The only ingredient that has changed in this recipe is the rice. We're swapping cauliflower rice for the old-school white rice and big facts: you won't miss it!

2 cups cauliflower rice, cooked (or 1 10-ounce bag frozen riced cauliflower) *please have this on hand before you get too excited about browning the ground beef!

1 medium yellow onion, chopped

6 large bell peppers (any color)

3 tablespoons olive oil

1½ pounds ground beef

2 garlic cloves, minced

1 teaspoon dried oregano

1 teaspoon paprika

1 teaspoon chili powder

1 teaspoon salt

¼ teaspoon pepper

1 14-ounce can crushed tomatoes

1 tablespoon tomato paste

1 cup Italian blend cheese, shredded

Preheat the oven to 400°

Cook the cauliflower rice. Chop the onion and prep the bell peppers.

Lay each pepper on its side and chop the stem off. Remove the seeds and membrane. Arrange the peppers in a baking dish that's small enough for them to stand upright. Grab a large pan and heat the oil over medium-high heat.

Brown the ground beef for 5–7 minutes, until it is no longer pink. The last thing you need is salmonella poisoning.

Add in the onion, garlic, oregano, paprika, chili powder, salt, and pepper.

Cook for 5 minutes or until the onion is tender. Take this time to reflect upon your day. Stir in the tomatoes and the tomato paste.

Turn the heat down to low.

Add the cauliflower rice and give it a stir.

Try to distribute the mixture into the bell peppers evenly, but don't obsess over it. Bake at 400° for 25 minutes.

Take the peppers out of the oven and sprinkle the cheese over the tops.

Bake for another 5 minutes or until the cheese melts. Dinner is ready! Enjoy it!

Store any leftovers in an airtight container in the refrigerator for up to 3 days.

Nutrition Per Serving
(1 stuffed pepper = 1 serving)

Calories: 410

Fat: 28.7g

Protein: 26.4g

Fiber: 3.6g

Total Carbs: 12.3g

Net Carbs: 8.7g

Steak Escape Skillet Dinner

Prep Time: 10 minutes

Cook Time: 15 minutes

Yield: 6

In 1982, self-proclaimed cheesesteak addicts Ken Smith and Mark Turner opened the first Steak Escape in Columbus, Ohio, to provide the world's mallgoers with something better than the ordinary sandwich. This recipe for a one-skillet Philly cheesesteak dinner is my breadless tribute to my favorite mall meal.

4 tablespoons butter, divided

1 medium-sized green bell pepper, sliced

1 medium red bell pepper, sliced

½ medium onion, sliced

1 ounce cremini mushrooms

2–3 teaspoons minced garlic

1½ pounds flank steak, thinly sliced

1 teaspoon Italian Stallion Seasoning (See recipe in Seasonings)

Salt & pepper to taste

7 slices provolone cheese

Melt two tablespoons of butter in a cast-iron skillet.

Add the bell peppers, onions, mushrooms, and garlic and sauté for 5 minutes, then remove from the pan.

Add the remaining butter and steak.

Season with Italian seasoning and salt and pepper.

Sear the steak on each side, then continue to cook on medium heat until it cooks thoroughly. Add the peppers, mushrooms, and onions back in and cook for another two minutes.

Set your oven to broil for the grand finale.

Add the provolone cheese to the top of the steak and veggies. Place the skillet in the oven for 2 minutes.

Serve hot and enjoy!

Nutrition Per Serving
(⅙ recipe = 1 serving)

Calories: 360

Fat: 22.3g

Protein: 34.4g

Fiber: 1.2g

Total Carbs: 5.1g

Net Carbs: 3.9g

It's Just Another Manic Monday Easy Meatloaf

Prep Time: 10 minutes

Cook Time: 40 minutes

Yield: 6

Put this meatloaf together on a Manic Monday or any other day of the week you need an easy dinner.

1 green bell pepper

½ onion

2 minced garlic cloves

1 pound ground beef or turkey

2 eggs

¼ cup grated Parmesan cheese

½ cup shredded cheddar cheese

½ cup almond flour or crushed pork rinds

1 tablespoon Worcestershire sauce

1 teaspoon salt

1 teaspoon black pepper

Sauce

1 tablespoon sugar-free Italian salad dressing

3 tablespoons sugar-free ketchup

¼ teaspoon fresh cracked black pepper

Preheat the oven to 375°.

In a food processor, pulse bell pepper, onion, and garlic cloves until minced.

(If you don't have a food processor, it's okay. You can dice these with a sharp knife.)

In a large bowl, use your hands to combine ground beef, eggs, parmesan cheese, cheddar cheese, almond flour, Worcestershire sauce, salt, and pepper.

Shape this into a loaf and place it in an oiled bread pan or baking dish. Bake for 25–30 minutes.

While the meatloaf is baking, grab a smaller bowl and whisk the Italian dressing, ketchup, and pepper together.

Take the meatloaf out of the oven, crank the temperature up to 425°. Drizzle sauce over the top of the meatloaf and bake for another 15 minutes. Store leftovers in an airtight container in the fridge for up to four days.

Nutrition Per Serving
(⅙ recipe = 1 serving)

Calories: 306

Fat: 21.9g

Protein: 19.4g

Fiber: 0.6g

Total Carbs: 3.5g

Net Carbs: 2.9g

Freeze-Frame Make-Ahead Chili

Prep Time: 10 minutes

Cook Time: 20 minutes

Yield: 6 servings

Whether you're looking for a make-ahead, freezer meal, or a family-friendly dinner, this Freeze Frame Chili has you covered.

Pairs well with sliced green onions, shredded cheddar cheese, a dollop of sour cream, and, of course, any J. Geils Band LP.

1 pound ground beef

½ small onion, chopped

4 teaspoons minced garlic

1 15-ounce can tomato sauce

1 14-ounce can diced tomatoes

1 cup water

2 tablespoons chili powder

1 tablespoon cumin

½ teaspoon salt

¼ teaspoon black pepper

Cook the ground beef, onion, and garlic in a large pot over medium-high heat until ground beef is browned.

Drain the fat or leave it in—it's up to you.

Add the tomato sauce, diced tomatoes, water, chili powder, cumin, salt, and pepper.

Bring this combination to a boil, then cut the heat to low and simmer for about 20 minutes. Top with sour cream, shredded cheddar cheese, green onions, or jalapeno slices.

Store any leftovers in an airtight container in the refrigerator for up to 5 days.

To Freeze: Freeze in an airtight container or heavy-duty freezer bag for up to 2 months.

Nutrition Per Serving
(1 cup = 1 serving)

Calories: 424

Fat: 31.1g

Protein: 27.8g

Fiber: 3g

Total Carbs: 8.5g

Net Carbs: 5.5g

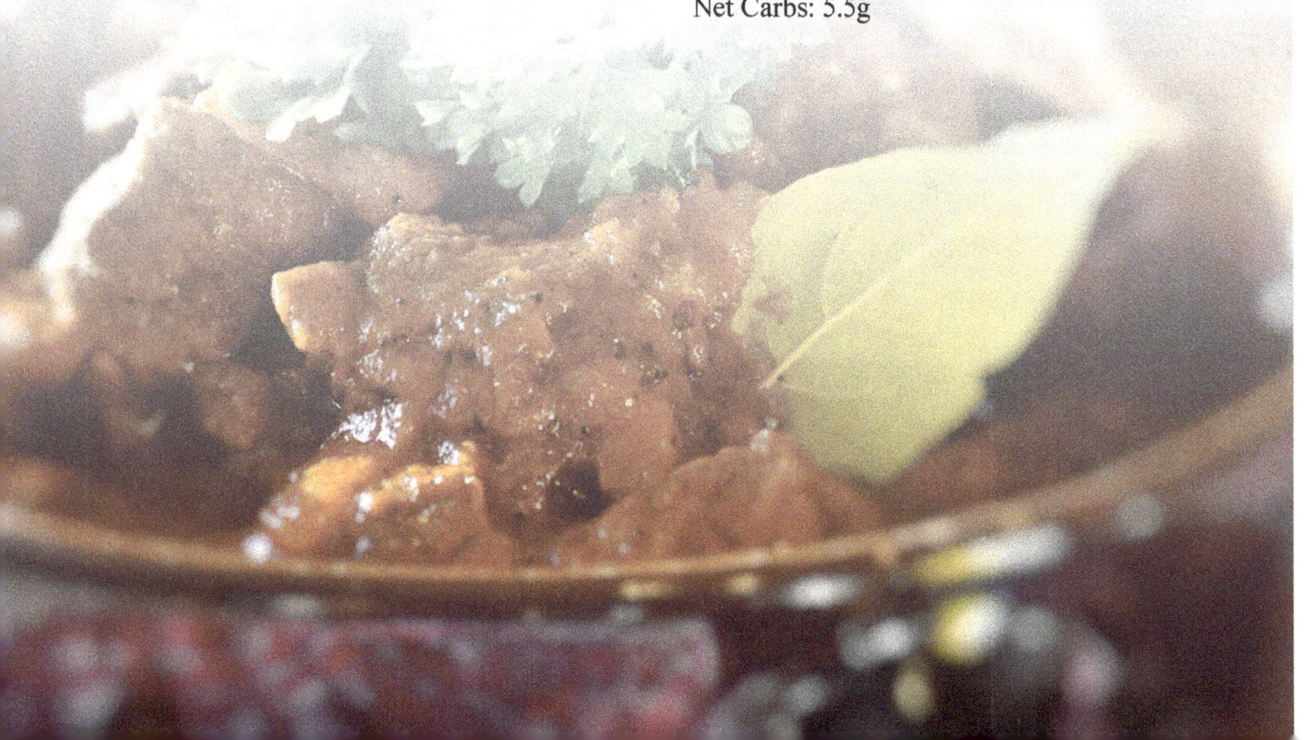

She Works Hard For the Money Cheeseburger Helper

Prep Time: 10 minutes

Cook Time: 20 minutes

Yield: 4

"Hamburger helper helps your hamburger help her make a great meal." But did it?

No, in reality, it suggested that a healthy whole meal needed a box of preservatives and carb-loaded macaroni noodles to sustain a family—not to mention the sexism involved. Still, I suppose help HIM make a great meal wouldn't have been so catchy.

Anyway.

You don't need any pre-packaged help (looking at you, macaroni) to make a family-friendly dinner fast.

This version is similar to the classic, with a few minor substitutions.

1 pound ground beef or ground turkey

1 8-ounce can tomato sauce

3 tablespoons dried minced onion

1 teaspoon garlic powder

½–1 teaspoon chili powder

½ teaspoon salt

½ teaspoon black pepper

1 14-ounce bag cauliflower florets

2 cups cheddar cheese, shredded

In a skillet over medium-high heat, brown ground beef until it is no longer pink. Add in tomato sauce, minced onion, garlic powder, chili powder, salt, and pepper. Simmer for around 8 minutes, stirring occasionally.

Add cauliflower florets, cover, and simmer for another 10 minutes until cauliflower is tender. Remove from heat and stir in cheddar cheese.

Serve with attitude.

Store leftovers in an airtight container in the refrigerator for up to 4 days.

Nutrition Per Serving
(1 cup = 1 serving)

Calories: 472

Fat: 36.2g

Protein: 29.2g

Fiber: 2g

Total Carbs: 7.8g

Net Carbs: 5.8g

Mexican Radio Taco Casserole

Prep Time: 15 minutes

Cook Time: 30 minutes

Yield: 8

Your days of running for the border—ahem, Taco Bell—may be over, but that doesn't mean you have to skip Taco Tuesday.

Pairs well with any song from the '80s with repetitive lyrics.

1 pound ground beef or turkey

2 tablespoons Homemade Taco Seasoning (See recipe in Seasonings) or store bought

6 eggs

1 cup heavy cream

3 minced garlic cloves

½ teaspoon salt

¼ teaspoon pepper

1 cup shredded cheddar cheese

½ cup diced tomatoes (optional for topping)

Preheat the oven to 350° and spray your favorite 9-inch baking dish with nonstick cooking spray. Grab your skillet and brown the ground beef (or turkey).

Once your ground beef (or turkey) has no signs of pink left, reduce heat to low and add the taco seasoning.

Stir and cook for another minute.

Then, add the taco meat to your baking dish and direct your attention to the layer that takes this dish to the next level.

Grab a large mixing bowl and combine the eggs, heavy cream, garlic, salt, and pepper. Pour this over the taco meat, top with shredded cheese, and bake for 30 minutes.

Serve topped with tomatoes, sour cream, chopped green onions, or cubed avocado. Store any leftovers in an airtight container in the refrigerator for up to 3 days.

Nutrition Per Serving
(1 cup = 1 serving)

Calories: 375

Fat: 28g

Protein: 24g

Fiber: 0.19g

Total Carbs: 2.14g

Net Carbs: 2g

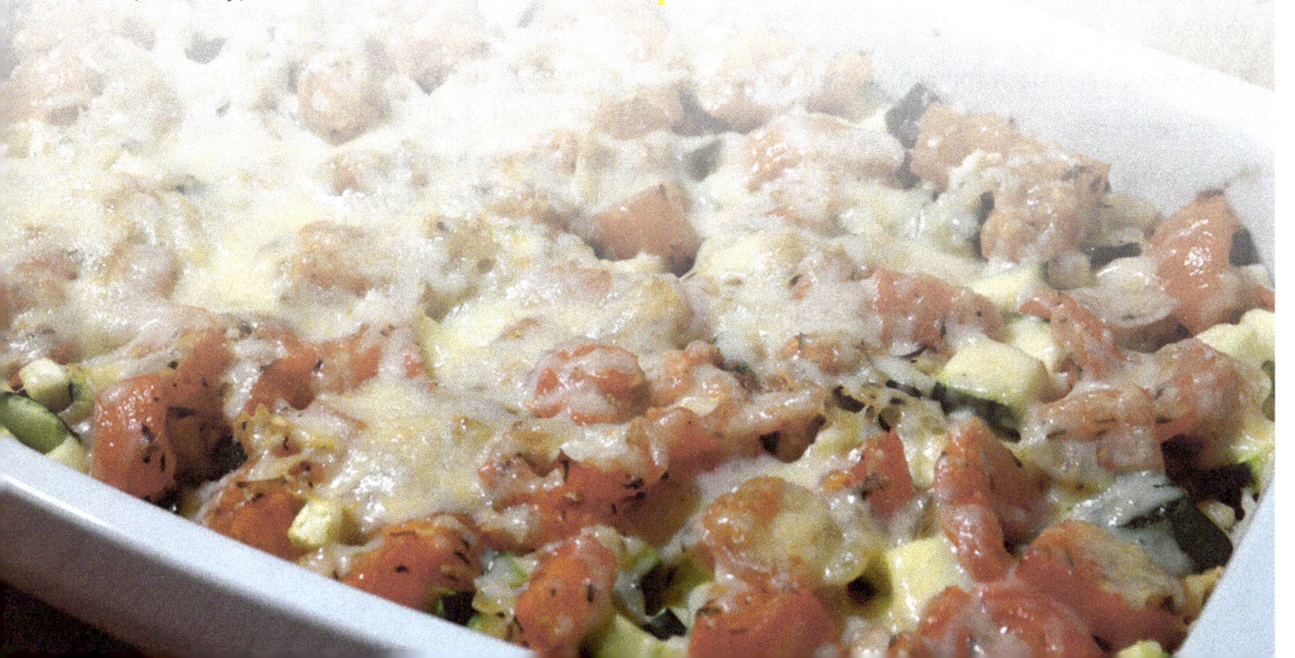

Keto Chicken Alfredo Casserole

Prep Time: 10 Minutes

Cook Time: 30 Minutes

Yield: 8

Note: You will need to have cooked chicken ready to go. You can boil it or bake it, or you can use a rotisserie—whatever you want. Just don't try to make this happen with raw chicken.

5 tablespoons butter

6–8 garlic cloves, minced

1 cup low sodium chicken broth

2½ cups heavy cream

1 teaspoon onion powder

1 teaspoon dried basil

1 teaspoon salt

½ teaspoon ground thyme

½ teaspoon red pepper flakes

½ teaspoon pepper

8 ounces cream cheese, softened and cut into cubes

½ cup onion, chopped

2 cups Parmesan cheese, grated and divided

2 12-ounce bags frozen cauliflower florets, thawed

1 10-ounce bag frozen spinach, thawed and dried

1 cup sour cream

1 cup Italian blend cheese, divided

3 cups cooked chicken, shredded (You can use a store-bought rotisserie).

Preheat the oven to 350° and grease a large casserole dish.

Grab a large skillet, set the heat on the stove to medium, and melt the butter. Whisk in the minced garlic and cook for 2 minutes, stirring regularly.

Next, turn the heat down to low and whisk in the chicken broth, heavy cream, and the spices: onion powder, dried basil, salt, ground thyme, red pepper flakes, and pepper.

Turn up the heat and whisk until the sauce starts boiling. Then reduce heat to low and simmer for around 8 minutes—stirring occasionally.

Add the cream cheese, onion, and 1 cup of Parmesan cheese and continue to cook until the cream cheese is melted.

Add the cauliflower florets and the spinach and cook on low for another 5 minutes until all the ingredients are stirred together, and the veggies are coated.

While that's cooking, combine the sour cream and Italian cheese in a small bowl. Transfer half of the sauce mixture into a greased casserole dish.

Cover with the shredded chicken.

Top the chicken with the sour cream and cheese combination (you'll need to spread this evenly over the chicken.)

Next, top with the remaining sauce mixture, top with the remaining Parmesan cheese. Bake for 20 minutes.

Serve and enjoy.

Leftovers keep in the fridge for up to 4 days in a covered dish or airtight container.

Nutrition Per Serving
(⅛ recipe = 1 serving)

Calories: 365

Fat: 24g

Protein: 31.4g

Fiber: 1g

Total Carbs: 5.9g

Net Carbs: 4.9g

I'll Stop The World and Melt With You Chicken Cordon Bleu

Prep Time: 15 minutes

Cook Time: 25 minutes

Yield: 8

Instead of going through the trouble of a DIY-breading route, this Chicken Cordon Bleu Casserole layers the classic ingredients to create a one-dish meal that is rich, creamy and, here's my favorite part, easy!

1 cup butter, melted

1 ounce cream cheese, softened

4 tablespoons lemon juice

2 tablespoons Dijon mustard

½ teaspoon salt

¼ teaspoon black pepper

1 cup cooked chicken, shredded

6 slices Swiss cheese

6 slices ham, chopped

Optional Topping:

2 ounces pork rinds

⅔ grated Parmesan

1 teaspoon garlic powder

¼ teaspoon salt

⅛ teaspoon black pepper

You can use chicken breasts, tenders, or rotisserie chicken—as long as it is cooked and shredded. Preheat the oven to 350° and prepare a casserole or baking dish with a little butter.

Make the sauce by combining melted butter, softened cream cheese, Dijon mustard, lemon juice, salt, and pepper with an electric mixer or by hand in a medium-sized bowl.

Add shredded chicken and stir.

Layer the shredded chicken combination, followed by the ham in the baking dish. Top with Swiss cheese.

Bake at 350° for 30 minutes.

Meanwhile, make the topping by placing pork rinds, Parmesan, garlic powder, salt, and pepper in a large Ziploc bag.

Crush and shake until it resembles bread-crumbs. Top the casserole with breadcrumbs and serve.

Store leftovers covered in the refrigerator for up to 5 days.

Nutrition Per Serving
(⅛ recipe = 1 serving)

Calories: 450

Total Fat: 34g

Protein: 27g

Fiber: 0.2g

Total Carbs: 2g

Net Carbs: 1.8g

Baked Fajita Casserole

Prep Time: 10 minutes

Cook Time: 30 minutes

Yield: 8

If you are planning dinner for your family or meal prepping, then you cannot go wrong with this Mexican-inspired low-carb casserole that is ready in 30 minutes or less!

2 large chicken breasts, boneless, skinless, cubed

8 ounces cream cheese, softened

⅓ cup tomato sauce

¼ cup chicken broth

1 teaspoon cumin powder

1½ teaspoons chili powder

1 teaspoon garlic powder

3 teaspoons paprika

½ teaspoon salt

¼ teaspoon pepper

4 bell peppers, red, yellow, green, cut into strips

1 onion, cut into slices

1 cup Mozzarella, shredded

Preheat the oven to 400° and prep a casserole dish.

In a medium bowl, combine cream cheese, tomato sauce, and chicken broth.

Place the cubed chicken into the casserole dish and top with cumin, chili powder, garlic powder, paprika, salt, and pepper. Stir to coat the chicken with the spices.

Add the cream cheese combination and stir to combine well. Top with bell peppers and onions.

Sprinkle Mozzarella cheese on top. Bake for 15–25 minutes.

Serve over cauliflower rice, zucchini noodles, or with nothing! (It's fabulous alone.)

Nutrition Per Serving
(⅛ recipe = 1 serving)

Calories: 393

Fat: 16.5g

Protein: 34g

Fiber: 1.5g

Total Carbs: 7.1g

Net Carbs: 5.6g

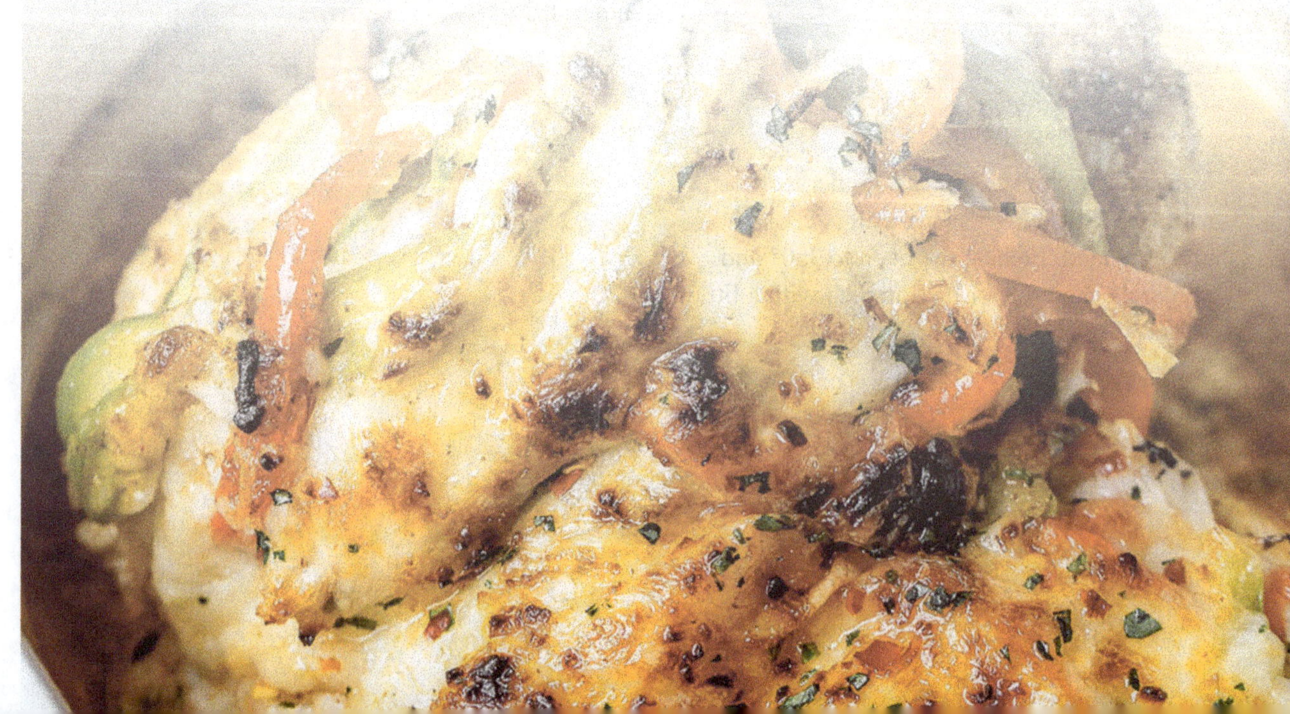

Got Brass ... In Crockpot Better Than Sex Chicken Soup

Prep Time: 15 minutes

Cook Time: 15 minutes

Yield: 8–10

Gives you all the benefits of sex—it's healthy, easy, and you can enjoy it every single day—plus you can refrigerate it when you're done! Make sure you start with cooked chicken, or you'll be pretty disappointed once you get to that step.

1 slices bacon, cooked & crumbled

2 tablespoons butter

½ cup onion, diced

2 teaspoons minced garlic

6 cups chicken broth

2 tablespoons What's Hiding In the Valley Ranch Seasoning (See recipe in Seasonings)

¼ teaspoon salt

¼ teaspoon crushed red pepper flakes

½ teaspoon pepper

1 bay leaf

1 cup shredded chicken, cooked and shredded

8 ounces cream cheese, softened

½ cup sharp cheddar cheese, shredded

2 cups broccoli (1 12-ounce bag frozen florets, thawed)

½ cup heavy cream

¼ cup chopped green onions

Grab a large soup pot or Dutch Oven and fry the bacon over medium heat. Remove the bacon once it's crispy, but don't throw out the grease—you'll need it!

Cut the heat down to low, add the butter to the pot and once it's melted, add the onions and garlic and cook for 2 minutes.

Next, add the chicken broth, ranch seasoning, salt, crushed red pepper flakes, pepper, and bay leaf. Crank up the heat—bring it to a rolling boil.

Cut the heat back to low and cook for 5 minutes.

Stir in the shredded chicken, followed by the cream cheese and cheddar cheese. Stir until the cheeses are melted and combined evenly with the chicken.

Add the broccoli and heavy cream and cook for another 2 minutes. Remove from heat, top with remaining bacon and green onions.

Serve, eat, and enjoy!

Store any leftovers in the refrigerator for up to 5 days.

Nutrition Per Serving
(1 cup = 1 serving)

Calories: 310

Fat: 23g

Protein: 29.1g

Fiber: 1g

Total Carbs: 5g

Net Carbs: 4g

Walk This Way Crockpot Shredded Chicken Chili

Prep Time: 10 minutes

Cook Time: 6 hours

Yield: 10

The collaboration of Run-D.M.C. and Aerosmith made music history in 1986. It was the first song to blend Hip hop and rock and earned the artists an MTV VMA Moonman and proved that trying something new and taking the risk of pushing boundaries pays off.

The takeaway? Your friends and family may not understand your new eating style, just like folks doubted the concept of Run-D.M.C. and Steven Tyler working. Do it anyway. Your results will do all the explaining for you.

1 tablespoon olive oil

2 teaspoons fresh lime juice

3 teaspoons garlic, minced

1 cup onion, diced

2 pounds chicken breasts

1 cup chicken broth

1 cup green chiles

1 teaspoon chili powder

1 teaspoon cumin

½ teaspoon cayenne powder

1½ cup heavy cream

8 ounces cream cheese

Heat olive oil, lime, and garlic on medium heat in a nonstick skillet and sauté onions for 2–3 minutes until they're transparent.

Set aside.

Add chicken, broth, green chiles, and all dry seasonings to your crockpot. Add in onions and garlic.

Set the crockpot for 6 hours on low. Or 4 hours on high.

Walk away and move on with your life for the next few hours.

After 4–6 hours, it's time to return to the kitchen to shred the chicken. All you have to do is stir it with a fork inside the crockpot.

No need for any extra dishes or work! That's it. Chicken shredded.

Last Step: Add cream cheese followed by heavy cream and cook for another 45 minutes to 1 hour. Store any leftovers covered in the fridge for up to five days.

Nutrition Per Serving
(1 cup = 1 serving)

Calories: 266

Fat: 16.4g

Protein: 23.3g

Fiber: 0.8g

Total Carbs: 6.1g

Net Carbs: 5.3g

Less Than Zero Garlic Butter Chicken Skillet

Prep Time: 5 minutes

Cook Time: 10 minutes

Yield: 4

This garlic butter chicken is perfect for nights when you have (less than) zero time to cook! Pairs well with the 1987 film starring Robert Downy, Jr. and/or a "Hazy Shade of Winter."

1 thin-cut chicken filets or 2 chicken breasts, halved

1–2 teaspoons Italian Stallion Seasoning (See recipe in Seasonings)

¼ teaspoon salt

¼ teaspoon crushed red pepper flakes (optional)

⅛ teaspoon pepper

1 tablespoon olive oil

2 tablespoons butter

4 garlic cloves, minced

Rinse chicken and pat it dry with a paper towel.

(If you're using thick chicken breasts, slice them in half.)

In a small bowl, combine Italian seasonings, salt, red pepper flakes, and pepper. Add this seasoning to the chicken.

Grab your favorite saucepan.

Add olive oil and set the stove to medium-high heat.

Add the seasoned chicken and cook for 4 minutes per side. Set aside on a plate. Reduce heat to low, add butter and sauté garlic for about a minute.

Add chicken and cook for another 2 minutes until chicken is cooked completely. Leftovers keep in the fridge for up to 4 days in a covered dish or airtight container.

Nutrition Per Serving
(¼ recipe = 1 serving)

Calories: 150

Fat: 10g

Protein: 12g

Fiber: 0g

Total Carbs: 1g

Net Carbs: 1g

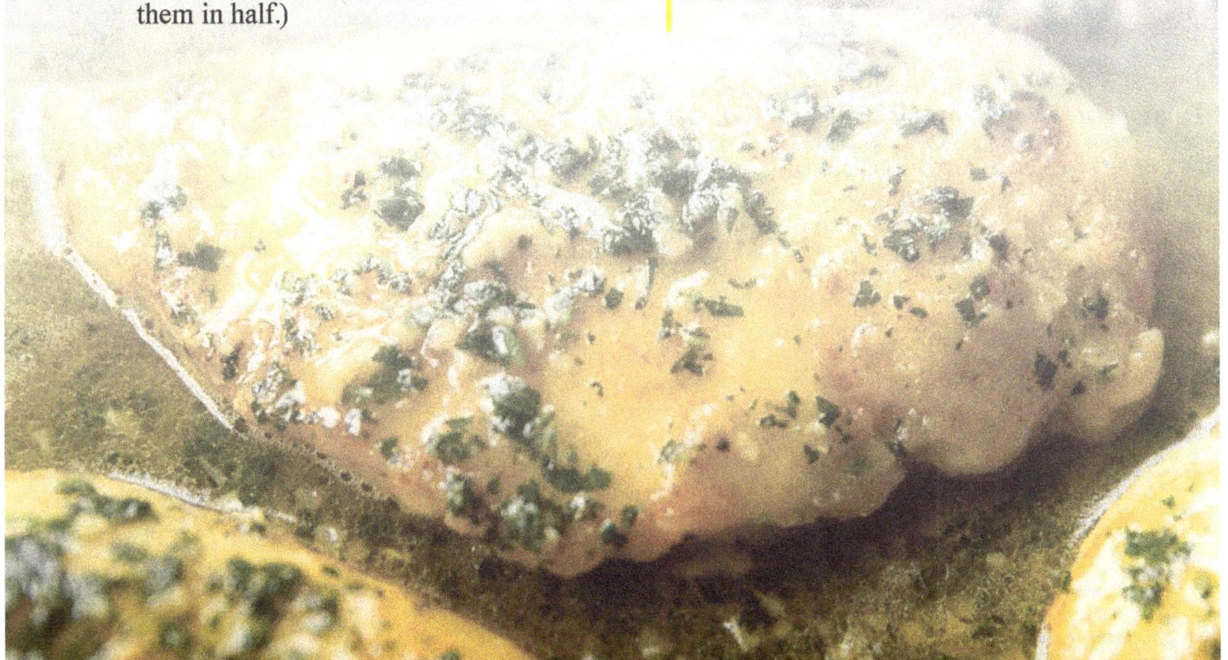

Toni Basil-Inspired Chicken Parmesan

Prep Time: 10 minutes

Cook Time: 30 minutes

Yield: 8

Chicken parmigiana, or chicken parm, is traditionally a carbohydrate loaded nightmare—breaded chicken usually served on top of pasta or in between two slices of bread—which is unnecessary. You can save yourself from the added sugars and carbs by swapping breadcrumbs with pork rinds and marinara with a sugar-free sauce and have a dinner Toni Basil would definitely cheer for.

Pairs well with "Hey Mickey" and pom-poms.

4 large chicken breasts, sliced in half

½ cup Parmesan cheese, grated

2 cups pork rinds, crushed

1 teaspoon onion powder

2 teaspoons garlic powder

4 eggs

1 cup sugar-free marinara sauce

2 cups shredded mozzarella cheese

2 tablespoons minced basil

Salt & pepper to taste

Preheat the oven to 350°. Line or spray a large baking sheet. You know the drill.

Slice the chicken breasts in half using a sharp knife–or use a dull butter knife if you're into torturing yourself.

Set to the side while you make the breading by mixing the Parmesan cheese, pork rinds, onion powder, and garlic powder in a food processor.

Set up a chicken prep assembly line by putting the breading in a dish next to the baking sheet. Then grab a large bowl and add the eggs.

Dip each piece of chicken into the egg, then the breading, then the cookie sheet. This process is known in the world of cooking as dredging, but we're keeping it real and calling it what it is: a pain in the (bleep).

Repeat until all eight pieces of chicken are breaded and in the pan.

Bake for 20 minutes, then drizzle the marinara sauce over the chicken, followed by mozzarella cheese.

Bake an additional 10 minutes, then serve topped with basil. "Hey Mickey" cheer, optional, but recommended.

Store leftovers in airtight containers for up to one week in the refrigerator.

To Freeze: Place in an airtight container and freeze for up to 2 months.

Nutrition Per Serving
(⅛ recipe = 1 serving)

Calories: 500

Fat: 18.7g

Protein: 75.6g

Fiber: 0.5g

Total Carbs: 2.6g

Net Carbs: 2.1g

Down In Kokomo Shrimp Kabobs

Prep Time: 15 minutes

Cook Time: 15 minutes

Yield: 2

Whether you're headed to Aruba, Jamaica, or to the couch to eat dinner, eating food on a stick will always make you happy. And if you're not a shrimp fan, you can always substitute the fish with chicken or steak.

12 jumbo shrimp

1 medium zucchini, sliced into 1-inch pieces

½ red onion, cut into 1-inch pieces

2½ tablespoons olive oil

Sea salt & pepper to taste

¼ cup lemon basil pesto

4 skewers

Preheat oven to 450°

Prepare a sheet pan by lining it with foil. Chop zucchini and onion.

You're working with four skewers with this one—that's three shrimp per skewer.

Divide the veggies accordingly and place them on each stick.

Now, put the skewers on your sheet pan and drizzle with olive oil-season with sea salt and pepper to taste.

Bake for 15 minutes at 450°, then brush each skewer with the pesto and serve.

Nutrition Per Serving
(1 kabob = 1 serving)

Calories: 284

Fat: 16g

Protein: 25g

Fiber: 2g

Total Carbs: 7g

Net Carbs: 5g

Baked Tilapia with Garlic Butter & Lemon

Prep Time: 10 minutes

Cook Time: 10 minutes

Yield: 4

What we have here is a one-pan dinner that's simple to put together and ready in 20 minutes. If tilapia isn't your jam, this easy dinner works with salmon or shrimp too!

4 6-ounce tilapia filets

5 tablespoons butter, melted

1 tablespoon fresh lemon juice

Zest of 1 lemon

¼ teaspoon crushed red pepper flakes

3 cloves garlic, minced

Kosher salt & black pepper to taste

1 lemon, sliced

Preheat the oven to 425° and prep a 9 X 13 baking dish with oil or nonstick cooking spray. Season tilapia with salt and pepper and place the filets in the baking dish.

In a small bowl, mix the butter, lemon juice, lemon zest, crushed red pepper, and garlic.

Drizzle the tilapia with butter combination, top with sliced lemon, and bake for 10–12 minutes until fish flakes with a fork.

Serve and enjoy!

Nutrition Per Serving
(¼ recipe = 1 serving)

Calories: 244

Fat: 16.4g

Protein: 23.6g

Fiber: 0.1g

Total Carbs: 1.2g

Net Carbs: 1.1g

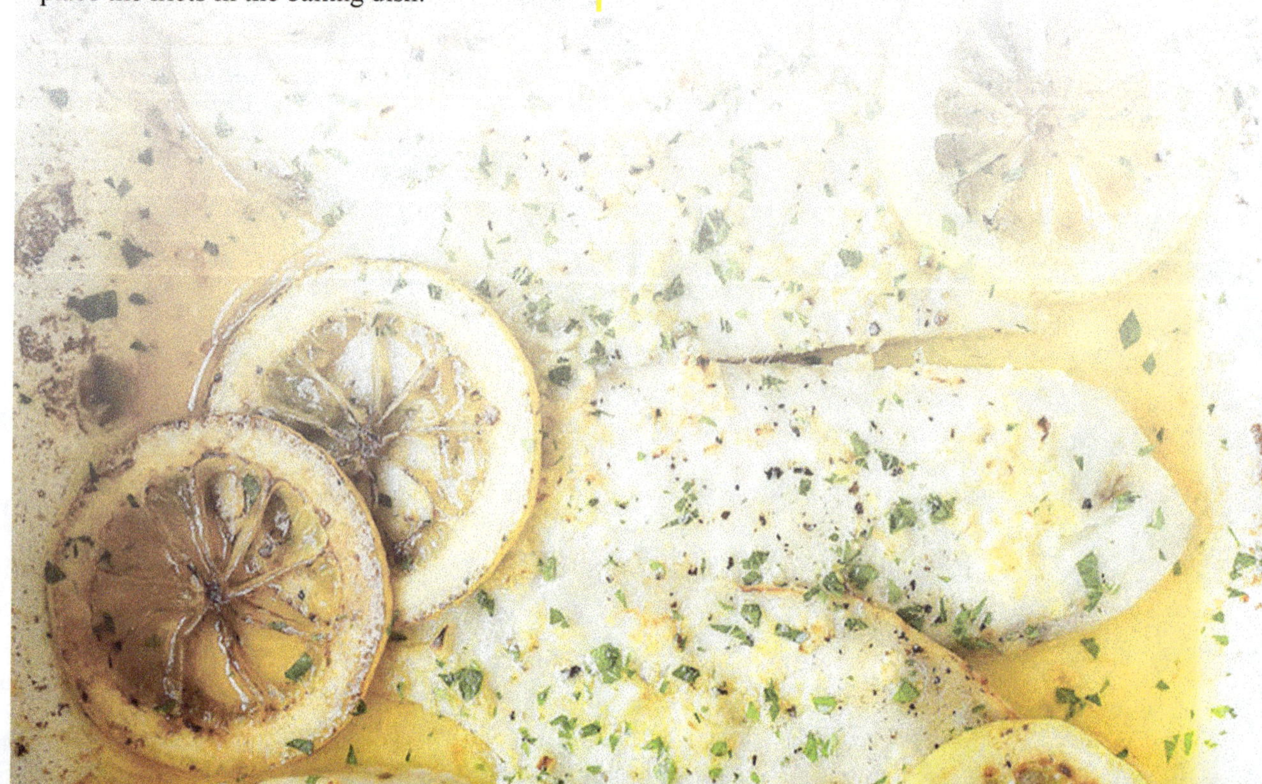

The Tide Is High But I'm Holding On Baked Salmon

Prep Time: 10 minutes

Cook Time: 15 minutes

Yield: 4

Because you're not the kind of girl who gives up just like that… but you are the kind of girl who needs dinner.

And it can't get easier than this four-ingredient main dish that's ready in less than 30 minutes. Pairs nicely with the 1980 tune by Blondie.

1 ½ pound salmon fillet

1.5 tablespoons olive oil

½ teaspoon sea salt

¼ teaspoon pepper

Place a cast-iron or ovenproof skillet in the oven before you preheat it to 450°. Season salmon with oil, salt, and pepper.

Now, carefully remove the hot skillet from the oven and put the salmon in, skin side down. Return to the oven and bake for 14–18 minutes.

Serve with gremolata or caper butter (both recipes are in the sauce section) or as is!

Nutrition Per Serving
(¼ recipe = 1 serving)

Calories: 295

Fat: 19g

Protein: 29g

Fiber: 0g

Total Carbs: 0g

Net Carbs: 0g

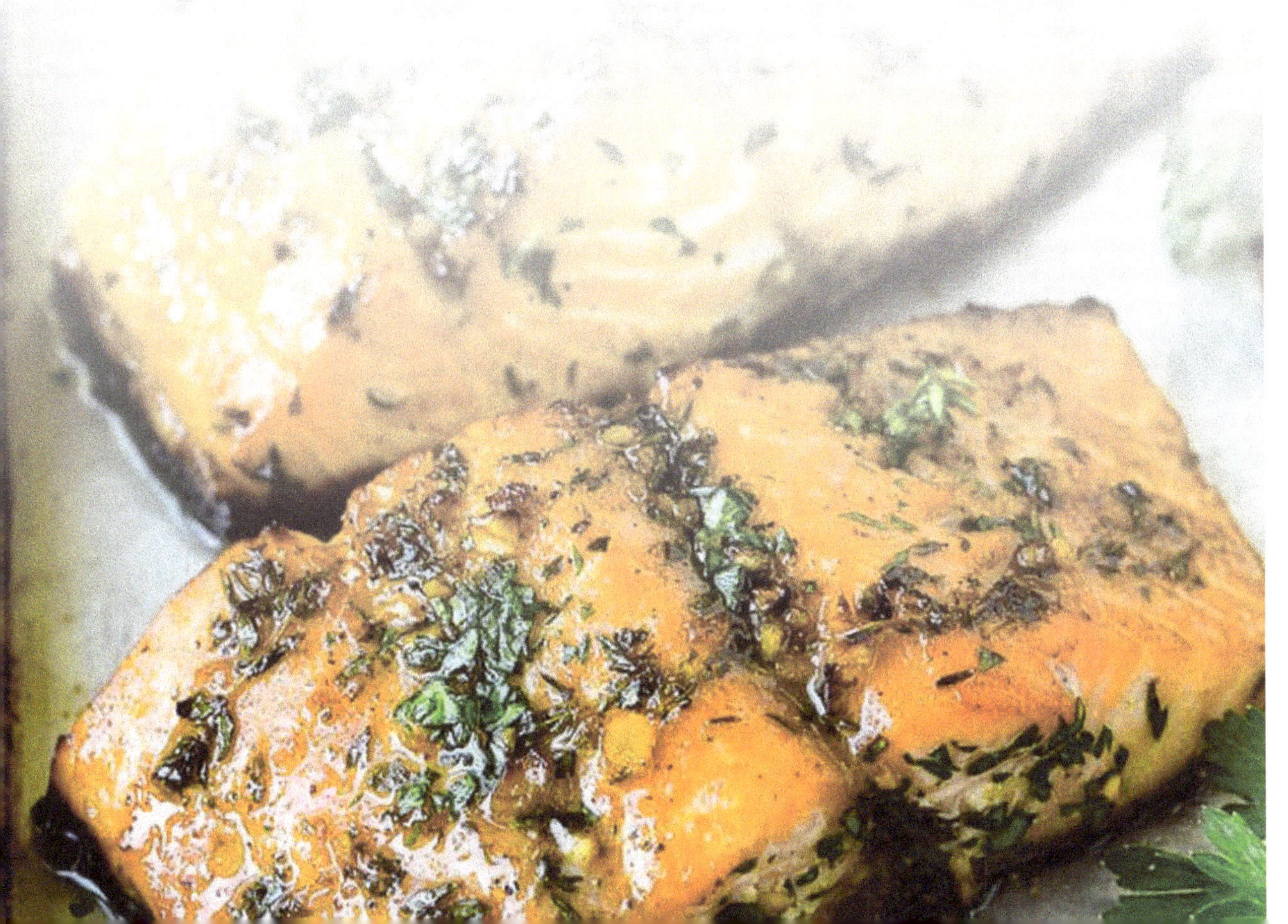

Spicy Blackened Mahi Mahi

Prep Time: 5 minutes

Cook Time: 8 minutes

Yield: 2

I took my daughter Savannah to the Bahamas when she graduated from high school, and one of the many things I loved about our trip was sampling all the spicy, authentic food. Which brings me to this blackened mahi mahi that tastes as if you put in a 5-star restaurant effort, but only takes ten minutes. Serve it with cauliflower rice, and you have a complete meal, with or without the ocean view.

2 teaspoons Louisiana Saturday Night Cajun Spice Seasoning (See recipe in Seasonings)

¼ teaspoon fennel seeds

⅛ teaspoon ground clove

¼ cup coconut oil or butter, melted

1 pound mahi mahi

½ lemon, sliced

Mix the spices and set aside.

Rinse the fish and pat dry with paper towels. Melt the butter.

Grab a large pan or cast-iron skillet and turn the stove up to high. Add the melted butter and the mahi mahi.

Coat both sides of the fish with the seasonings and sear on high heat for 2–3 minutes per side. Serve topped with lemon slices.

Oven-Baked Option

You can bake this dish in a foil-lined sheet pan at 400° for 10–12 minutes.

Nutrition Per Serving
(½ recipe = 1 serving)

Calories: 274

Fat: 12.2g

Protein: 38.2g

Fiber: 1.8g

Total Carbs: 2.1g

Net Carbs: 0.3g

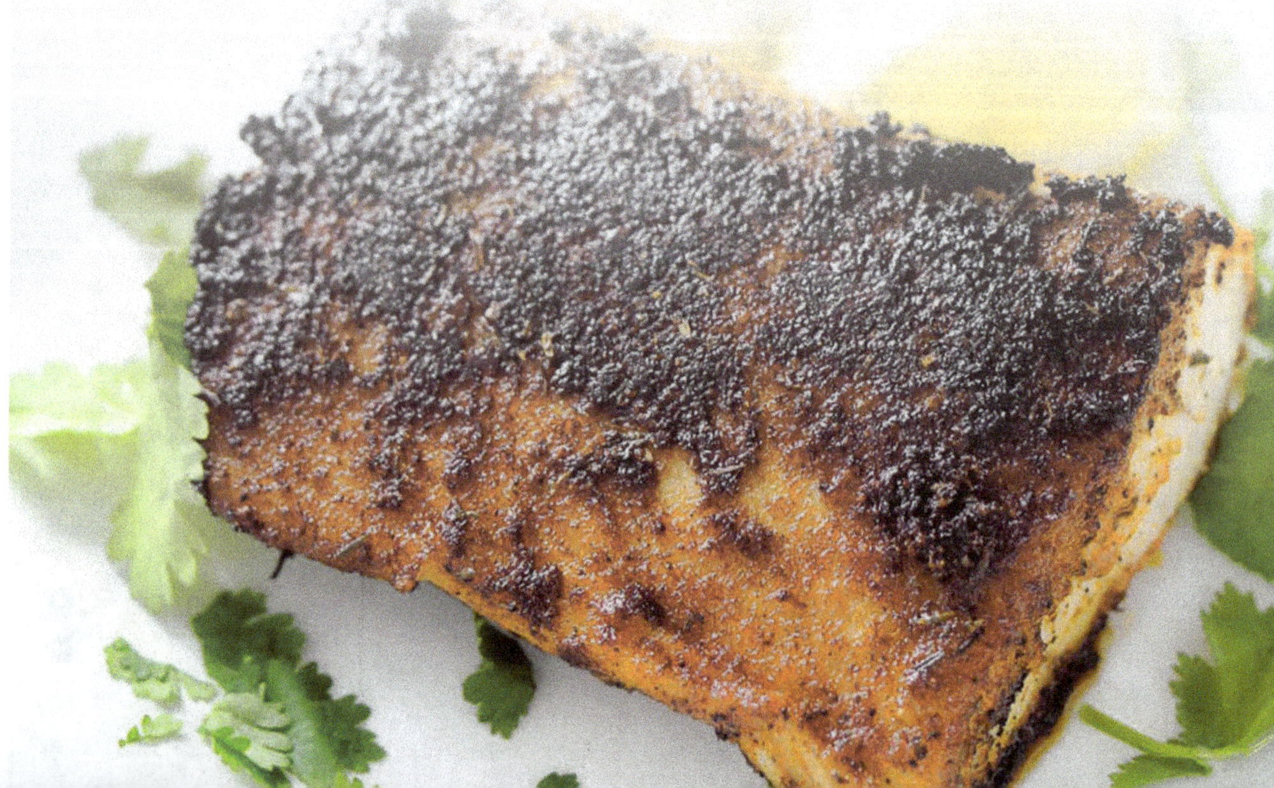

Kiss My Shrimp & Loaded Cauliflower Grits

Prep Time: 15 minutes

Cook Time: 15 minutes

Yield: 5 servings

This recipe may not be on the short-order side timewise, but I promise if you're looking for a comfort food style meal without the carbs, this one is hard to beat.

Pairs well with any Alice episode.

2 lbs shrimp, peeled & deveined

1 thick-cut strips of bacon, cooked and crumbled

¾ cup white button mushrooms, sliced

1 8-ounce block sharp cheddar cheese

1 8-ounce block pepper jack cheese

1 12-ounce bag riced cauliflower

1 cup heavy whipping cream

5 tablespoons salted butter

1 lemon, sliced

1 bunch green onions, chopped

Rinse the shrimp and remove the tails. De-vein if you want to take it that far. Fry the bacon and keep the grease—you'll need it.

Set the bacon aside and resist the temptation to eat it all right there. Rinse and slice the mushrooms.

Grate cheddar & pepper jack cheese (Pre-shredded will work—just know the manufacturer adds preservatives to keep it pretty on the shelf, which adds a few carbs.)

Cook the cauliflower rice

In a medium-large saucepan on low heat, add the cheese to the cauliflower rice. Stir in heavy cream.

In another saucepan, sauté shrimp, mushrooms, lemon juice, butter, and around two tablespoons bacon drippings until shrimp is golden brown.

Final Step: Combine cauliflower rice + shrimp (or serve the shrimp over the cauliflower rice) Top with green onions.

Boom. You just made comfort food. Give yourself a high-five. Or have a cocktail. And eat.

Nutrition Per Serving
(1 cup = 1 serving)

Calories: 763

Fat: 46.7g

Protein: 54.3g

Fiber: 0.7g

Total Carbs: 6.3g

Net Carbs: 5.6g

And now, here's a little 1980's-style motivation brought to you by… Rocky Balboa.

The '80s brought us more than big shoulder pads and preservatives; we got not one, but two Rocky movies, Rocky III and Rocky IV. Everyone remembers Sylvester Stallone's portrayal of Rocky, but what many folks don't know is that he is the real inspiration.

Before Stallone's script for the original Rocky was purchased, the man was beyond broke. As in, homeless and had to sell his dog broke. He'd been offered $300,000.00 for his script by a studio but turned it down because they wouldn't agree to let him star in the movie.

In other words, he chose to be homeless over selling out. He believed in himself—in his ideas—and did not compromise even when life got hard.

You're going to encounter hardship along your journey—that's inevitable. Whatever you do, don't stop believing in yourself or your dreams. You are capable of much more than you realize.

When the studio agreed to let Stallone star in the movie, they gave him a $35,000.00 advance, and he did buy his dog back—for $15,000.00. The Rocky franchise went on to make history—grossing $225 million.

Appetizers & Snacks

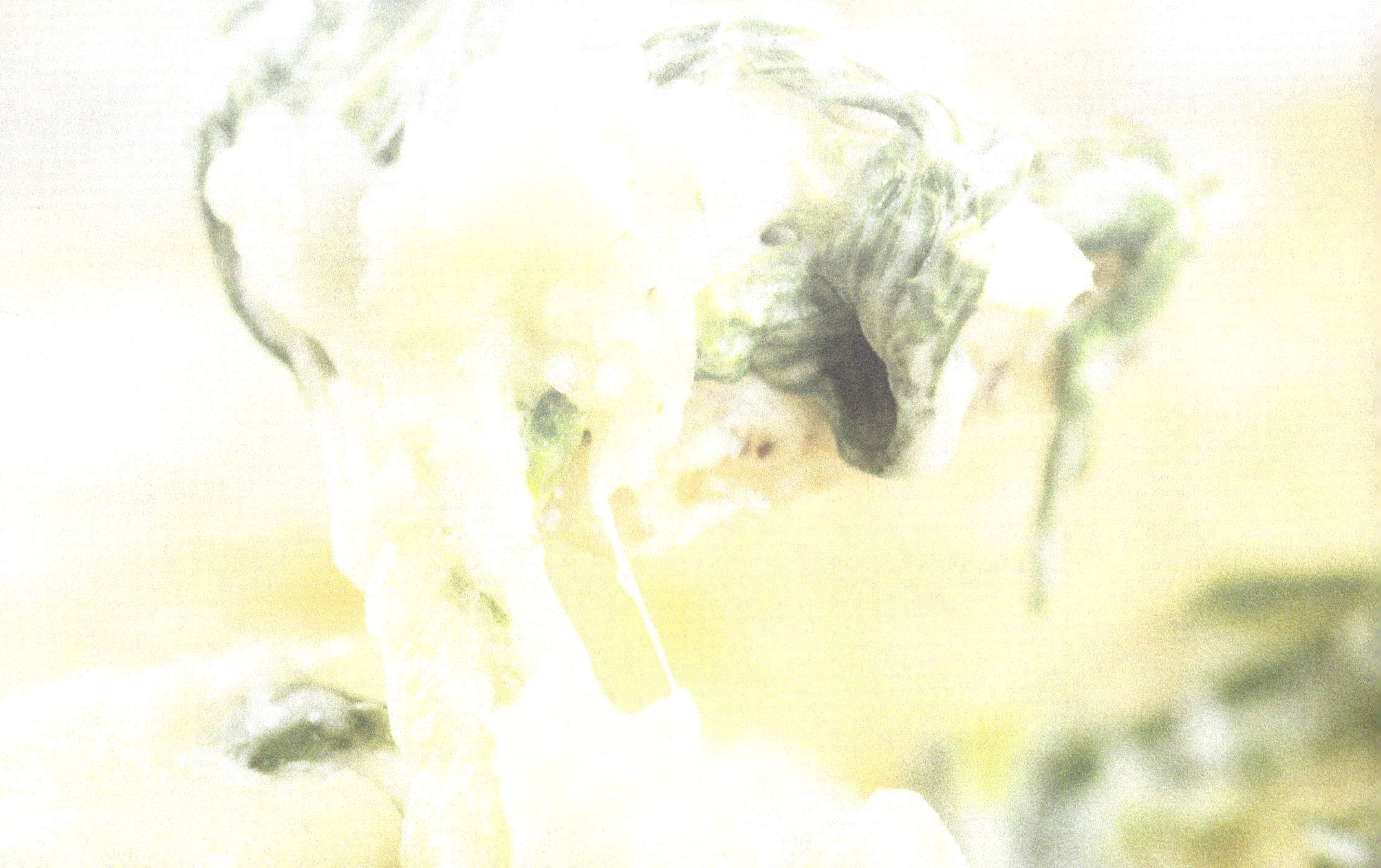

You Spin Me Right Round Spinach Dip

Prep Time: 10 minutes

Cook Time: 20 minutes

Yield: 14

Was the 1984 hit by Dead or Alive about a relationship going nowhere or was it a veiled reference to the spin the sugar industry used to vilify fat?

These are the things that make you go, hmm.

This one is as good as it gets. It's perfect for a party, tailgating, or anytime you need to get your spinach on. Oh, and if you don't care for spicy? No problem! Just omit the Tabasco and red pepper—they're fab, but they are not deal-breakers.

4 tablespoons butter

½ cup onion, diced

1 teaspoon minced garlic

2 10-ounce packages frozen chopped spinach, thawed and dried

1 cup (8 ounces) sour cream

8 ounces cream cheese, softened

1 cup Monterey Jack cheese, divided

1 cup grated Parmesan cheese, divided

1–2 teaspoons Tabasco sauce (optional)

¼ teaspoon salt

¼ teaspoon red pepper flakes

Preheat the oven to 350° and grease your favorite 2-quart baking dish.

Now throw or carefully place the butter in a large skillet, set the heat to medium, and sauté the onion and garlic for about 5 minutes until it's soft.

Stir in spinach, sour cream, cream cheese, ½ cup Monterey Jack, and ½ cup Parmesan. Then add Tabasco, salt, and red pepper flakes.

Feel free to take it for a taste test drive and add extra salt or Tabasco if necessary. Stir until it's all mixed up, and you almost can't stand it anymore.

Remember the greased baking dish? Well, it's time to use it.

Pour the spinach mixture into the dish, top it off with what's left of the Monterey and parmesan, and bake for 10 minutes.

Serve with sliced veggies, cheese crisps, or keto crackers.

Nutrition Per Serving
(½ cup= 1 serving)

Calories: 219

Fat: 19.7g

Protein: 7.1g

Fiber: 1.1g

Total Carbs: 4.8g

Net Carbs: 3.7g

Killer Crab Dip

Prep Time: 10 minutes

Cook Time: 20 minutes

Yield: 12

Warning: If you bring this dip to a party, three things will happen: you will be asked to bring it again, at least four people will ask for the recipe, and you will not have any left to take home and eat while you watch Netflix. So, you may want to make two just in case.

¼ cup green onions, chopped

1 tablespoon butter

1 teaspoon minced garlic

8 ounces cream cheese, softened and cubed

¼ cup sour cream

¼ cup mayonnaise

1 cup cheddar cheese, shredded

1 tablespoon Worcestershire

1 tablespoon lemon juice

½ teaspoon cayenne pepper

¼ teaspoon black pepper

½ teaspoon salt

16 ounces lump crabmeat

Melt butter in a large skillet over medium heat. Sauté green onions for a minute or two until they're soft. Add the garlic and give it a stir. Then add cream cheese and stir until it's melted.

In a separate large bowl, mix sour cream, mayonnaise, cheddar cheese, Worcestershire, and lemon juice. Then add the cayenne pepper, black pepper, and salt.

By now, the cream cheese should be nice and melted—so add that to the sour cream mixture, followed by the crabmeat.

Transfer to a casserole dish and bake at 350° for 20 minutes—top with chopped green onions.

Serve and enjoy.

Store any leftovers in the fridge for up to 5 days.

Nutrition Per Serving
(¼ cup = 1 serving)

Calories: 190

Fat: 15.4g

Protein: 10.5g

Fiber: 0g

Total Carbs: 2.1g

Net Carbs: 2.1g

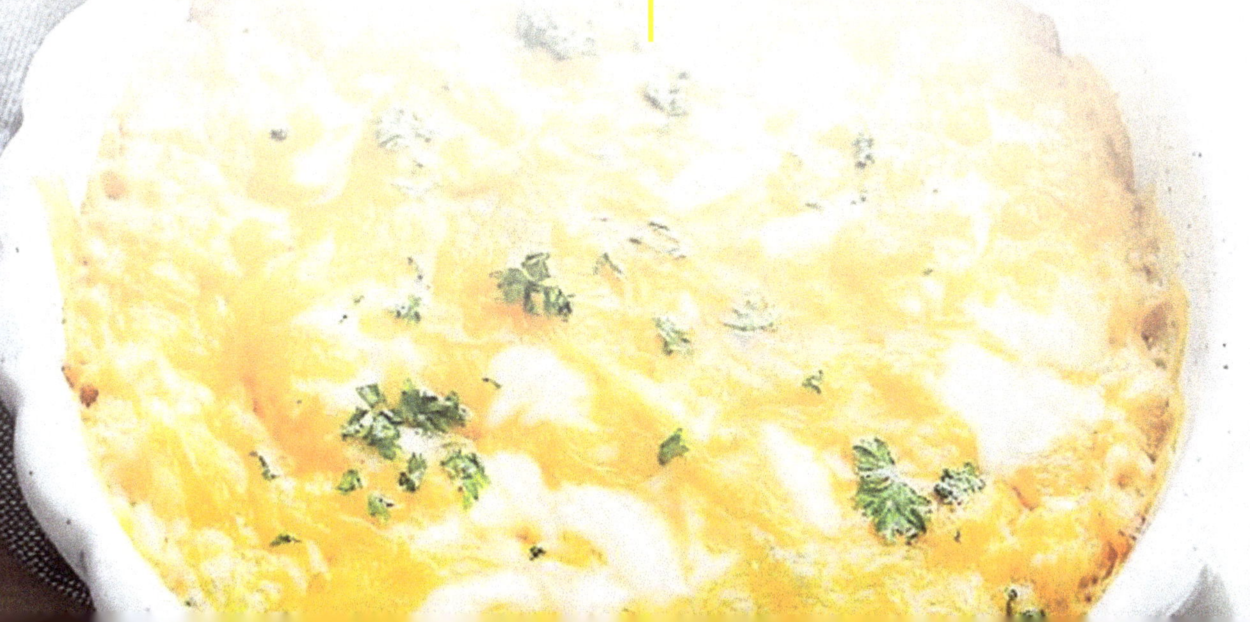

My Girl Wants to Party All the Time BLT Dip

Prep Time: 10 minutes

Cook Time: 5 minutes

Yield: 8

If you're hosting a party or need something to take because showing up empty-handed to a soiree is not what you're about—here's a fab dip you can whip up quick so you can focus on what's important: contouring and figuring out what you're going to wear.

Pairs well with that one song Eddie Murphy did in 1985.

1 pound bacon, fried crispy and chopped

1 cup lettuce, chopped

1 cup tomatoes, chopped

¼ cup green onions, chopped

8 ounces cream cheese, softened

¾ cup sour cream

2 tablespoons What's Hiding In the Valley Ranch Seasoning (See recipe in Seasonings)

Rinse and chop up the lettuce, tomatoes, and green onion

s.

In a medium-sized bowl, combine the softened cream cheese, sour cream, and ranch seasoning with a hand mixer.

You could try doing it with a spoon, but you'll be there for a while, and you may not achieve the right consistency.

(You will also probably get very angry, especially if you're in a hurry.)

Now, spread the cream cheese mixture in an even layer into the bottom of a 9-inch baking dish. Top with lettuce, tomatoes, bacon, and green onions.

Serve with fresh veggies or three-ingredient crackers.

Store any leftovers in an airtight container in the refrigerator for up to three days.

Nutrition Per Serving
(½ cup = 1 serving)

Calories: 235

Fat: 22g

Protein: 5g

Fiber: 0g

Total Carbs: 3g

Net Carbs: 3g

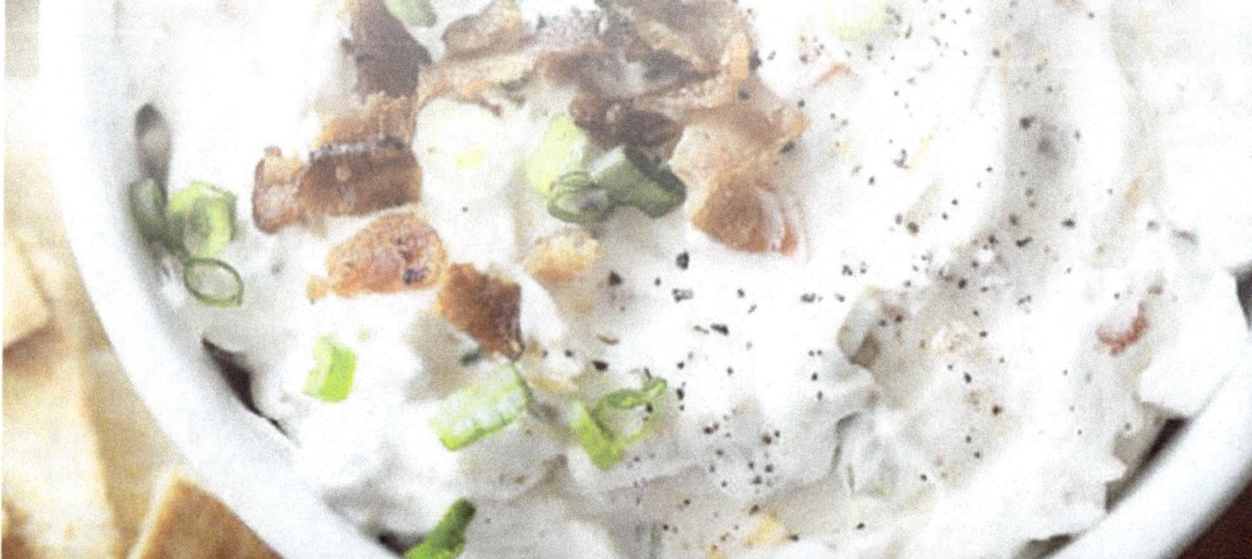

Easy Party Cheese Ball

Prep Time: 15 minutes + 1 hour to chill

Cook Time: 5 minutes

Yield: 10 (Serving size is about 2 teaspoons)

16 ounces (2 8-ounce packages) cream cheese, softened

1 cup shredded cheddar cheese (I like sharp, but you do you)

2 tablespoons What's Hiding In the Valley Ranch Seasoning (See recipe in Seasonings)

¼ cup green onions, chopped

1 cup pecans, chopped

¾ cup bacon bits

Combine the cream cheese, cheddar, and ranch.

You can do this easily in a food processor and save your arm a workout. If you don't have a food processor—go get one. I'll wait.

Just kidding! You can mix this by hand, but it's going to take a little longer to combine.

Now, using your hands, shape the cheese into a ball, wrap it in plastic wrap and let it chill in the refrigerator for about an hour or until it's firm.

Meanwhile, rinse and chop the green onions and pecans.

In your favorite medium bowl, combine the green onions, pecans, and bacon bits. Roll the cheese ball into this mixture until it's coated.

Wrap it up tightly in plastic wrap and refrigerate it until you are ready to serve with pork rinds, bell pepper slices, celery sticks, or keto crackers.

Keep any leftovers in an airtight container in the fridge for up to 5 days.

Nutrition Per Serving
(2 teaspoons = 1 serving)

Calories: 280

Fat: 27.3g

Protein: 6.4g

Fiber: 1.1g

Total Carbs: 4.5g

Net Carbs: 3.4g

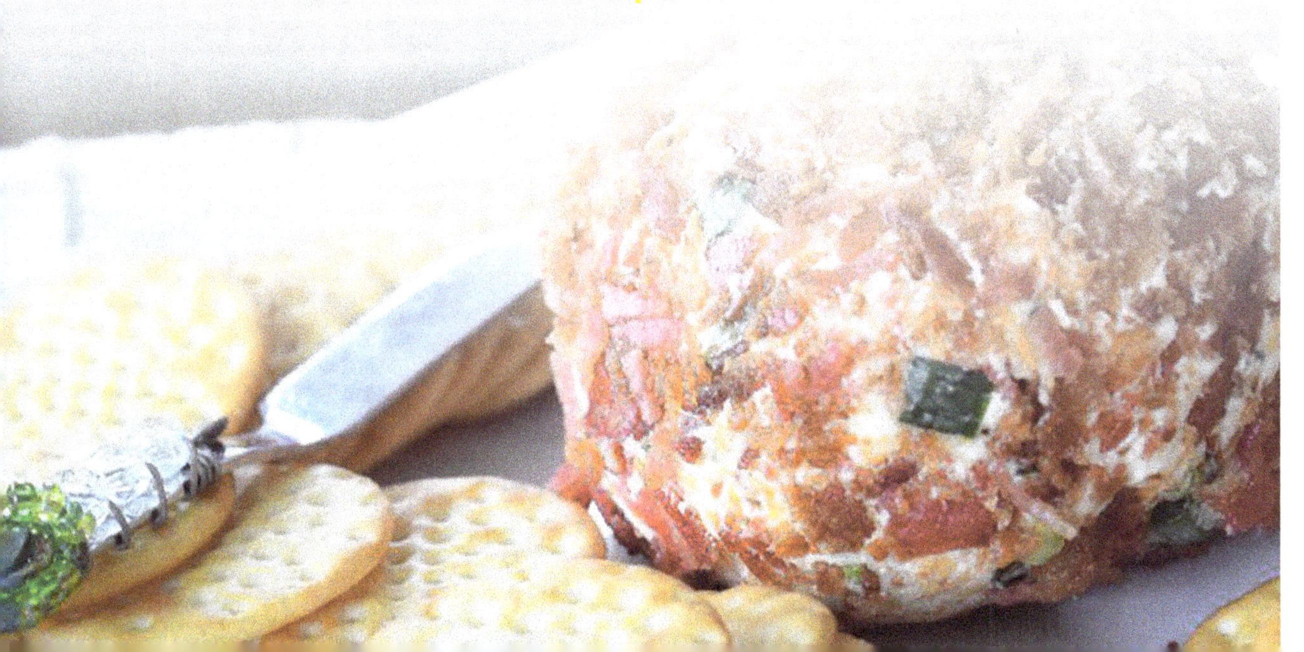

Devil Inside Deviled Eggs

Prep Time: 15 minutes

Cook Time: 15 minutes

Yield: 12

The combination of bacon and pickle relish in this recipe makes both keto-aficionados, and never-diet-types swoon at parties. They're almost as flawless as Michael Hutchence's hair in the '80s.

6 large eggs

5 slices bacon, crumbled

¼ cup mayonnaise

1 teaspoon prepared yellow mustard

1 tablespoon dill pickle relish

Salt & pepper

2 tablespoons green onions, chopped (optional, garnish)

Paprika (optional, garnish)

Position the eggs in a medium-sized pan and cover with enough water to boil. Bring to a boil for 15 minutes to let the egg yolks firm.

Rinse eggs in cold water, then crack the shells and peel under running cold water. Slice each egg in half and carefully remove the yolks. Remember, presentation is everything. (Just kidding, I don't care if you don't.) In a separate bowl, mash the egg yolks with a fork.

Then add mayonnaise, mustard, relish, salt, pepper, and two-thirds of the bacon.

Spoon the yolk combination into the egg halves and top with remaining bacon crumbles, chopped green onion, and paprika.

Pro Tip: Put the yolk mixture into a large Ziploc bag & seal. Then use scissors to snip off a corner of the bag to fill each egg.

Store any leftovers in the fridge in an airtight container for up to 3 days.

Nutrition Per Serving
(3 eggs = 1 serving)

Calories: 290

Fat: 25.8g

Protein: 14.3g

Fiber: 0.1g

Total Carbs: 2g

Net Carbs: 2g

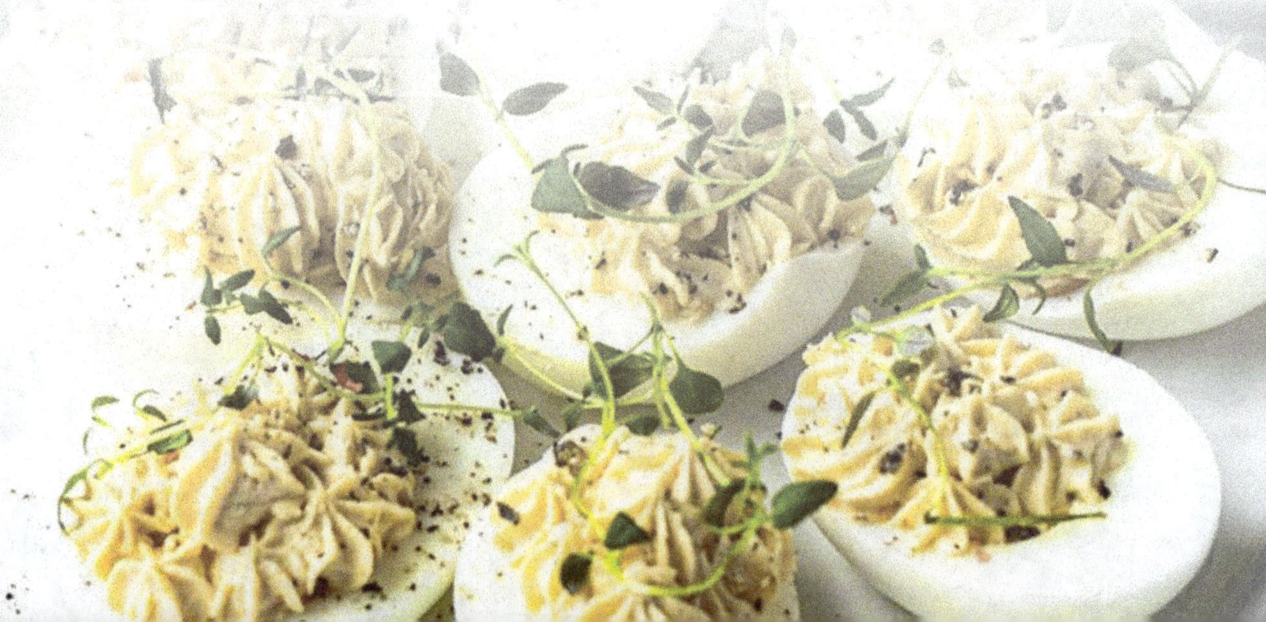

Balsamic Tomato & Mozzarella Kabobs

Prep Time: 15 minutes

Cook Time: 0

Yield: 20

There's something about fresh mozzarella balls, especially when combined with grape tomatoes and balsamic dressing. It's like the best part of salad on a stick!

Warning: This calls for a 30-minute marinade time, which you can ignore if you need to.

2 tablespoons olive oil

2 tablespoons balsamic vinegar

1 teaspoon Italian Stallion Seasoning (See recipe in Seasonings)

¼ teaspoon kosher salt

¼ teaspoon fresh black pepper

20 fresh mozzarella balls*

(*If you cannot find fresh mozzarella balls, you can substitute with cubed mozzarella.)

20 cherry tomatoes

24 basil leaves

20 wooden skewers

In a medium bowl or whatever you have available, combine olive oil, balsamic vinegar, Italian seasoning, salt, and pepper.

Add mozzarella balls and toss to coat each one as evenly as possible. Marinate for at least 30 minutes in the fridge.

Rinse the tomatoes and basil. Pat dry with a paper towel.

Now thread each skewer in this order: tomato—basil leaf—mozzarella ball—basil leaf—tomato. Repeat until you have 20 skewers.

Keep this covered in the fridge until you're ready to serve.

Nutrition Per Serving
(1 kabob = 1 serving)

Calories: 95

Total Fat: 8g

Protein: 5g

Fiber: 0g

Total Carbs: 1g

Net Carbs: 1g

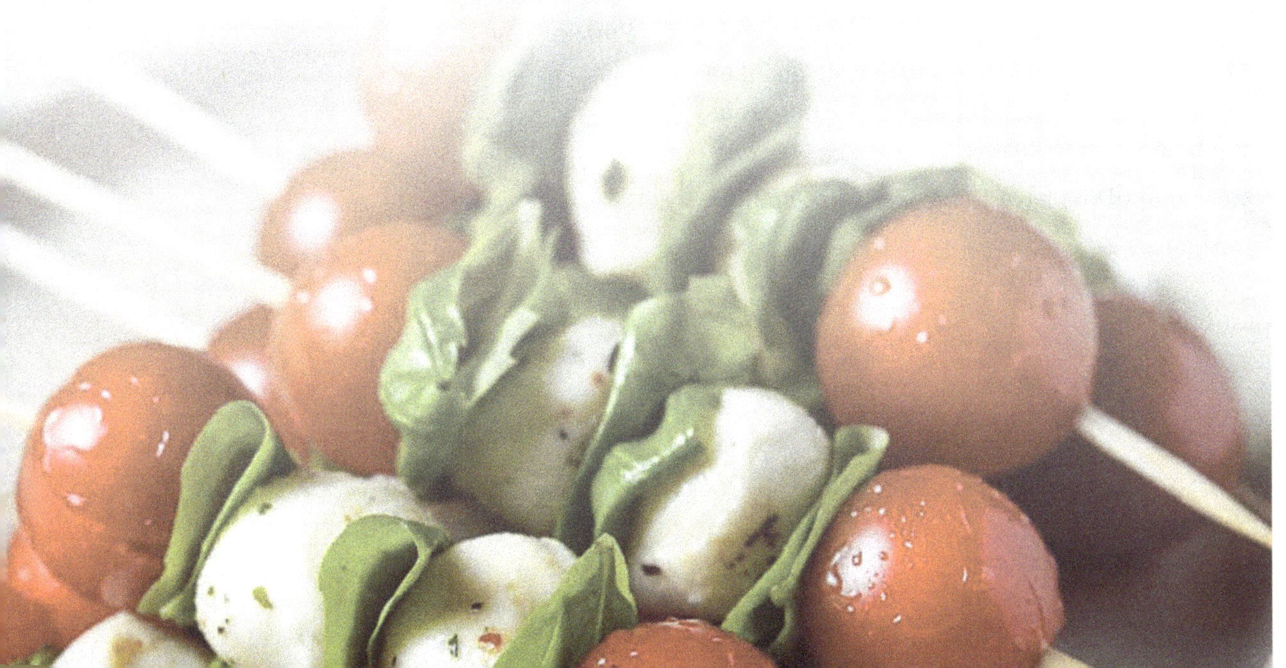

Supersonic Low Carb Mozzarella Sticks

Prep Time: 5 minutes

Cook Time: 5 minutes + 1 hour freeze time

Yield: 12

This time next month you'll be at your class reunion. Unstoppable on the dance floor.

With or without J.J. Fad.

Until then, occupy your devastating hunger with this low carb version of the old school classic.

6 Mozzarella cheese sticks, halved

1 cup almond flour

4 tablespoons Parmesan cheese, grated

4 teaspoons Italian Stallion Seasoning (See recipe in Seasonings)

1 teaspoon garlic powder

1 teaspoon sea salt

1 egg

½ cup coconut oil or 2 tablespoons olive oil

Cut cheese sticks in half.

Combine almond flour, parmesan cheese, Italian seasoning, garlic powder, and salt in a large bowl or extra-large freezer bag.

In a medium-sized bowl, lightly beat the egg.

Dip each mozzarella stick into the egg and then dredge into the almond flour mixture or toss in the freezer bag to coat.

Repeat until you have 12 breaded Mozzarella sticks.

Arrange the cheese sticks on a parchment paper-lined pan with enough room in between, so they do not touch.

Put the pan in the freezer for at least an hour, which keeps the cheese from melting during cooking.

To pan-fry: Heat coconut oil or olive oil in a medium pan over high heat. Once your skillet is hot, fry the cheese sticks in a single layer for about 1–2 minutes.

To bake: Bake on a lined cookie sheet in a 400° oven for 5 minutes, then flip the cheese sticks and bake for another 5 minutes.

To air fry: Air fry at 400° for 8 minutes.

Store any leftovers in the refrigerator for up to 4 days.

To Freeze: Freeze before cooking. After the cheese sticks are flash-frozen, transfer to a heavy-duty Ziploc bag and store in the freezer for up to 3 months.

Nutrition Per Serving
(1 cheese stick = 1 serving)

Calories: 190

Total Fat: 14.7g

Protein: 5.5g

Fiber: 0.3g

Total Carbs: 2.2g

Net Carbs: 1.4g

Buffalo Stance Chicken Dip
(crockpot, oven, open field, or nightclub)

Prep Time: 10 minutes

Cook Time: 25 minutes

Yield: 10–12

Whether you're planning a party or a girl's night at home, you will love this spicy dip that takes grazing to another level. Pairs well with a sassy state of mind.

1/2 cup celery, chopped

2 cups chicken breasts, cooked and shredded (or rotisserie chicken)

12 ounces cream cheese

1 cup cheddar

1 cup Monterey Jack

1 cup crumbled blue cheese + 2 tablespoons (Separated)

1 cup Franks hot sauce

Optional Garnish:

Chopped green onions

Sliced jalapenos

Crumbled bacon

Crumbled blue cheese

Oven Instructions:

Preheat to 375°

Rinse & chop celery.

Boil chicken and shred it with a hand mixer or use diced or shredded rotisserie chicken. In a saucepan or the microwave, melt the cream cheese until smooth.

Add in the Monterey Jack, 1 cup blue cheese, celery, hot sauce, and chicken and stir until all of the cheeses are melted.

Transfer everything into your favorite casserole dish.

Bake for 25 minutes – sprinkle remaining blue cheese on top.

Crockpot/Slow Cooker Instructions:

Combine ingredients & set on low – 3 hours or high for 60 – 90 minutes.

Nutrition Per Serving
(½ cup = 1 serving)

Calories: 355

Fat: 26.5g

Protein: 25.7g

Fiber: 0g

Total Carbs: 2.7g

Net Carbs: 2.6g

Rock Your World Guacamole

Prep Time: 20 Minutes

Cook Time: 45 minutes + at least 1 hour to let the flavor develop

Yield: 6

3 Haas Avocados, peeled and seeded

1 lime, juiced (2 tablespoons)

½ teaspoon kosher salt

½ teaspoon cumin

¼ teaspoon cayenne pepper

½ onion, finely chopped

2 Roma tomatoes, diced

1 tablespoon cilantro or parsley, chopped

1 garlic clove, minced

½ Jalapeno pepper, seeded and diced (optional)

Scoop the avocado into a mixing bowl and toss with lime juice. Drain excess lime juice into a small bowl or cup to use later.

Add salt, cumin, and cayenne pepper and mash together with a potato masher or a fork until you've got a fabulous, chunky texture.

Add chopped onion, diced tomatoes, cilantro, garlic, jalapeno, and ½ tablespoon lime juice. Stir and cover with heavy-duty plastic wrap.

Then walk away for at least an hour to let the flavor develop. That's right, leave it right there on the counter and walk away. Taste after an hour and add salt and lime juice if needed.

Store any leftovers covered in the refrigerator.

Nutrition Per Serving
(2 tablespoons = 1 serving)

Calories: 172

Total Fat: 15g

Protein: 2g

Fiber: 7g

Total Carbs: 11g

Net Carbs: 4g

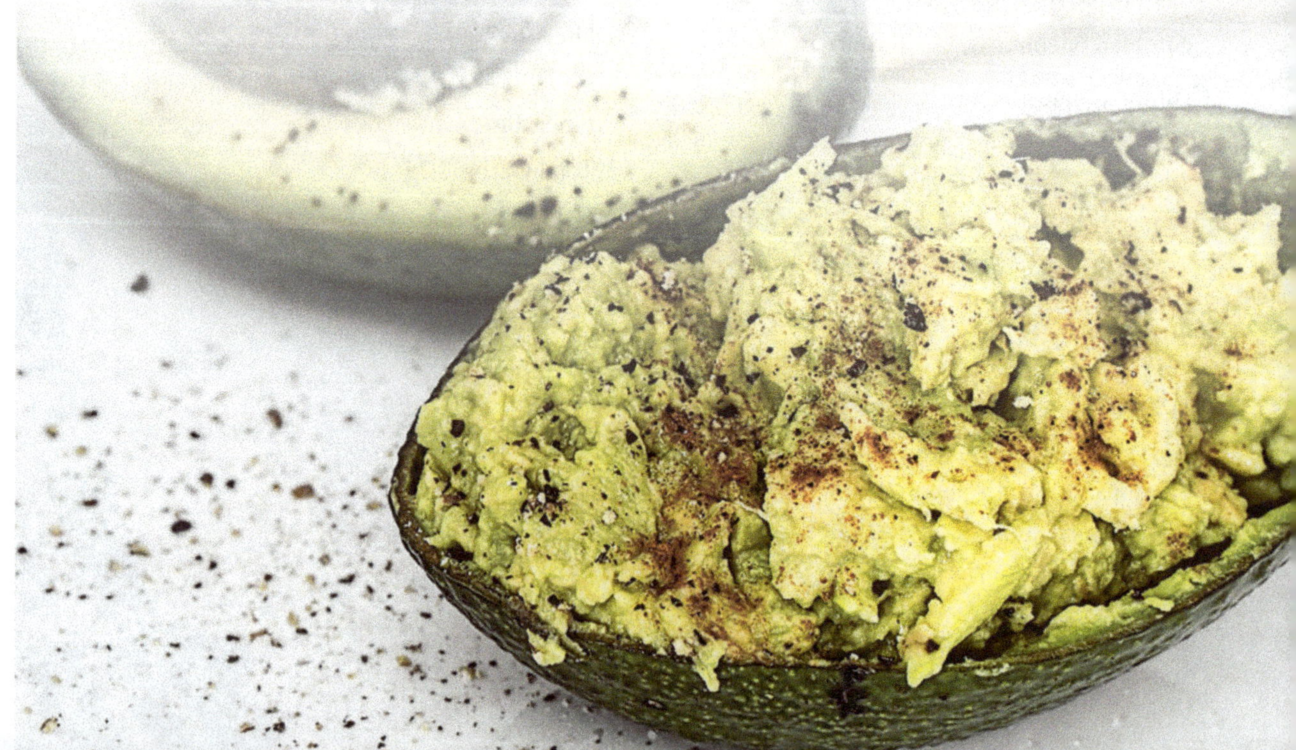

In It to Win It Bacon Asparagus Roll-Ups

Prep Time: 10 minutes

Cook Time: 10 minutes

Yield: 2 dozen

Anytime you mix bacon and cream cheese, you cannot lose.

12 Asparagus spears, trimmed (take a little off the bottom to get rid of the bitter-tasting part) and halved

12 slices of bacon, cut into thirds

8 ounces cream cheese, softened

½ teaspoon garlic powder (or 1 clove garlic, minced)

½ teaspoon kosher salt

¼ teaspoon black pepper

Preheat the oven to 400° and line a baking sheet with parchment paper.

Trim and cut the asparagus spears, then boil them for 5 minutes. Transfer asparagus from boiling water to a large bowl filled with cold water to cool them off.

Fry the bacon over medium-high heat until it is cooked on each side but not crispy. Be careful not to overcook.

In a small bowl or food processor, combine cream cheese, garlic, salt, and pepper.

Now, spread 1–2 teaspoons of the cream cheese mixture onto each slice of bacon. Then add an asparagus spear and roll it up until the bacon ends meet.

Arrange the roll-ups on the baking sheet and bake for 5 minutes until the cheese is warmed and the bacon is crisp.

Nutrition Per Serving
(2 roll ups = 1 serving)

Calories: 111

Total Fat: 9.1g

Protein: 6g

Fiber: 0.2g

Total Carbs: 1.2g

Net Carbs: 1

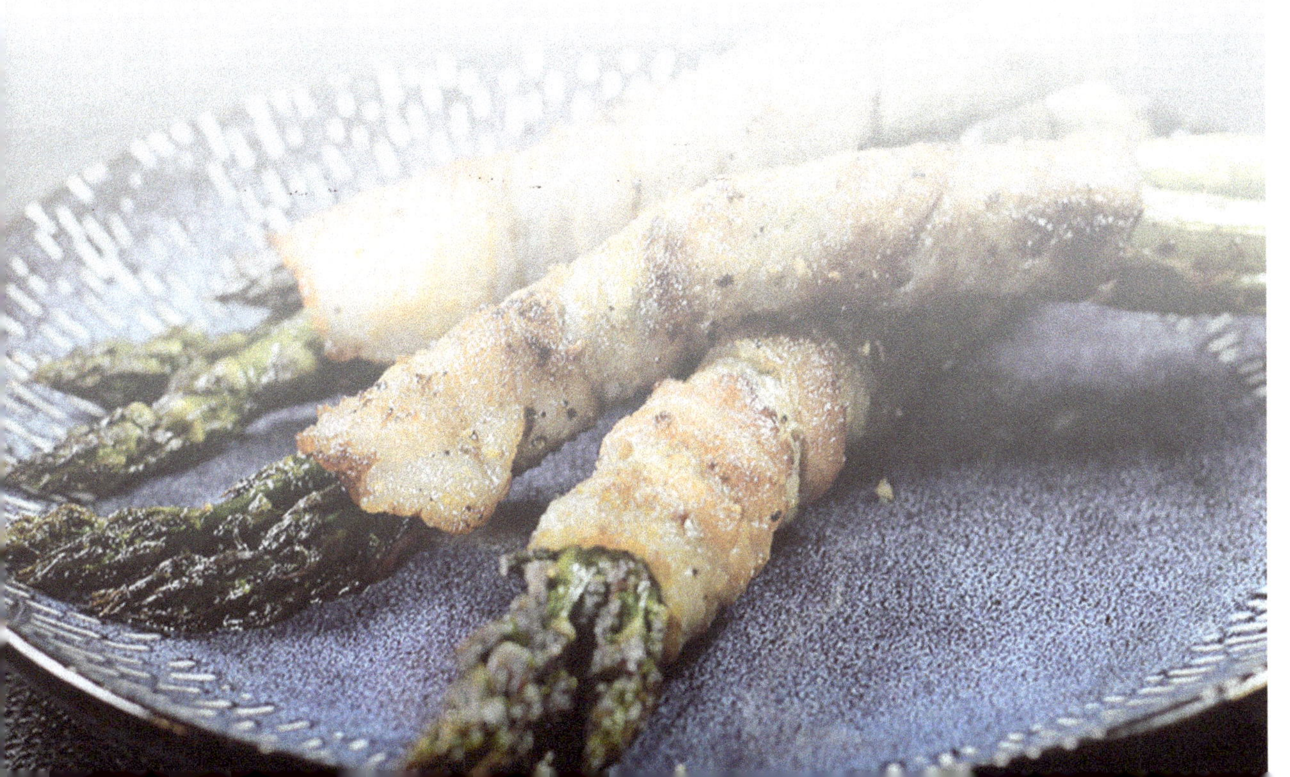

Sausage Balls

Prep Time: 10 minutes

Cook Time: 20 minutes

Yield: 50+

Fortunately, you don't need an advanced culinary or science degree or a lot of special ingredients to make this classic staple low carb.

8 ounces cream cheese, softened

1 pound ground breakfast sausage

1 cup blanched almond flour

1 ½ cups shredded cheddar cheese

1 tablespoon baking powder

1 clove garlic, minced

Preheat the oven to 375° and line a baking pan with parchment paper. Cut the softened cream cheese into small pieces.

In a large bowl, combine raw sausage, almond flour, shredded cheddar, cream cheese, baking powder, and garlic.

Use a mini cookie scoop, a tablespoon, or your hands, to form each sausage ball—shoot for 1 inch a piece.

Bake at 375° for 20 minutes.

Store in the refrigerator for up to 3 days.

To Freeze: Let sausage balls cool after baking, then flash freeze them for an hour. Transfer to a heavy-duty freezer bag or container and freeze for up to 6 months.

Nutrition Per Serving
(4 balls = 1 serving)

Calories: 317

Total Fat: 28g

Protein: 13g

Fiber: 1g

Total Carbs: 5g

Net Carbs: 4g

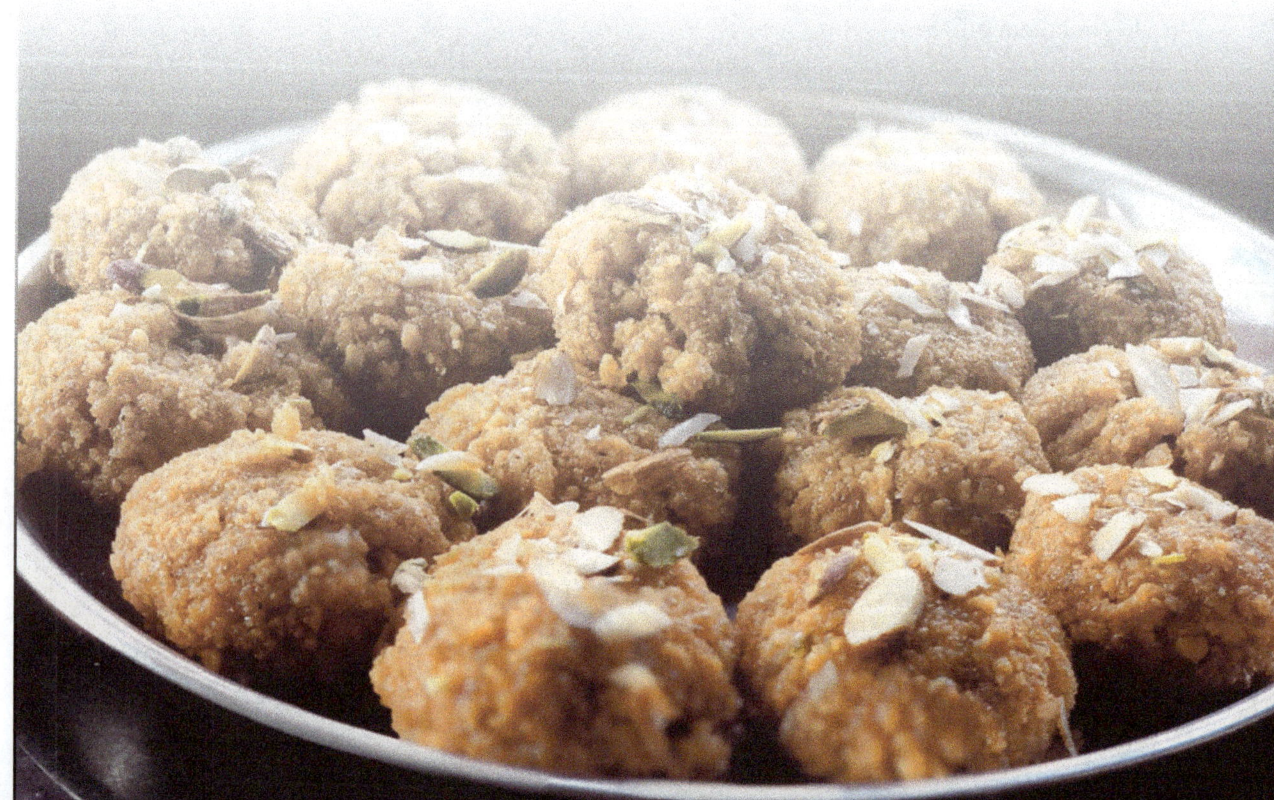

Roll It Up My Homeboy Ham & Cheese Pinwheels

Prep Time: 15 minutes

Chill Time: 2 hours

Yield: 24

These Pinwheels are an old school favorite that you can throw together in minutes. Playing Success-n-Effect's "Roll It Up My Homeboy" is optional, but highly recommended.

1 8-ounce package cream cheese, softened

¼ pound Genoa salami (about 8-10 slices)

1 tablespoon prepared horseradish

7 slices of ham

7 dill pickle spears

In a food processor, blend cream cheese, salami, and horseradish. Process for about 2 minutes until smooth.

Arrange ham slices on a pan and equally distribute the cream cheese mixture on each. Now place a dill pickle spear in the center of each piece of ham and roll tightly.

Wrap in plastic wrap and refrigerate for 2-3 hours. Cut into 1-inch bites and serve.

Nutrition Per Serving
(1 pinwheel = 1 serving)

Calories: 34

Total Fat: 3g

Protein: 2g

Fiber: 0g

Total Carbs: 1g

Net Carbs: 1g

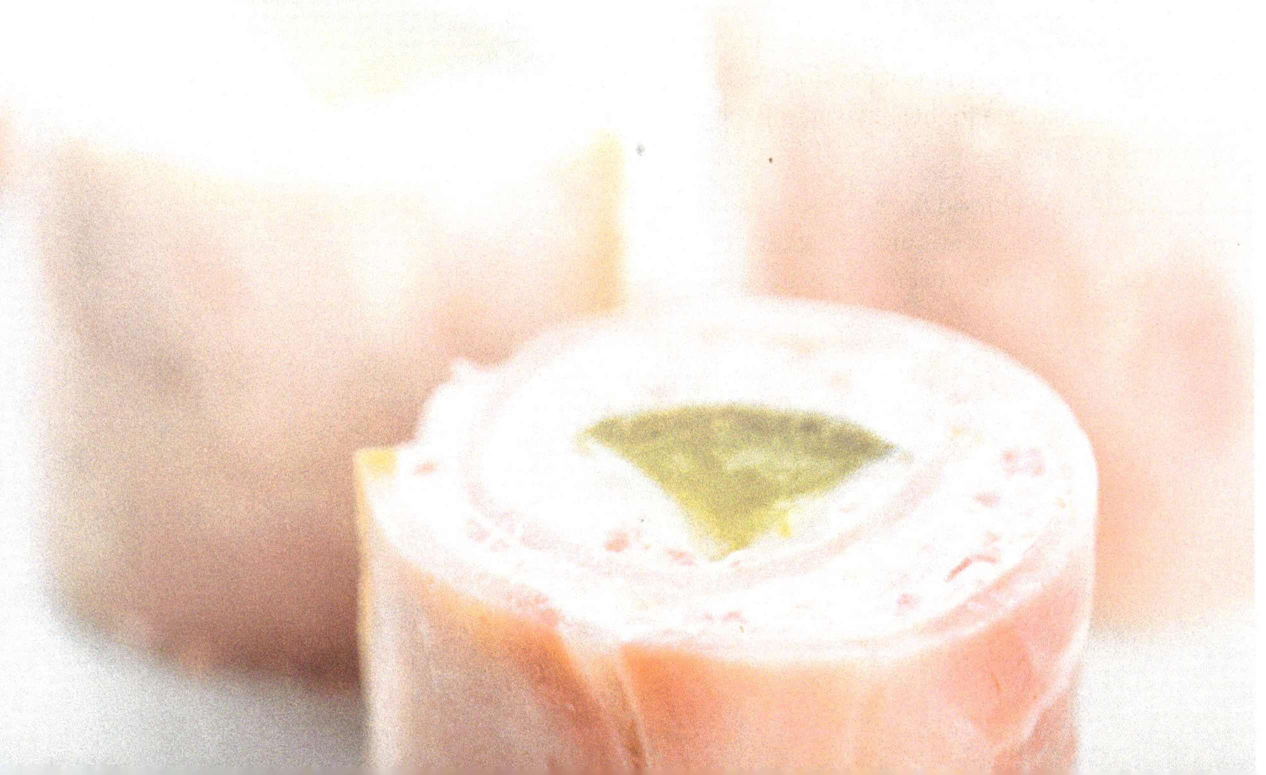

The Secret of My Success 3-Ingredient Party Crackers

Prep Time: 15 minutes

Cook Time: 25 minutes

Yield: 40

Ok, so after going a few months on keto without a single cracker in my life, I decided to up my low carb baking game and ventured out into the world of crunch. Because all good dips need a vehicle to your mouth, and sometimes a sliced veggie just won't cut it. This three-ingredient cracker recipe is the closest thing you're going to get to a legit crunchy cracker. And topped with flaked sea salt, the texture is spot on.

Pairs well with any dip, and the 1987 film starring Michael J. Fox that reminds us sometimes the good guys—and gals—finish first.

1 cup almond flour

1 tablespoon ground flaxseed

½ teaspoon of sea salt

3 tablespoons water

½ teaspoon pink Himalayan salt or flaked sea salt (optional—but recommended for topping)

Preheat the oven to 350° and prep a large baking pan with 2 sheets of parchment paper. (One for lining the pan and one for helping you roll out the dough.)

Next, combine the almond flour, flaxseed, salt, and water in a bowl and stir until dough forms. Now you're ready to roll that dough out onto the lined pan.

Use your hands to form the dough into a square, then cover with the second sheet of parchment paper and use a rolling pin to spread it out.

The goal here is to create a uniform layer that is around ⅛ inch thick. Do not grab a ruler and measure this—just keep it in mind.

Once your dough is spread out, discard the parchment paper and top with sprinkled Pink Himalayan or flaked sea salt.

Then grab your pizza cutter or a knife and cut the dough into small squares. Now it's time to bake! Place the dough into the oven and bake for 20-25 minutes. Cool and serve.

Store any leftovers in an airtight container or bag at room temperature for up to 4 days.

Nutrition Per Serving
(10 crackers = 1 serving)

Calories: 175

Fat: 15g

Protein: 6g

Fiber: 4g

Total Carbs: 7g

Net Carbs: 3g

It Takes Two Ingredients to Make Easy Cheese Crisps

Prep Time: 5 minutes

Cook Time: 8 minutes

Yield: 30 crisps

I wanna rock right now…

These cheese crisps are the perfect 10-minute chip, cracker, or crouton substitute. Use these as a vehicle for guacamole, crab dip, or whenever you need something with crunch.

Since there are several different ways you can make these crisps, I'm going to tell you about all of them. I recommend you go with whatever works for you.

The Easiest Way To Make Cheese Crisps

Go to the deli section and buy a party-sized package of assorted pre-sliced cheeses.

They are already perfectly sized and sliced, and all you have to do is arrange the slices about 2 inches apart on parchment paper and put them in the oven.

Make sure you leave enough room between the slices, or you'll end up with one sheet pan size crisp—which is not the worst thing in the world; you can still eat it, but it's not pretty.

If you want to add seasoning, go for it.

Everything Bagel and What's Hiding In the Valley Ranch Seasoning (See recipes in Seasonings) are my favorites.

Preheat the oven to 400° and line a baking pan with parchment paper. Arrange cheese slices at least 2 inches apart and bake for 8-10 minutes. Transfer to a paper towel to cool to absorb any oil.

Using Shredded Cheese

You can also make these with your choice of shredded cheese and seasonings. Here's the 411.

1 cup shredded cheddar cheese

1 cup shredded Parmesan

1½ teaspoons seasoning

Preheat the oven to 400° and line a baking pan with parchment paper.

Mix the cheeses and then dollop portions of cheese onto the wax paper. You can go rogue and throw the cheese on the pan with reckless abandon or dollop 30, evenly sized portions on the pan.

It's up to you.

Try to space each about 2 inches apart, or you'll end up with a solid pan of cheese. Sprinkle seasoning of choice on each and bake for 6-8 minutes.

Move to cool on paper towels to absorb excess oil. Store in an airtight container.

Nutrition Per Serving
(6 crisps = 1 serving)

Calories: 158

Fat: 11.9g

Protein: 11.2g

Fiber: 0

Total Carbs: 1.2g

Net Carbs: 1.2g

5-Minute Parmesan Chaffle Garlic Bread

Prep Time: 2 Minutes

Cook Time: 3 Minutes

Yield: 2

Here's my favorite savory twist on the basic cheddar and egg chaffle. (Yes, chaffle—with a C. It's a low carb waffle—not a typo.) Think of them as your go-to swap for garlic bread. Or use them as sandwich bread. Or dip them in sugar-free marinara sauce for a snack or appetizer.

½ cup mozzarella

1 tablespoon grated Parmesan cheese

1 egg

1 minced garlic clove or ¼ teaspoon garlic powder

½ teaspoon Italian Stallion Seasoning (See recipe in Seasonings)

¼ teaspoon baking powder

Turn on your mini waffle iron and spray it with a little coconut oil or your favorite keto-friendly nonstick spray.

In a small bowl, combine the mozzarella cheese, Parmesan cheese, egg, garlic, Italian seasoning, and baking powder.

Place half the batter in the mini waffle maker for 2-3 minutes. Repeat with the remaining batter. (You can add bacon, top with chives or green onions, and a dollop of cream cheese instead of butter.) Use these for sandwiches or snacks or eat for breakfast.

Store in an airtight container in the refrigerator for up to 5 days. Reheat in a toaster, skillet, or oven.

To Freeze: Place each chaffle in a freezer bag separated with wax paper, so they don't stick together.

Defrost in the microwave or overnight.

Reheat in a toaster, skillet, oven, or your air fryer set at 300° for 2-3 minutes.

Nutrition Per Serving
(1 chaffle = 1 serving)

Calories: 155

Fat: 10.7g

Protein: 12.3g

Fiber: 4g

Total Carbs: 2.4g

Net Carbs: 1.8g

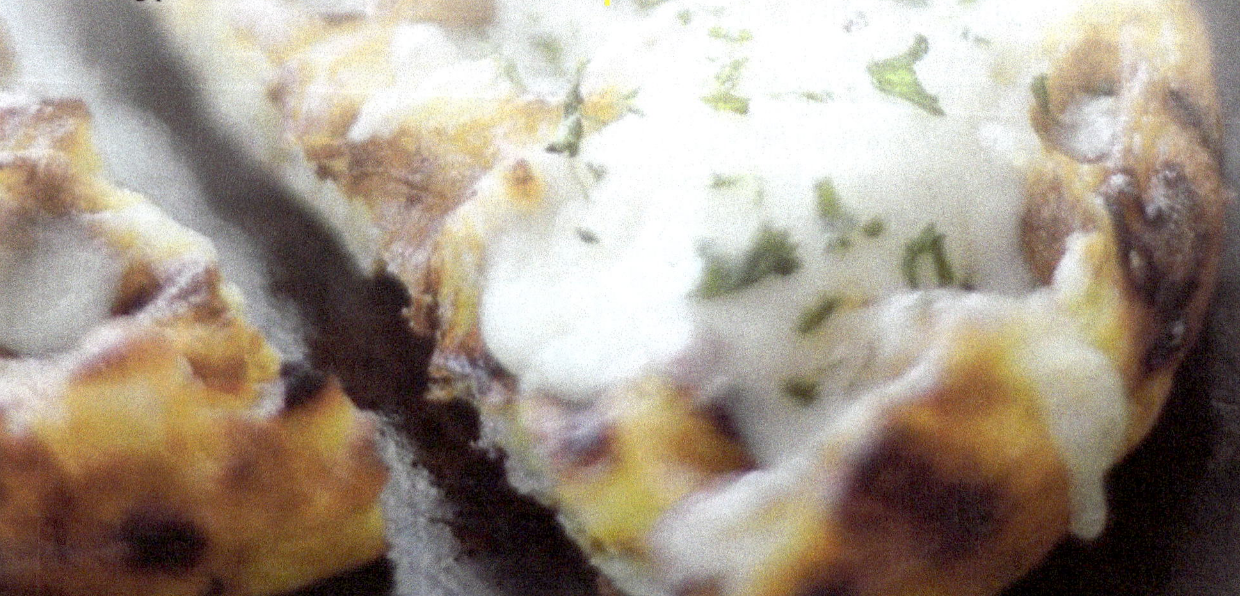

Bread

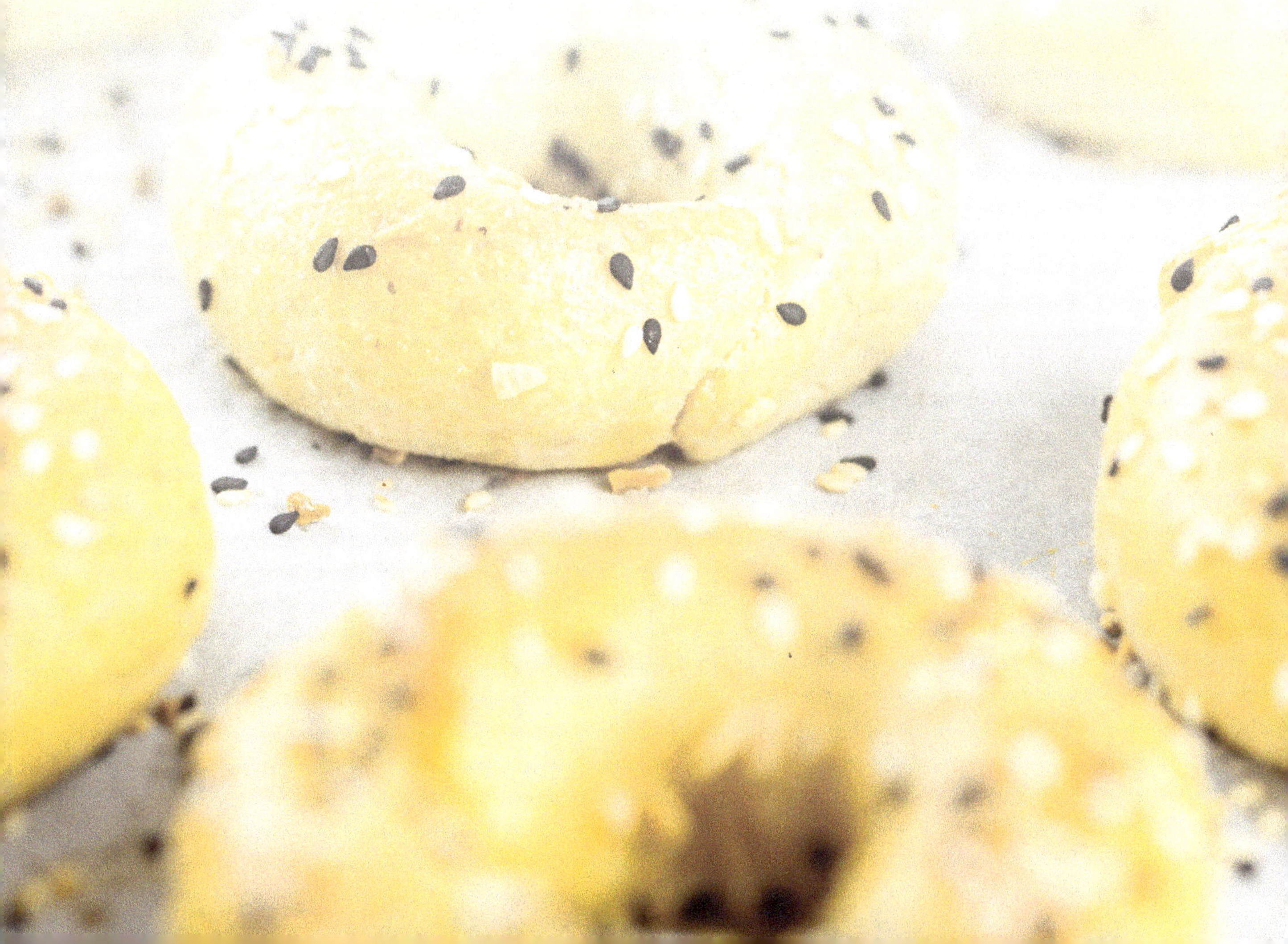

When I See You Smile 90-Second Bad English Muffins

Prep Time: 2 minutes

Cook Time: 90 seconds

Yield: 1

Junior high. 1989.

The dance that changed everything.

The cafe-gym-a-torium was decked out with dim lighting, a disco ball, and a DJ that had thus far failed to unite the class.

It's 10:30 P.M. with 30 minutes left.

Just as you were giving up hope, you hear it.

The synthesized piano ignites butterflies in your stomach. This is your moment.

A last-minute touch up with Bonnie Bell.

He crosses the gym floor. Asks you to dance. And at that moment, all's right with the world. Make this muffin happen in moments.

Don't give up when you've gotten this far.

Pairs well with any Bad English album, couple skates, and junior high nostalgia.

1 tablespoon coconut oil

3 tablespoons almond flour

½ tablespoon coconut flour

½ teaspoon baking powder

Dash of sea salt

1 egg

Combine ingredients in a microwave-safe ramekin or mug. Microwave for 90 seconds.

Give it a minute or so to cool and remove.

Slice it in half and toast it in the toaster or the oven. Top with butter.

Nutrition Per Serving

(1 muffin = 1 serving)

Calories: 307

Fat: 27g

Protein: 12g

Fiber: 4g

Total Carbs: 8g

Net Carbs: 4g

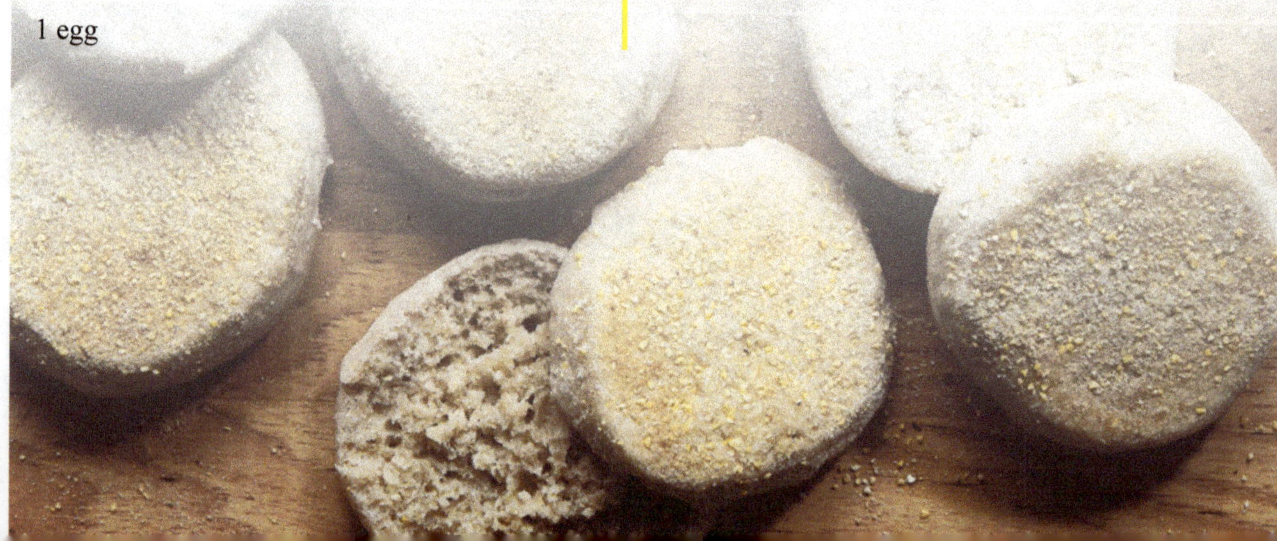

Cloud Bread

Prep Time: 20 minutes

Cook Time: 30 minutes

Yield: 12

Cloud bread is one of the easiest low carb bread swaps for sandwich bread, toast, and rolls. Also known as Oopsie Rolls, this bread has a light and fluffy texture.

Bonus: It's easy to make—no kneading required!

Note: Cloud bread often looks like meringue fresh out of the oven. Give it a few hours after baking before you judge the texture—it takes a few hours to get the legit bread texture.

3 eggs (whites and yolks separated)

⅛ teaspoon cream of tartar

1 ounce cream cheese or Mascarpone cheese, softened & cubed

1 teaspoon Italian Stallion Seasoning (See recipe in Seasonings)

⅛ teaspoon salt

Preheat the oven to 300°

Line a baking sheet with parchment paper and grease lightly with cooking spray.

Place egg whites and cream of tartar in a medium-sized mixing bowl. Using a hand mixer on high, beat until stiff peaks form. (The cream of tartar helps stabilize the eggs, so they hold their shape.) In a separate bowl, combine egg yolks, cream cheese, Italian Stallion seasoning, and salt. Blend with a mixer until smooth.

Now, gently fold the egg whites into the egg yolk mixture.

Using a large spoon or ¼ cup, scoop the mixture into six even rounds on the paper-lined baking sheet. Leave a little room between them because they will flatten and spread in the oven.

Bake at 300° for 20-30 minutes.

Since oven times vary, keep an eye on them starting at the 20-minute mark. When they're ready, the tops will be golden and firm.

Let the bread cool before removing it from the parchment paper. (You may want to use a spatula or a knife to separate it.)

To Freeze: Cool completely. Then flash freeze by placing it in the freezer for two hours. If your baking pan doesn't fit in your freezer, arrange the bread on a plate lined with parchment paper—(with no overlap!)

Store in the freezer separated by parchment paper sheets in an airtight container or heavy-duty freezer bag for up to 3 months.

Thaw overnight and reheat in the toaster.

Nutrition Per Serving
(1 roll = 1 serving)

Calories: 88

Fat: 7.9g

Protein: 2.9g

Fiber: 0g

Total Carbs: 0.7g

Net Carbs: 0.7g

Just Roll With It Cheddar Garlic Biscuits

Prep Time: 10 minutes

Cook Time: 25 minutes

Yield: 15

I'm no Betty Crocker, and I'm certainly not Steve Winwood either, but I have to say I was proud of myself after nailing these. I was going for a Red Lobster cheddar bay biscuit thing, but since buttermilk is out of the question, I improvised (ahem, rolled with it) and used cream cheese and cheddar. The result was a hit three days in a row. I count that as a win.

Roll with it, baby.

8 ounces cream cheese, softened

2 eggs

1 cup sharp cheddar cheese, shredded

6 cloves garlic, minced

½ teaspoon onion powder

½ teaspoon garlic powder

2½ cups almond flour

½ cup heavy cream

½ cup water

Preheat the oven to 350°. Grease 15 wells of a muffin pan.

Use an electric or stand mixer to combine the cream cheese and the eggs. Then add the cheese, garlic, onion powder, and garlic powder.

Once you have all those ingredients combined, add the almond flour, followed by the heavy cream and water.

Mix until all the ingredients are combined, and the dough is as lump-free as possible. Distribute into the greased wells of a muffin pan and bake for 20–25 minutes.

Cool and serve.

Nutrition Per Serving
(1 biscuit = 1 serving)

Calories: 252

Fat: 16.7g

Protein: 9.4g

Fiber: 0.6g

Total Carbs: 5g

Net Carbs: 4.4g

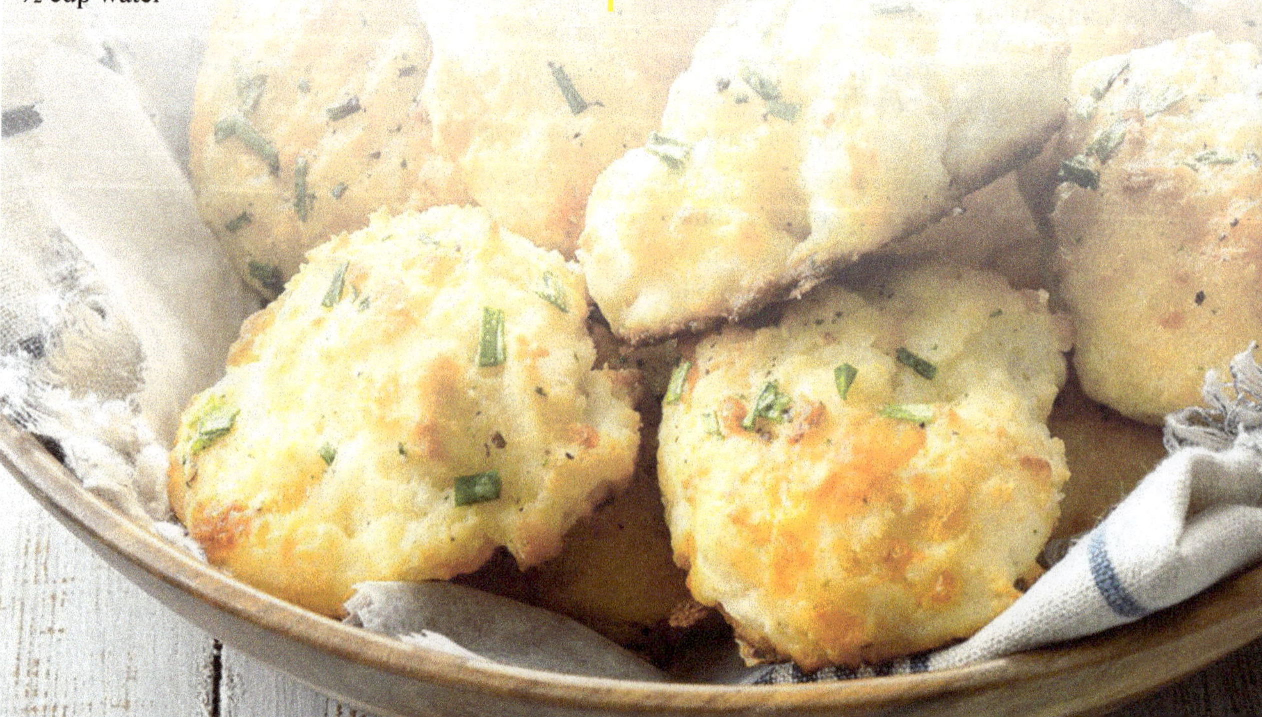

Soul To Soul Buns

Prep Time: 15 minutes

Cook Time: 35 minutes

Yield: 12

Let's take it to a slow jam—all the way back to 1989 when Motown legends The Temptations released "Soul to Soul"—a song about the need for connection. A friend. True love. Someone with whom we can share our stories, and yes, even our souls.

We all need someone we connect with on a spiritual level—a human bond we can rely on when our heart craves the comfort of that kind of extraordinary love.

This Soul Bun recipe will tide you over while you wait for yours.

8 ounces cream cheese, softened

3 tablespoons butter, melted

2½ tablespoons avocado oil

1½ tablespoons heavy whipping cream

2 eggs

1 egg white only

1 cup + 3 tablespoons whey protein powder, unflavored

1½ teaspoons baking powder

½ teaspoon xanthan gum

½ teaspoon garlic powder

¼ teaspoon baking soda

¼ teaspoon salt

¼ teaspoon cream of tartar

Homemade Everything Bagel Seasoning (See recipe in Seasonings) or sesame seeds

Grease a 12 cavity whoopie pie pan or muffin top pan with butter and preheat your oven to 350°.

In a large mixing bowl, beat together cream cheese, butter, avocado oil, whipping cream, eggs, and egg white.

In a separate bowl, combine protein powder, baking powder, xanthan gum, garlic powder, baking soda, salt, and cream of tartar. Do your best to get all the lumps out.

Channel your general frustrations to make this time go by faster. Now, add this mixture into the cream cheese combo ¼ cup at a time. Stir until you're confident it's combined. (It will look like cake batter.) Distribute batter into your pan of choice evenly.

Sprinkle the tops with Everything Bagel seasoning or sesame seeds. Bake for 15-25 minutes.

The buns will be golden brown and slightly firm to touch. (I baked mine in a whoopie pie pan for 17 minutes.)

Keep an eye on your buns because they will go from almost done to burned FAST. Cool before removing from the pan.

Nutrition Per Serving
(1 bun = 1 serving)

Calories: 175

Fat: 14.42g

Protein: 9.34g

Fiber: 0g

Total Carbs: 2.5g

Fathead Dough Pizza Crust

Prep Time: 15 minutes

Cook Time: 15 minutes

Yield: 1 pizza crust—8 slices

1½ cups full-fat mozzarella cheese, shredded

2 tablespoons full-fat cream cheese, cubed

1 egg

¾ cup almond flour

¼ teaspoon garlic powder

¼ teaspoon oregano

Preheat the oven to 425°.

Grab your favor-
ite medium-sized, microwave-safe bowl and mix the mozzarella and cream cheese. Microwave it for 30 seconds, then stir it and microwave it for another 30 seconds or until the cheese is melted.

Stir in the almond flour, egg, and oregano.

When the ingredients are combined, throw the spoon in the sink and get ready to get your hands dough dirty.

We're about to knead the dough—and if you're not familiar with the term, don't be intimidated. It's just a fancy way of saying squeeze the dough like it's a stress ball.

It will start to become more dough-like within a minute. Once it has reached dough consistency, form it into a ball. Remind yourself of how amazing you're going to feel after you make low carb pizza a thing. Place that ball of dough on the pan and spread it into a square with your hands.

Cover it with the second sheet of paper and grab your rolling pin. If you don't have a rolling pin, use a can. Channel your inner MacGyver and come up with something—you don't have to be fancy.

Roll whatever you're using until you have a thin, even crust. Poke a few holes in the crust with a fork to prevent a bubbling situation later.

Bake for 12-14 minutes at 425°

Remove from the oven, top with 1 cup sugar-free sauce, cheese, and whatever toppings you like (pepperoni, sausage, veggies), then bake for five more minutes.

Store the (unbaked) dough wrapped tightly in plastic wrap in the refrigerator for up to one week. Store the (baked) crust in the fridge for up to one week.

To Freeze Dough: Freeze the dough by forming it into a ball and wrapping it tightly in plastic wrap. When you're ready to use it, thaw and roll.

To Freeze Crust: You can also freeze the baked crust by wrapping it in plastic wrap for up to 3 months. When you're ready to use it, just pop it into the oven—no thawing necessary!

Nutrition Per Serving
(1 slice = 1 serving)

Calories: 138

Fat: 8.2g Protein: 7g

Fiber: 0.3g

Total Carbs: 2.4g

Net Carbs: 2.1g

Rising Up, Straight to the Top Zucchini Bread

Prep Time: 20 minutes

Cook Time: 45 minutes

Yield: 8

Sylvester Stallone was Rocky. He had the guts. And the glory. And the eye of the tiger.

Much like Sly's epic journey to win the heavyweight championship title, this zucchini bread will help you rise to the top.

Do not allow your cravings to defeat you. You are a champion.

1½ cups almond flour

¼ cup oat fiber

½ teaspoon baking powder

½ teaspoon baking soda

1 teaspoon ground cinnamon

½ teaspoon ground nutmeg

½ teaspoon ginger powder

½ teaspoon salt 3 eggs

¼ cup salted butter (softened)

½ cup granulated erythritol

1 cup zucchini, shredded

Prep a 9 X 5 loaf pan with oil or line it with parchment paper. Preheat the oven to 325°

In a medium bowl, combine almond flour, oat fiber, baking powder, baking soda, cinnamon, nutmeg, ginger, and salt.

In a separate large bowl, use a hand mixer to combine the eggs, butter, and erythritol. Make sure they're well combined. (You may need to scrape the sides of the bowl.)

Now, with the mixer set on low, add the flour combo. Stir in the zucchini with a spoon.

Pour the batter into the loaf pan and bake for 45 minutes or until a toothpick inserted into the center comes out clean.

Cool for 10 minutes in the pan.

Then remove from the pan and let the bread cool completely before slicing and serving. Store leftovers in an airtight container in the fridge for up to 5 days.

Nutrition Per Serving
(⅛ recipe = 1 serving)

Calories: 267

Fat: 22.8g

Protein: 8.6g

Fiber: 8.5g

Total Carbs: 11.2g

Net Carbs: 2.7g

One-Ingredient Parmesan Cheese "Chips"

Prep Time: 5 minutes

Cook Time: 5 minutes

Yield: 25

What's the point of a fabulous dip if there's nothing to dip with? These Parmesan cheese crisps are a fabulously simple alternative to chips, and they're easy to customize with your favorite herbs and spices. Just sprinkle 'em on before baking.

1 cups Parmesan cheese, grated

Prep a baking sheet with parchment paper and preheat the oven to 400° Grab a tablespoon and dollop the Parmesan cheese onto the pan. Repeat. Leave an inch between dollops, or you'll end up with a solid sheet of cheese (which is edible, but not at all chip-sized.)

Bake for 3-5 minutes.

Nutrition Per Serving
(5 crisps = 1 serving)

Calories: 152

Fat: 11g

Protein: 11g

Fiber: 0g

Total Carbs: 1g

Net Carbs: 1g

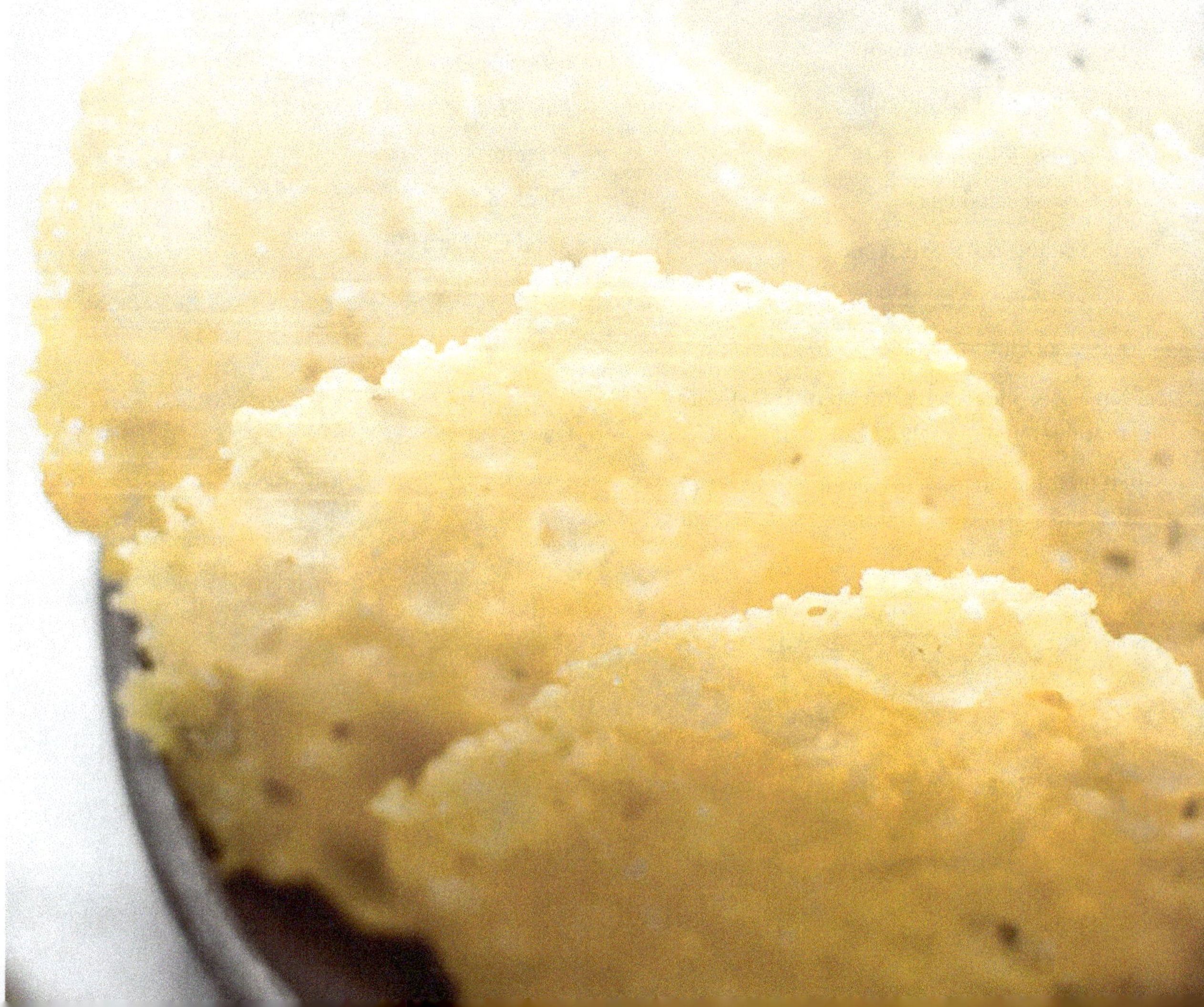

Everything But the Carbs Bagels

Prep Time: 15 minutes

Cook Time: 14 minutes

Yield: 8

When you're not a pro in the kitchen, making bagels happen—and making them look remotely like the "real thing" is a little tricky, but nowhere near as hard as living without them. Using a combination of Fathead dough, a little baking powder, and the low-key addictive Everything Bagel seasoning, you can make a legit tasting low carb bagel.

Note: You need a good mixer for this. I'm warning you upfront—if you attempt mixing this by hand, you may end up super mad and frustrated.

Tip: Give yourself at least 30 minutes between creating the dough and working with it. Almond flour dough needs to chill, and so do you. You'll both perform better after a little break.

1 cup mozzarella cheese

2 ounces (4 tablespoons) cream cheese

2 cups blanched almond flour

4 eggs (divided)

1 tablespoon baking powder

3 tablespoons Homemade Everything Bagel Seasoning (See recipe in Seasonings) or Sesame seeds

Preheat the oven to 400° and line a baking sheet with parchment paper.

In a microwave-safe bowl, combine the mozzarella cheese and cream cheese. Melt in the microwave for 1–2 minutes—stirring every 30 seconds.

Combine the almond flour, two eggs, and baking powder—in a food processor or with a handheld electric mixer.

Stir in melted cheeses.

Lightly coat your hands with cooking oil or wet them with a little water, so you don't end up with a sticky dough finger situation and knead this combination until it starts to look like dough.

If you're having dough issues—you may need to reheat it in the microwave for a few seconds. The cheese needs to be hot to cooperate.

Divide dough into eight rolled lines. Then create a circle with each to form a bagel shape. Whisk the remaining egg.

Brush the tops of each bagel with the remaining egg and top with Everything Bagel seasoning or sesame seeds and bake at 400° for 15–20 minutes.

Store any leftovers in the refrigerator for up to 5 days. Freeze in heavy-duty freezer bags for up to 3 months.

Nutrition Per Serving
(1 bagel = 1 serving)

Calories: 327

Fat: 19g

Protein: 15.3g

Fiber: 1.3g

Total Carbs: 7.3g

Net Carbs: 4.4g

Coconut Flour Tortillas

Prep Time: 5 minutes

Cook Time: 10 minutes

Yield: 12

These coconut flour tortillas are perfect for Taco Tuesday, and Wednesday, and Thursday. I mean, why limit taco night to once a week?

½ cup coconut flour

6 eggs

1¼ cup unsweetened almond milk

½ teaspoon cumin

¾ teaspoon sea salt

1 tablespoon gelatin powder, unflavored

Grab your favorite mixing bowl and whisk all the ingredients until smooth. Walk away for a minute or two to let it thicken. Take this time for a bathroom break or think about that vision board you never seem to get around to making.

Now, grab a small skillet and set heat to medium-high. Add a drop of cooking oil and add ¼ cup's worth of batter.

Cook until bubbles form in the center and the edges are golden brown (similar to making pancakes) Flip and cook for another 1–2 minutes.

Repeat until you've used all the batter, or you're too tired to go on. Store any leftovers in the fridge for up to 3 days.

Tip: Place paper towels or wax paper between them so they won't stick together.

Nutrition Per Serving
(1 tortilla = 1 serving)

Calories: 55

Fat: 4g

Protein: 5g

Fiber: 3g

Total Carbs: 4g

Net Carbs: 1g

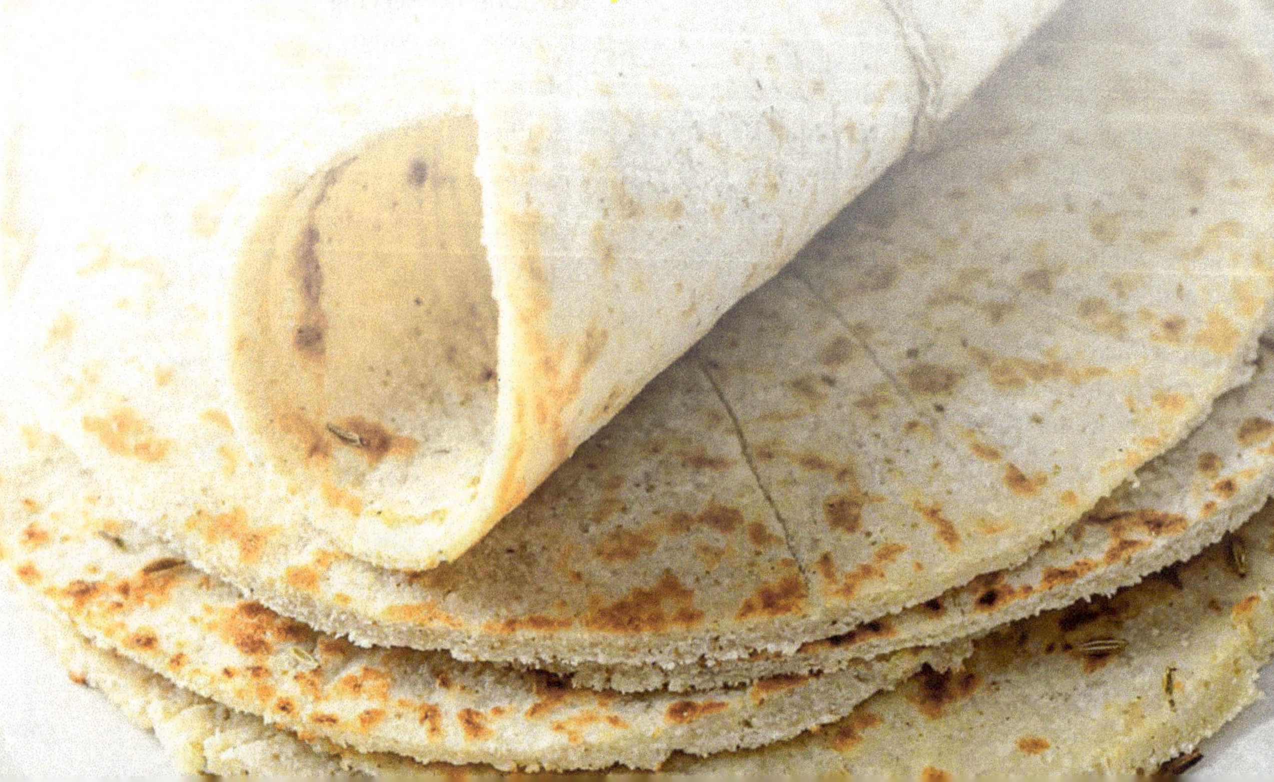

Sweet Dreams Cinnamon Muffins

Prep Time: 10 minutes

Cook Time: 14 minutes

Yield: 12 muffins

In 1983 the Eurythmics reminded us that sometimes you could travel the world while what you've been looking for is right in front of you.

Make these muffins ahead (or at the last minute) anytime you need to dream a sweet dream, kick back and chill. They bring just the right amount of spice and sweetness.

Pairs well with the Eurythmics or any Annie Lennox track.

1½ cups blanched almond flour

1 tablespoon baking powder

1 tablespoon ground cinnamon + 1 teaspoon ground cinnamon, divided

2 eggs

½ cup granular erythritol

2 tablespoons salted butter, softened 1 tablespoon heavy whipping cream

½ teaspoon vanilla extract

Prep a muffin tin with cooking spray, butter, oil, or muffin liners and preheat the oven to 350° In a small bowl, combine almond flour, baking powder, and 1 tablespoon cinnamon.

In a separate medium-sized bowl, whisk the eggs, then add the erythritol, butter, heavy cream, vanilla, and the remaining teaspoon of cinnamon.

Stir until combined.

Slowly stir in the almond flour mixture until combined. Pour the batter into the muffin pan—filling each cup ¾ full. Bake for 12–14 minutes.

Let the muffins cool before removing them from the pan. Store any leftovers in the fridge for up to a week.

Nutrition Per Serving
(2 muffins = 1 serving)

Calories: 218

Fat: 19.2g

Protein: 7.4g

Fiber: 3.4g

Total Carbs: 6.3g

Net Carbs: 2.9g

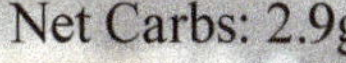

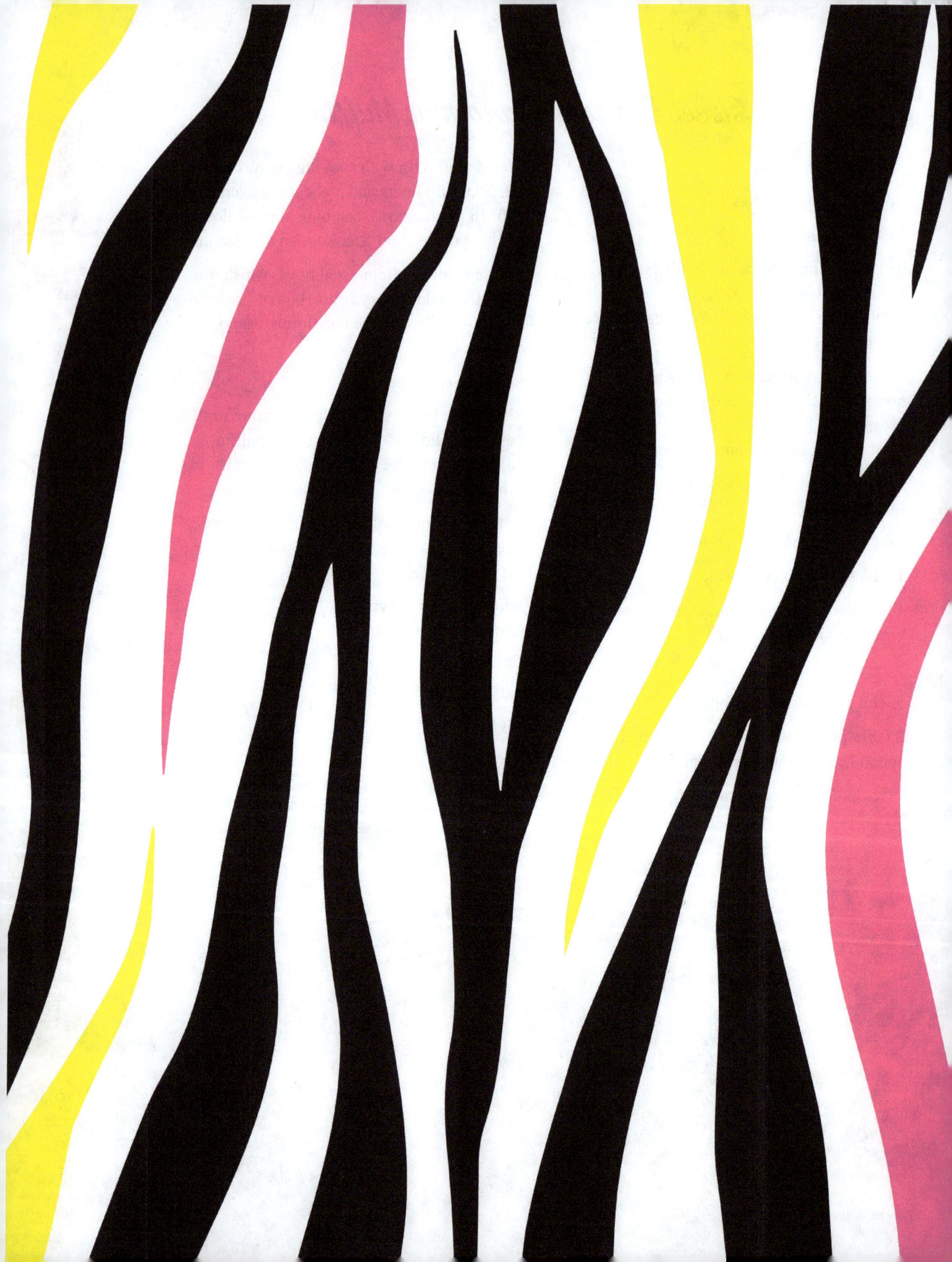

Sides

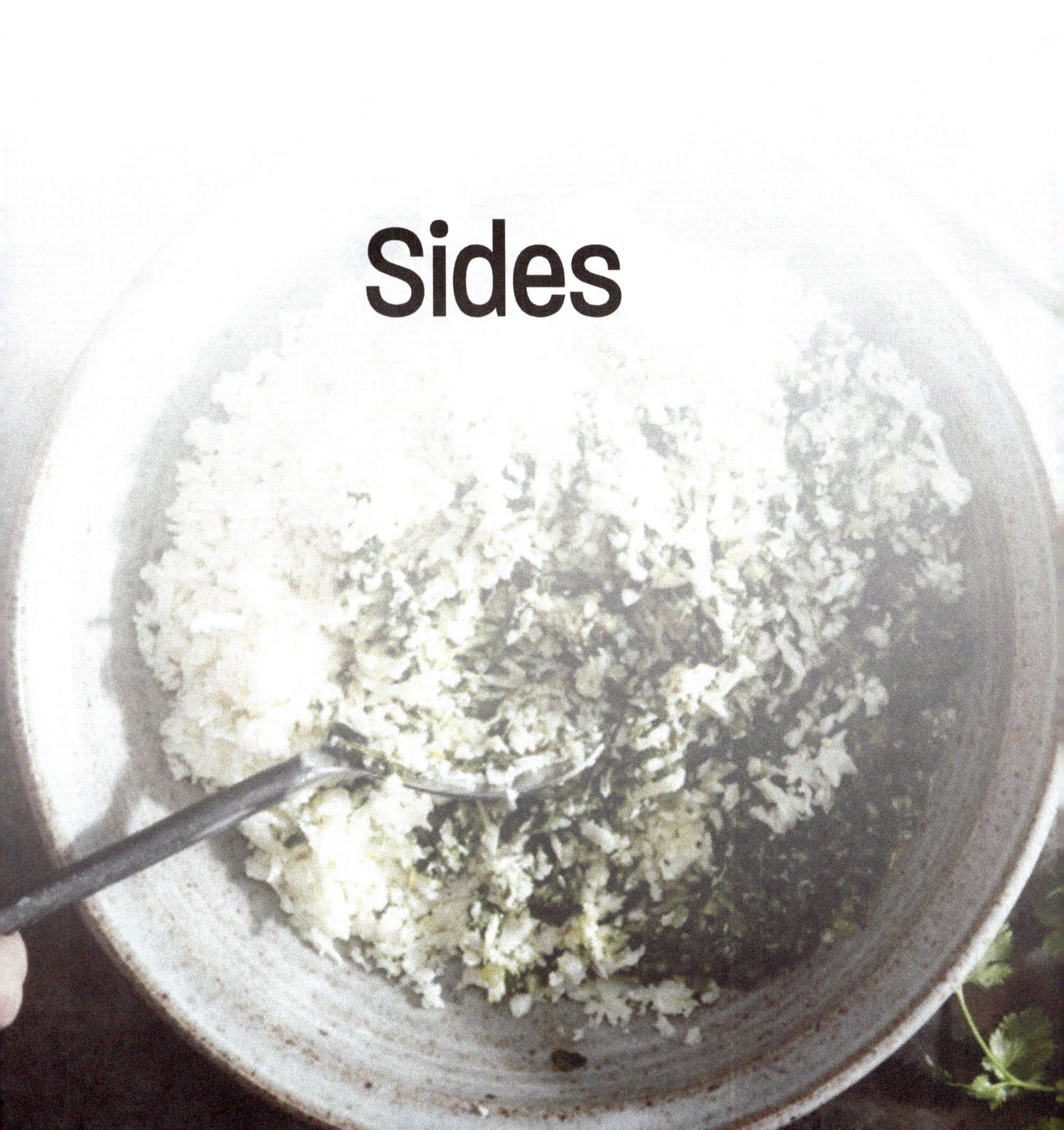

I Can't Believe It's Not Real Cauliflower Potato Salad

Prep Time: 10 minutes

Cook Time: 10 minutes

Yield: 6

If you remember the 1981 alternative-to-butter-margarine-spread, I Can't Believe It's Not Butter, then you are familiar with the feeling of being fooled by a fake that was supposed to be healthy. This mock potato salad made with a simple cauliflower swap for potatoes is legit healthy and as close as you can get to the "real thing" without sacrificing flavor or taste.

4 hard-boiled eggs, chopped

½ cup dill pickle relish

2 stalks celery, chopped

¼ cup green onions, chopped

1 cup mayonnaise

1 tablespoon yellow mustard

½ teaspoon sweet paprika

½ teaspoon garlic powder

½ teaspoon salt

¼ teaspoon pepper

2 10-ounce bags frozen cauliflower florets, cooked & dried

2 slices bacon, cooked & crumbled (optional)

In a large mixing bowl, combine eggs, relish, celery, onions, mayonnaise, mustard, paprika, garlic powder, salt, and pepper.

Add the cauliflower and mix well.

Chill in the fridge for at least 2 hours before serving. Top with bacon crumbles and serve.

Store covered in the refrigerator for up to 4 days.

Nutrition Per Serving
(1 cup = 1 serving)

Calories: 282

Fat: 29g

Protein: 3.2g

Fiber: 1.1g

Total Carbs: 3.8g

Net Carbs: 2.4g

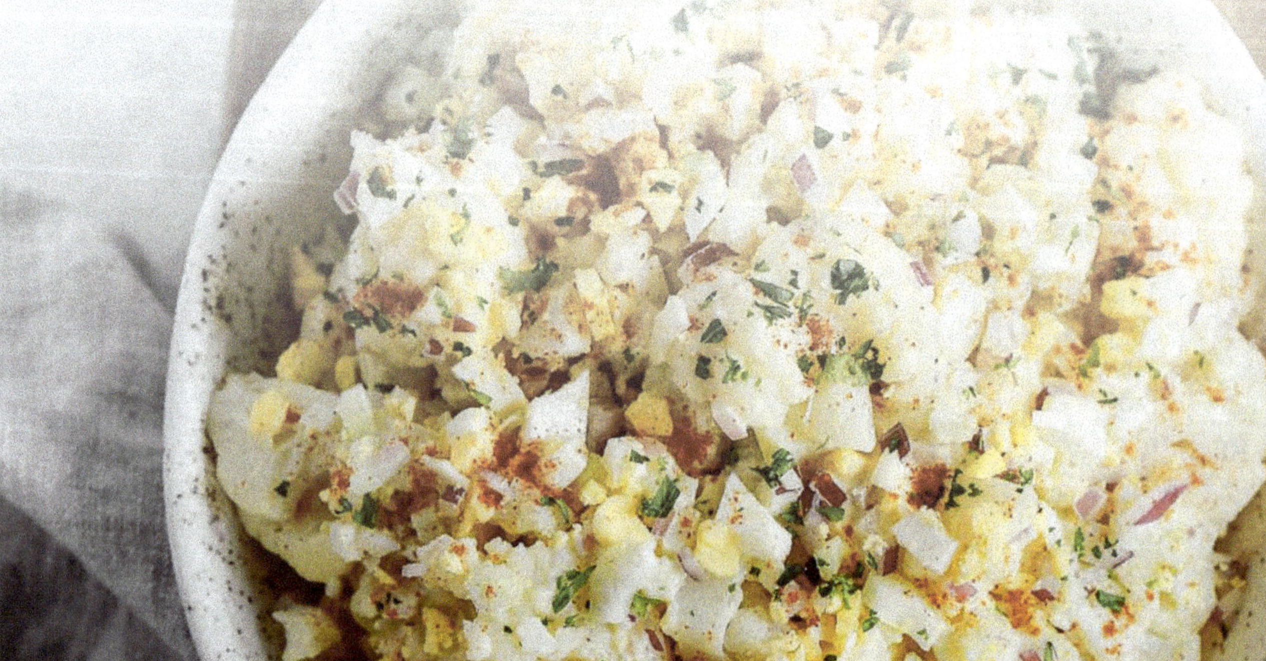

Karma Chameleon Cauliflower

Prep Time: 10 minutes

Cook Time: 20 minutes

Yield: 8

Cauliflower was not my favorite vegetable as a kid, and I was a kid who loved veggies. But there was something about the bland, white cauliflower that made me think of it as broccoli's unfortunately dull cousin who showed up on my plate as a space filler. Thankfully, as I've gotten older, I have gotten wiser, and my idea of cauliflower has shifted from bland to blank canvas.

Roasting cauliflower brings out its sweetness. It makes a fabulous side dish for roasts, steaks, lamb, chicken, and some fish dishes.

1 head of cauliflower (about 8 cups worth)

¼ cup olive oil

5-6 cloves garlic, chopped

2 teaspoons fresh thyme, chopped (you can sub ground thyme)

2 teaspoons kosher salt

¼ teaspoon crushed red pepper

Preheat the oven to 450° and prep a large baking pan with oil or nonstick cooking spray.

Prepare the cauliflower: remove any green leaves. Slice the head in half, remove the core, and divide it into florets as best you can by hand.

Chop into bite-sized florets.

Combine the olive oil, garlic, and red pepper in a large bowl and add in the florets, tossing to combine.

(If you'd prefer to attempt this on the baking sheet to save yourself the trouble of using a new dish, you can, but you will run the risk of uneven distribution of spices. It's up to you to weigh the pros and cons. Remember what Boy George said: Every day is like survival.)

Add salt and thyme and toss again.

Transfer cauliflower to the baking pan and roast for 10 minutes, toss it and continue roasting for ten more minutes.

You'll know it's done when the cauliflower will be tender and golden around the edges. Store in an airtight container in the fridge for up to 3 days.

Reheat in the oven set at 375° for 15 minutes.

Nutrition Per Serving
(1 cup = 1 serving)

Calories: 62

Fat: 4.1g

Protein: 2.2g

Fiber: 2.2g

Total Carbs: 6g

Net Carbs: 3.8g

I'm All Out Of Carbs Cauliflower Rice

Prep Time: 10 minutes

Cook Time: 10 minutes

Yield: 4

Chances are rice has been a staple in your favorite casseroles, one-dish main courses, and soups for as long as you can remember. You may feel a hint of sadness thinking of this old standby ingredient. You may feel a sense of loss—and that's okay. Feel it and move on. I will make this breakup easier for you by giving you a few healthy substitute recipes that will change your tune.

I haven't counted lately, but there are over 100 ways to prepare cauliflower rice. Here are my two favorites, starting with the most basic.

1 medium head cauliflower (4 cups)

½ teaspoon of sea salt

¼ teaspoon black pepper

2 tablespoons butter or olive or coconut oil

Core the head of cauliflower and cut the florets into bite-sized pieces. Place the florets into a food processor to shred the cauliflower. If you don't have a food processor, you can use a cheese grater.

Grab a large skillet and heat the butter or oil over medium-high heat. When the butter or oil is melted, add the cauliflower and cook for ten minutes until tender. Then add salt and pepper and serve.

Alternative Cooking Method: Microwave

Place cauliflower rice, butter or oil, salt, and pepper in a covered medium microwave-safe dish. Cook for 5 minutes.

Give it 2–3 minutes to sit before opening, then stir and serve.

Nutrition Per Serving
(1 cup = 1 serving)

Calories: 78

Fat: 6.1g

Protein: 2.1g

Fiber: 2.2g

Total Carbs: 5.4g

Net Carbs: 3.2g

* You can buy cauliflower rice fresh or frozen from most grocery stores. Or you can make it at home—it's up to you. The easiest way to get the job done is by using a food processor.

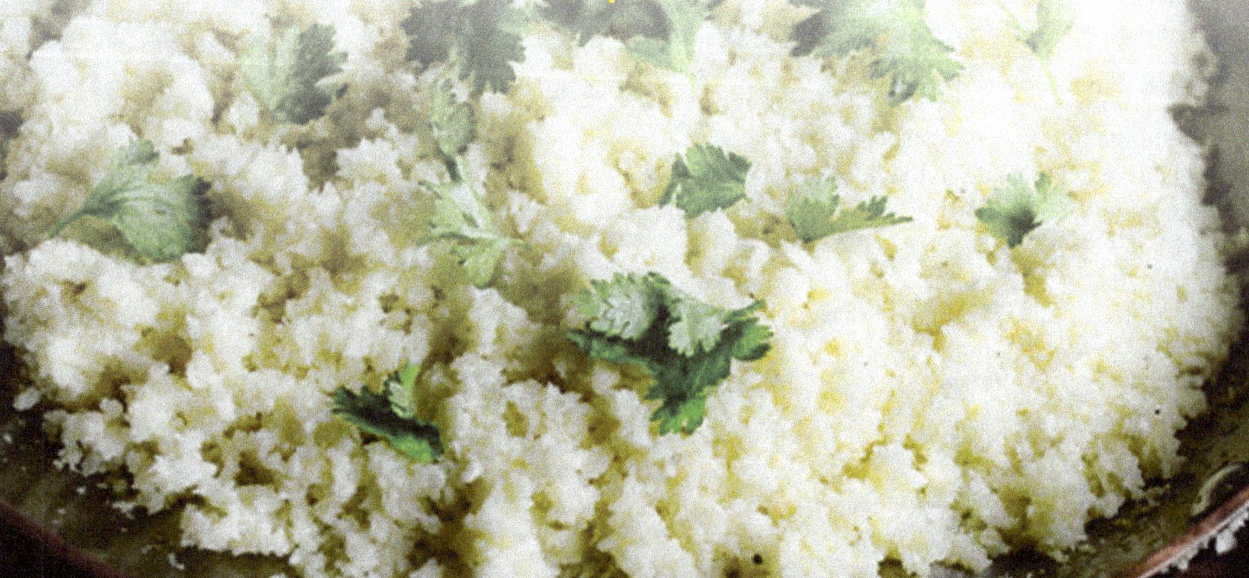

Easy Cheesy Cauliflower Rice

Prep Time: 5 minutes

Cook Time: 10 minutes

Yield: 4

When you need a quick dish that doesn't take a ton of effort or ingredients, this cheesy cauliflower recipe will be your ride or die side dish.

2 tablespoons butter

1 head of cauliflower (4 cups riced cauliflower)

½ teaspoon kosher salt

¼ teaspoon black pepper

¼ teaspoon garlic powder

½ cup shredded cheddar cheese

¼ cup cream cheese

Optional Topping:

4 slices of bacon, cooked and crumbled

¼ cup green onions, chopped

Stovetop Instructions:

Melt the butter in a large skillet over medium-high heat.

Add rice cauliflower and cook for ten minutes, stirring occasionally. Add salt, pepper, garlic powder, cheddar, and cream cheese.

Cook until the cheese is melted.

Serve topped with crumbled bacon, butter, chopped green onions, or nothing—you don't have to top it with anything. Sometimes less is more.

Microwave Instructions:

Put riced cauliflower, butter, salt, pepper, and garlic powder in a microwave-safe bowl and cook for 4 minutes.

Stir it and microwave for another 2 minutes.

Stir in the cheddar cheese and microwave for another 2 minutes. Remove from the microwave and stir in the cream cheese.

It's ready. Eat it.

Nutrition Per Serving
(1 cup = 1 serving)

Calories: 138

Fat: 11g

Protein: 6g

Fiber: 3g

Total Carbs: 5g

Net Carbs: 2g

Creamy Cucumber Salad

Prep Time: 30 minutes

Chill Time: 0

Yield: 6

Peeled and chopped cucumbers are the stars of this creamy German salad recipe with sour cream and fresh dill.

2 English cucumbers, peeled and chopped

½ red onion, sliced

¾ cup sour cream

2 tablespoons Apple Cider vinegar

3⅓ tablespoons fresh dill, chopped

½ teaspoon Sea salt

¼ teaspoon black pepper

½ teaspoon granulated sugar substitute (optional)

Rinse, peel and chop cucumbers, then let them dry on a paper towel for around 20 minutes to soak up moisture. Chop the red onion.

In a large bowl, whisk sour cream, vinegar, dill, salt, pepper, and granulated sugar substitute. Fold in the cucumbers and onion. Serve chilled.

Store any leftovers in an airtight container in the refrigerator for up to 5 days.

Nutrition Per Serving
(½ cup = 1 serving)

Calories: 57

Fat: 2.9g

Protein: 2.3g

Fiber: 1.2g

Total Carbs: 5.6g

Net Carbs: 4.4g

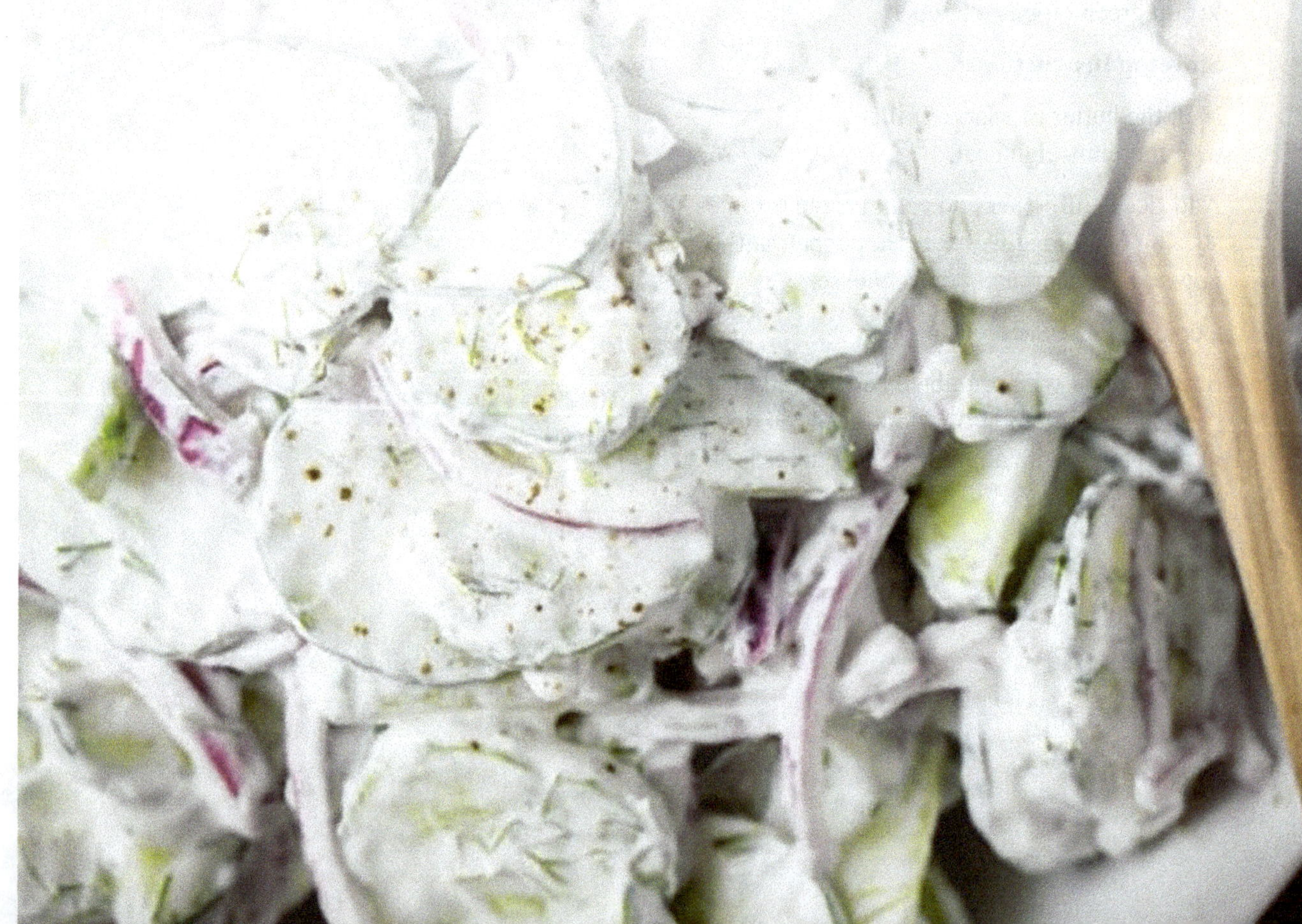

Easy Sauteed Asparagus

Prep Time: 5 minutes

Cook Time: 5 minutes

Yield: 4

A simple side dish that's perfect in a pinch with a garlic-infused oil that sounds fancy (and tastes delicious.)

2 cloves garlic

2 tablespoons olive oil

1 bunch asparagus (about 2 cups)

Kosher salt & black pepper to taste

Peel and smash garlic with a chef's knife. If you don't have a chef's knife, do not feel bad. Just grab a freaking sharp knife and move on. Or use minced garlic instead.

Heat olive oil in a medium-sized skillet on medium-high heat. Add garlic and brown for about 2 minutes.

Remove the garlic from the skillet and throw it over your left shoulder. Or into the trash can. You can thank it for serving its purpose.

Trim the ends from the asparagus and sauté it in the oil for 5 minutes. Season with salt and pepper.

Serve and enjoy.

Nutrition Per Serving
(1/2 cup = 1 serving)

Calories: 77

Total Fat: 7.1g

Protein: 1.6g

Fiber: 1.5g

Total Carbs: 3.3g

Net Carbs: 1.8g

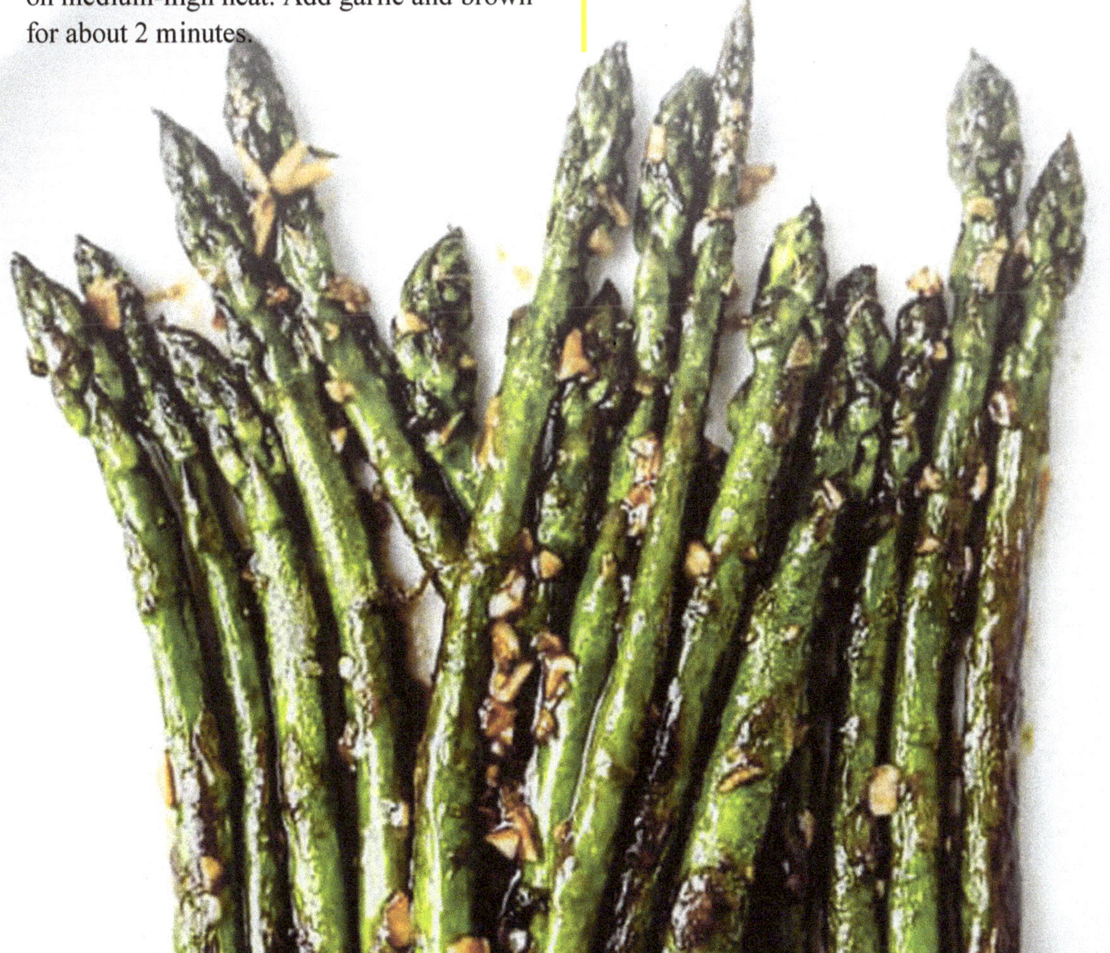

Easy 20-Minute Creamed Spinach

Prep Time: 5 minutes

Cook Time: 15 minutes

Yield: 6

If you're using fresh spinach: 1 pound of fresh cooks down to around 1 ½ cups worth, the equivalent of 1 10-ounce package frozen.

1 10-ounce bag frozen spinach

1 teaspoon butter

¼ cup onion, diced

1 clove garlic, minced

2 ounces cream cheese

⅓ cup heavy cream

½ cup Parmesan cheese, grated

Salt & pepper

Start by thawing the frozen spinach in the microwave. Remove any excess water with paper towels or cheesecloth. In a large saucepan, melt butter over medium heat.

Sauté onions for 4 minutes or until tender. Add the garlic and sauté for another minute. Stir in cream cheese and heavy cream.

Turn up the heat and simmer for 2–3 minutes or until thickened. Add in spinach and stir.

Serve topped with grated Parmesan.

Nutrition Per Serving
(½ cup = 1 serving)

Calories: 185

Fat:18.4g

Protein:3.4g Fiber: 0.4

Total Carbs: 2.5g

Net Carbs: 2.1g

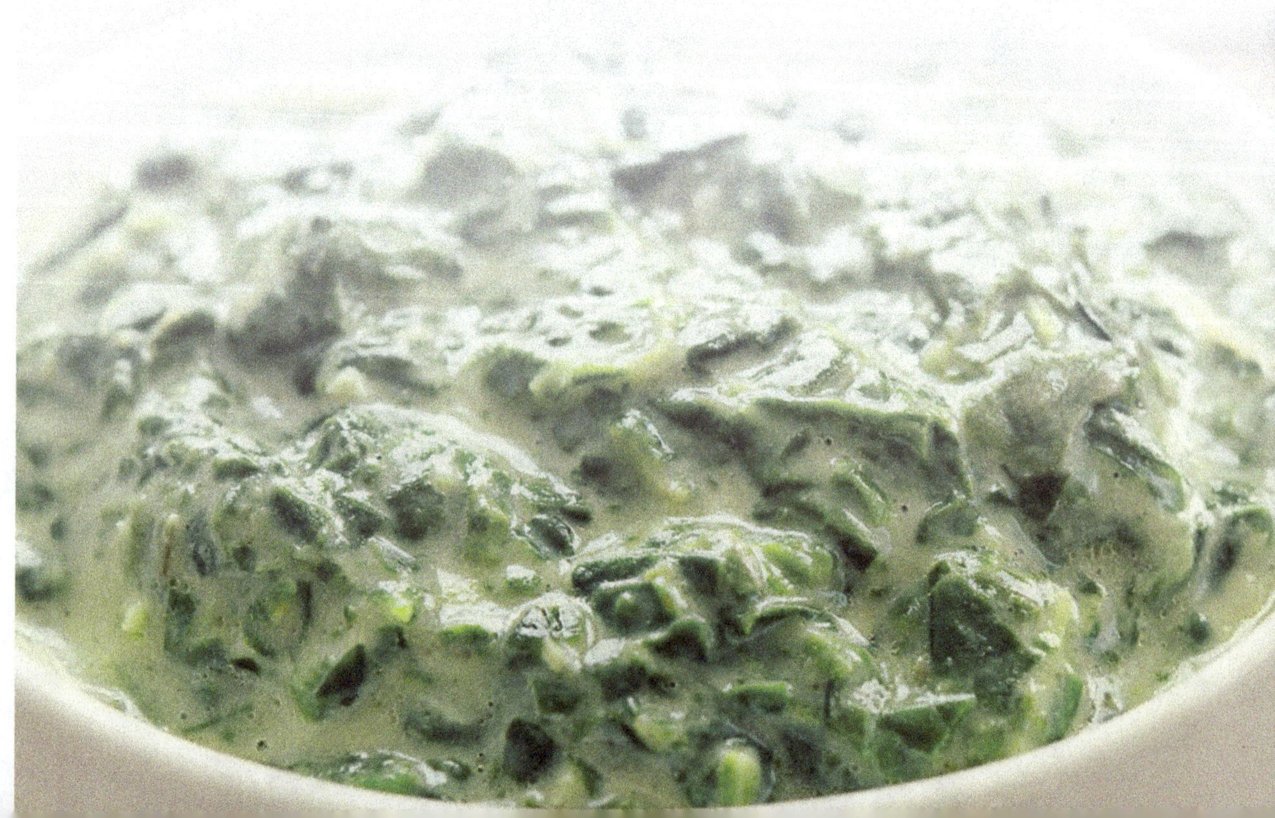

Brussels Sprouts with Bacon

Prep Time: 10 minutes

Cook Time: 30 minutes

Yield: 8

1½ pounds brussels sprouts

½ cup pecans, chopped

1 stick butter

6 slices bacon, cooked

¼ cup olive oil

We're starting by rinsing and chopping the sprouts—assuming you didn't buy pre-washed.

Now I know, making a commitment to chopping for the next 8 minutes may sound like a nightmare to some of you, but trust me, it is worth the effort.

Not to make this too complicated, but depending on the sprouts' size, you may have to chop a few into fourths to get the flavor right.

Put the ½ cup chopped pecans on standby. If you're using whole pecans, make life easier, and crush them with a rolling pin between two pieces of wax paper.

Melt half a stick of butter in the microwave and add the pecans. Walk away as fast as you can before you eat the bowl.

Next, fry your bacon.

Add in ½ of a stick of butter and a cup of Brussels sprouts.

Then go ahead and pour the olive oil over the top and sauté—make sure each sprout gets covered. Gradually add in more sprouts until they're all in the pan and coated evenly.

Sauté for around 10 minutes.

Serve topped with the buttered pecans.

Nutrition Per Serving
(1 cup = 1 serving)

Calories: 300

Fat: 30.3g

Protein: 4.9g

Fiber: 2.3g

Total Carbs: 5.2g

Net Carbs: 2.9g

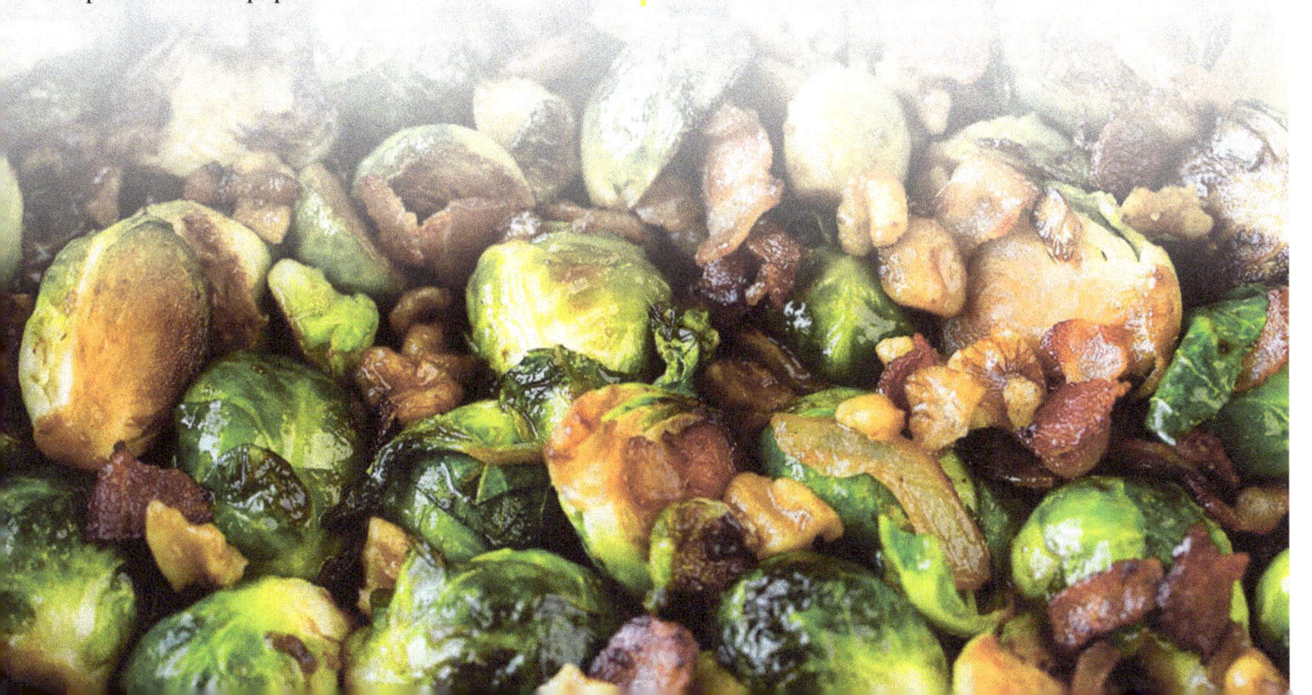

Zoodles with Pesto

Prep Time: 15 minutes

Cook Time: 5 minutes

Yield: 2

Full disclosure: while this zoodle recipe is a little extra, because, ahem, you are going all-in by creating pasta from a vegetable – rest assured it is worth the effort.

Zucchini Noodles:

2 medium zucchinis

1 tablespoon olive oil

¼ teaspoon black pepper

¼ cup Parmesan cheese, grated

Pesto:

1½ cups fresh baby spinach

½ cup fresh basil

¼ cup olive oil

¼ cup walnuts, chopped

1 garlic clove, minced

Dash of salt

Slice the zucchini with a julienne peeler or with a spiralizer.

Add the ingredients for the pesto to a food processor and pulse until smooth.

Heat olive oil in a large pan over medium-high heat. Add the zucchini noodles (zoodles) and cook for 5 minutes. Remove from heat, add the pesto and toss until all the zoodles are coated. Top with Parmesan cheese.

Nutrition Per Serving
(½ recipe = 1 serving)

Calories: 336

Fat: 34.6g

Protein: 7.1g

Fiber: 1.7g

Total Carbs: 3.7g

Net Carbs: 2g

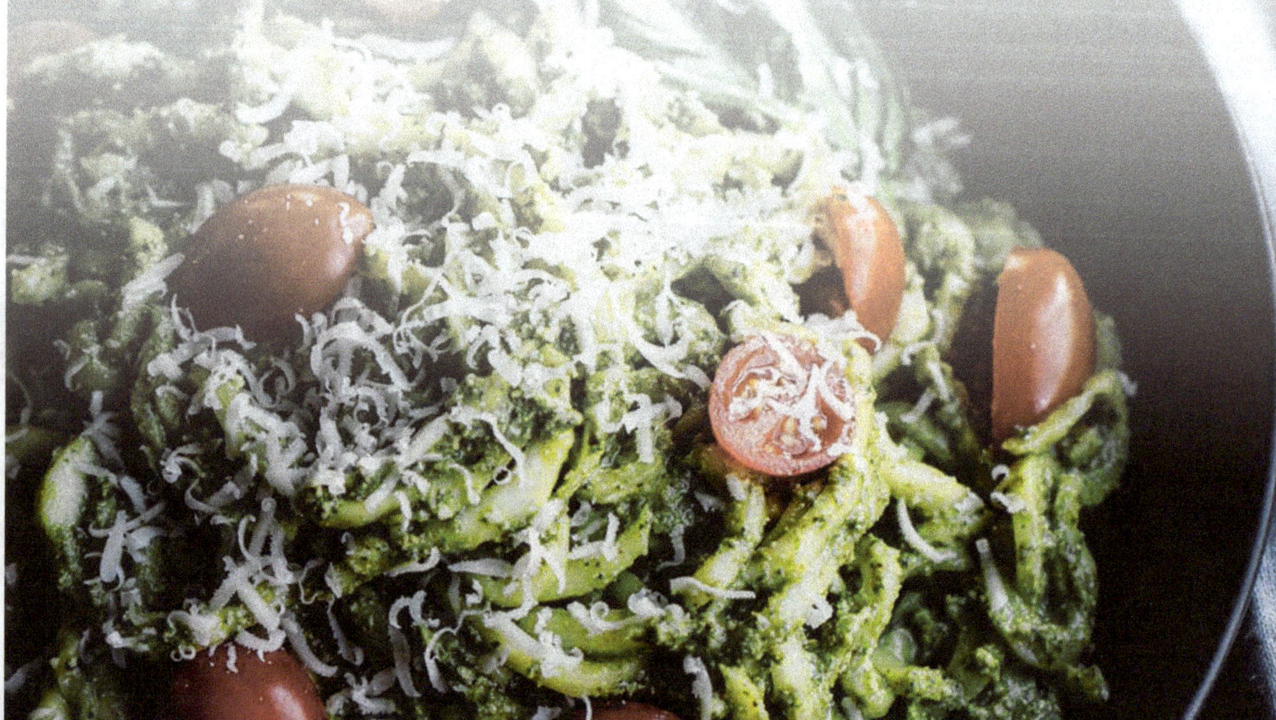

Antipasto Salad

Prep Time: 10 minutes

Cook Time: 0 minutes

Yield: 8

Antipasto is the traditional first course of a formal Italian meal. Since we are breaking conventional rules, feel free to enjoy this salad as an appetizer or the main event.

1 heart romaine lettuce chopped (7 cups)

2 cups cherry tomatoes, sliced

4 tablespoons extra virgin olive oil

½ teaspoon sea salt

¼ teaspoon black pepper

¼ cup fresh basil

6 ounces thinly sliced prosciutto

1 ounces Genoa salami—cut into bite-sized pieces

1 5-ounce package mini pepperonis

½ cup pepperoncini peppers, drained

1 14-ounce can of artichoke hearts, drained

½ cup black olives

8-ounce package fresh mozzarella balls

Rinse and chop romaine lettuce and tomatoes.

In a small bowl, whisk olive oil, salt, pepper, and basil together.

In a separate, large bowl, toss the lettuce, tomatoes, prosciutto, salami, pepperoni, peppers, artichoke hearts, olives, and mozzarella balls.

When you're ready to serve, toss with olive oil dressing.

Nutrition Per Serving
(1 cup = 1 serving)

Calories: 345

Fat: 30g

Protein: 14g

Fiber: 1g

Total Carbs: 3g

Net Carbs: 2g

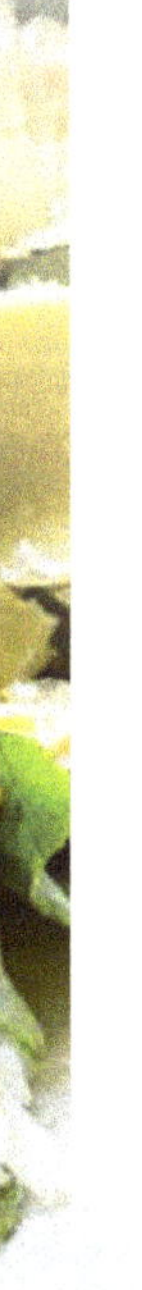

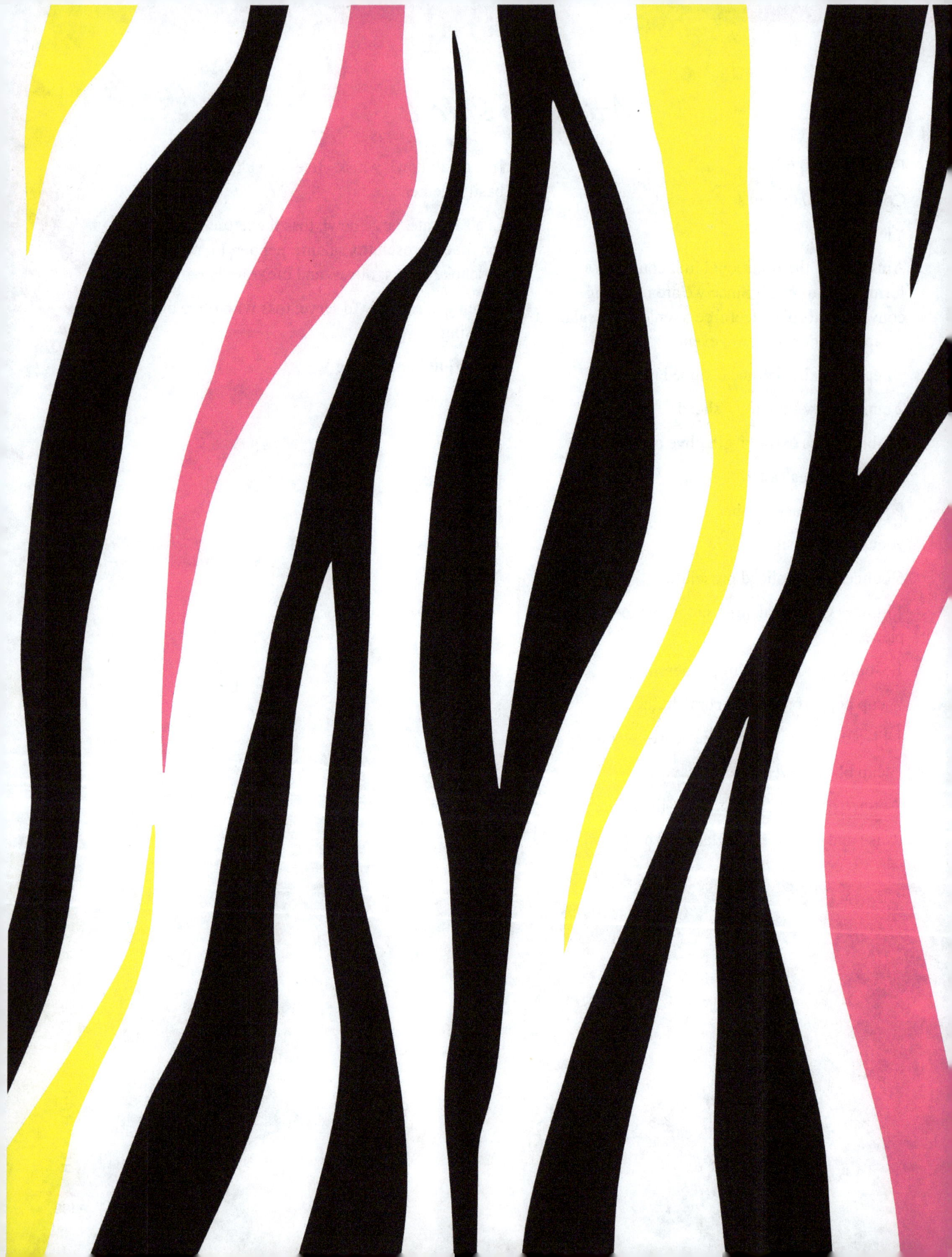

Sauces

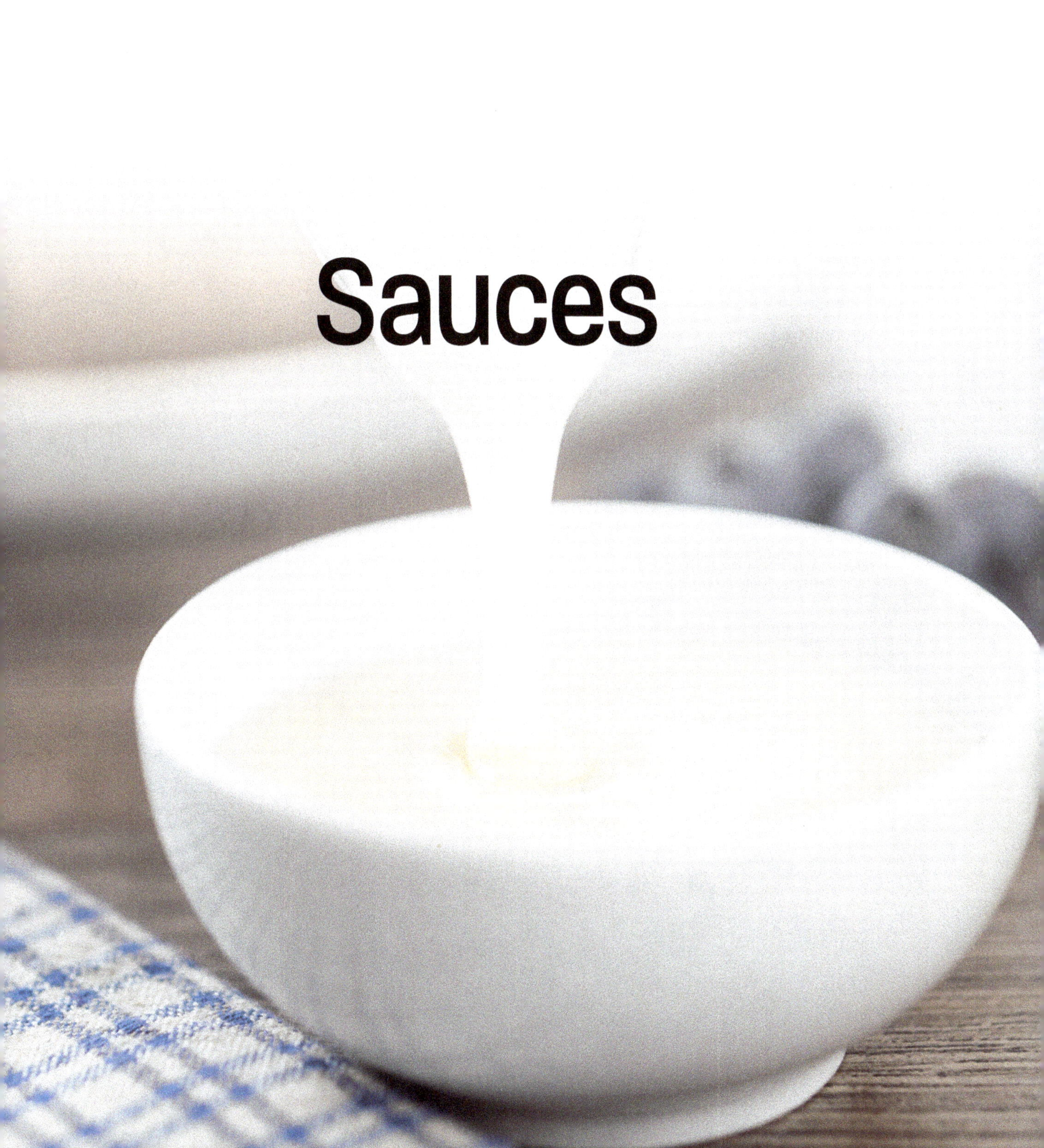

What's Hiding In the Valley Ranch Dressing

Prep Time: 5 Minutes

Cook Time: 5 Minutes

Yield: 12

Skip the preservatives and the hard-to-say ingredients on traditional Ranch dressing and DIY the salad dressing that doubles as a dip for veggies.

1 cup mayonnaise

½ cup sour cream

2 teaspoons lemon juice

2 teaspoons dried parsley

1 teaspoon dried dill

1 teaspoon dried chives

½ teaspoon onion powder

½ teaspoon garlic powder

½ teaspoon sea salt

¼ – ½ teaspoon black pepper

¼ cup unsweetened almond milk or coconut milk or heavy cream (Add This Last!)

Combine the ingredients in a mason jar with a lid or a bowl and store in the refrigerator for up to four days.

Nutrition Per Serving
(2 tablespoons = 1 serving)

Calories: 156

Fat: 17g

Protein: 0.4g

Fiber: 0g

Total Carbs: 1g

Net Carbs: 0.9g

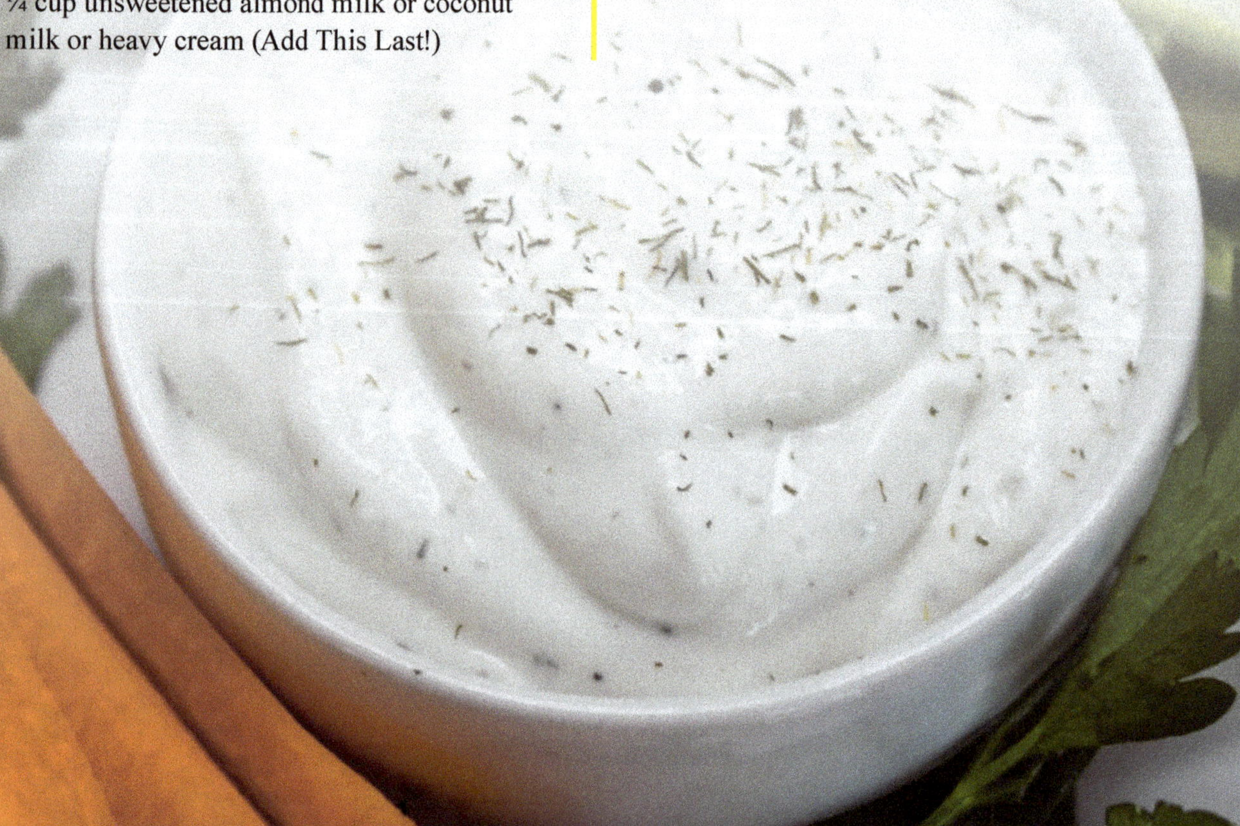

Just Make It At Home Keto Italian Vinaigrette

Prep Time: Less than 5 minutes

Cook Time: 30 minutes

Yield: 10

This recipe doubles as a marinade for veggies and pairs nicely with women who never use the phrase "pairs nicely" in conversation.

1 cup light virgin olive oil

1 tablespoon Italian Stallion Seasoning (See recipe in Seasonings)

4 tablespoons red wine vinegar

1 tablespoon Dijon mustard

½ teaspoon salt

¼ black pepper

Save yourself washing a dish and combine everything in a container with a lid and shake the hell out of it. This is a fabulous way to release anger, and doubles as a decent upper arm exercise.

For best results, allow at least 30 minutes to develop. You can store any leftovers in the fridge for up to 7 days.

Nutrition Per Serving
(2 tablespoons = 1 serving)

Calories: 198

Fat: 22g

Protein: 0g

Fiber: 0g

Total Carbs: Less than 1

Net Carbs: Less than 1

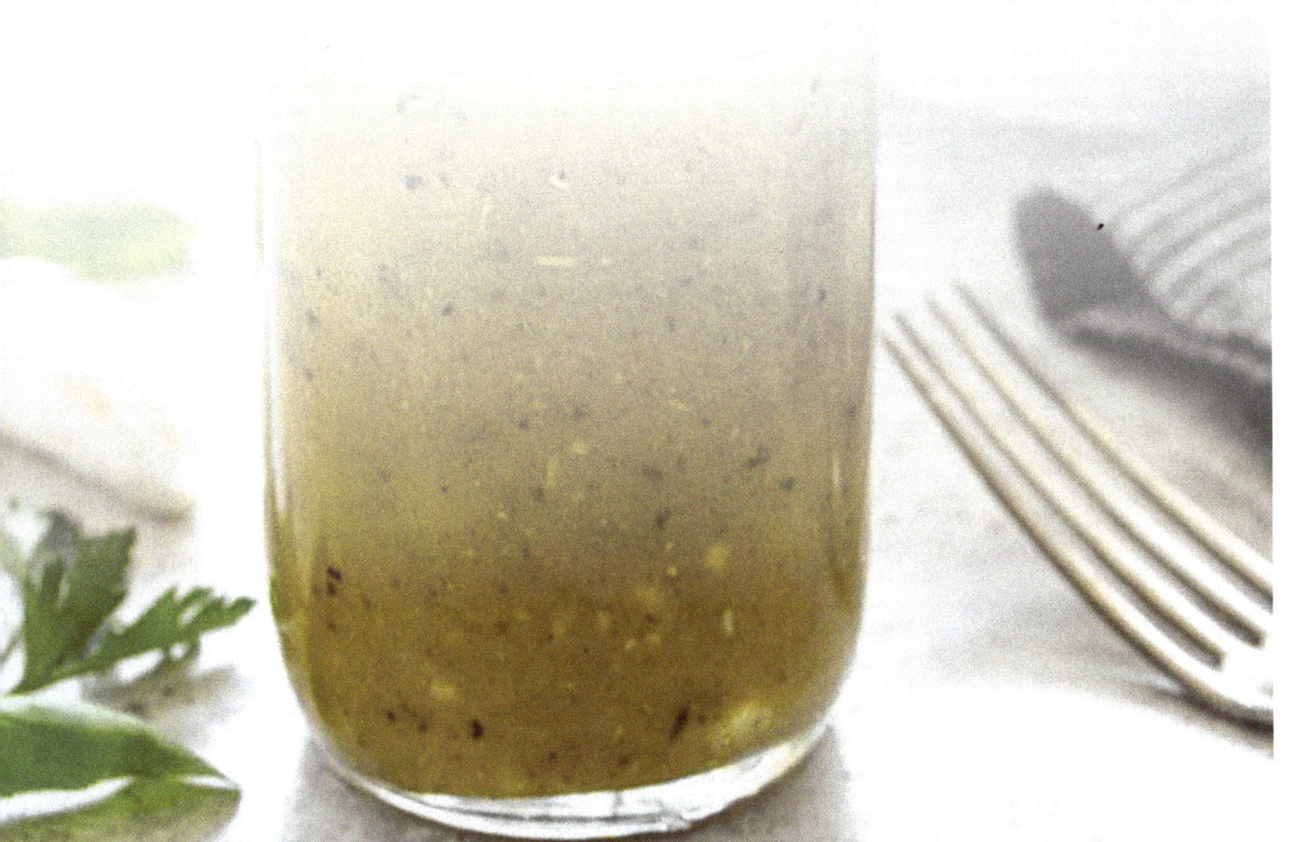

Carpe Diem Caesar Salad Dressing

Prep Time: 5 minutes

Cook Time: 0

Yield: 6

Will a salad dressing make your life amazing? I have no idea, but I'll tell you this, making small adjustments to the ingredients in your food and taking small steps each day toward your goal will 100% help you get there. Don't forget to seize the day.

¾ cup mayonnaise

⅓ cup Parmesan Cheese (grated)

1–3 teaspoons minced garlic (depending on how much you love garlic)

1½ teaspoons Dijon mustard

1 teaspoon lemon juice

1 teaspoon anchovy paste

½ teaspoon black pepper (or more to taste)

Combine all the ingredients in a medium-size bowl until fully blended. Serve immediately or store in an airtight container in the refrigerator for up to a week.

Nutrition Per Serving
(2 tablespoons = 1 serving)

Calories: 227

Total Fat: 24g

Protein: 2.3g

Fiber: 0

Total Carbs: 0.3g

Net Carbs: 0.3g

Blue Cheese Dressing (Or Dip)

Prep Time: 5 minutes

Chill Time: 1 hour

Yield: 18

Blue cheese (or Bleu if you're feeling fancy or French) is a whole mood, and an acquired taste. I prefer it stuffed into an olive at the bottom of a dirty martini, but it also works in a salad dressing.

Bonus: It doubles as a dip and a sauce for steaks and chicken.

½ cup crumbled blue cheese

1 cup mayonnaise

1 tablespoon sour cream (full fat)

½ cup heavy whipping cream

1 tablespoon lemon juice

¼ teaspoon Worcestershire sauce

½ teaspoon kosher salt

¼ teaspoon black pepper

1 tablespoon parsley, chopped

Grab a medium-sized bowl and combine the blue cheese, mayonnaise, sour cream, heavy cream, lemon juice, Worcestershire sauce, salt, pepper, and parsley. Serve chilled.

Store this dressing in an airtight container in the fridge for up to 4 days.

Nutrition Per Serving
(2 tablespoons = 1 serving)

Calories: 126

Fat: 12.9g

Protein: 1.9g

Fiber: 0g

Total Carbs: 0.7g

Net Carbs: 0.3g

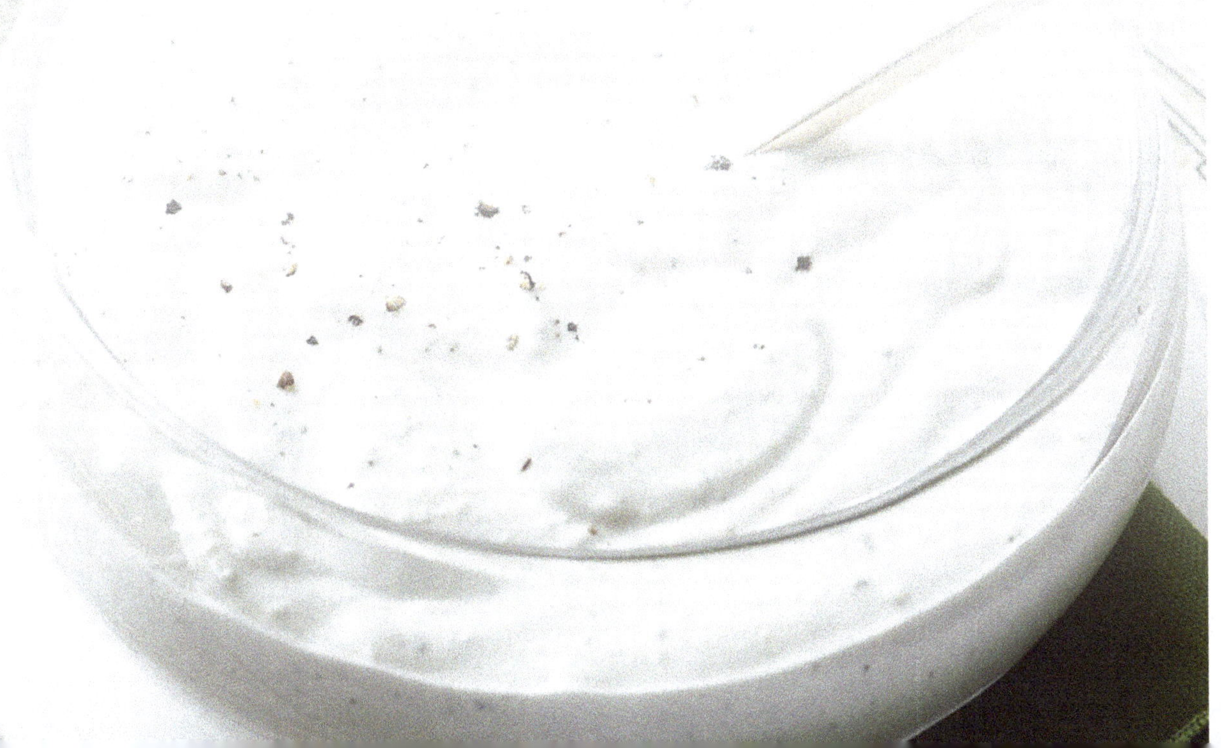

Legit Low Carb Hollandaise Sauce

Prep Time: 10 minutes

Cook Time: 10 minutes

Yield: 8

This Hollandaise sauce reminds me of Brennan's in New Orleans. Their eggs benedict is off the chain incredible. You can recreate a keto-friendly eggs benedict with this sauce or use it to top a steak!

4 egg yolks

1 tablespoons lemon juice

1 tablespoon cold water

½ cup butter, melted

1 pinch of cayenne pepper

1 pinch of sea salt

1 dash hot sauce (optional)

Stovetop Instructions:

Combine egg yolks, lemon juice, and cold water in a medium-sized glass or stainless-steel mixing bowl.

Whisk until the eggs are light and foamy.

In a double boiler, whisk the eggs over low heat, and add melted butter slowly. Whisk until the sauce has thickened.

Remove from heat and whisk in cayenne pepper, salt, and hot sauce.

If you don't have a double boiler: Bring a few tablespoons of water to a simmer in a large saucepan. Place the bowl containing the egg yolks directly over the simmering water—without letting the bottom of the pan touch the water. Keep this sauce covered and warm until ready to serve.

Store in an airtight container in the refrigerator for up to 2 days.

Microwave Instructions:

Whisk egg yolks, lemon juice, cayenne pepper, salt, and hot sauce in a microwave-safe bowl until smooth.

Slowly add the melted butter while continuing to stir. Heat this combination in the microwave for 15 seconds, then whisk. Microwave for another 10 seconds and whisk until smooth. The Hollandaise sauce will thicken as it cools.

Nutrition Per Serving
(2 tablespoons = 1 serving)

Calories: 130

Total Fat: 13.7g

Protein: 1.5g

Fiber: 0g

Total Carbs: 0.6g

Net Carbs: 0.6g

Mystic (Sugar-Free) Pizza Sauce

Prep Time: 5 minutes

Cook Time: 10 minutes

Yield: 12

This sugar-free, low-carb-friendly pizza sauce was 100% inspired by necessity—traditional pizza sauces contain too much sugar to even be considered as healthy.

Pairs well with the 1988 coming of age movie staring Julia Roberts.

1 8-ounce can tomato sauce

1 6-ounce can tomato paste

½ teaspoon dried basil

½ teaspoon dried oregano

½ teaspoon onion powder

½ teaspoon garlic powder

¼ teaspoon Sea salt

Grab your favorite saucepan and combine all of the ingredients. Simmer on low heat for 15 minutes, stirring occasionally.

Nutrition Per Serving
(2 tablespoons = 1 serving)

Calories: 185

Fat: 0.1g

Protein: 0.9g

Fiber: 0.9g

Total Carbs: 3.9g

Net Carbs: 3g

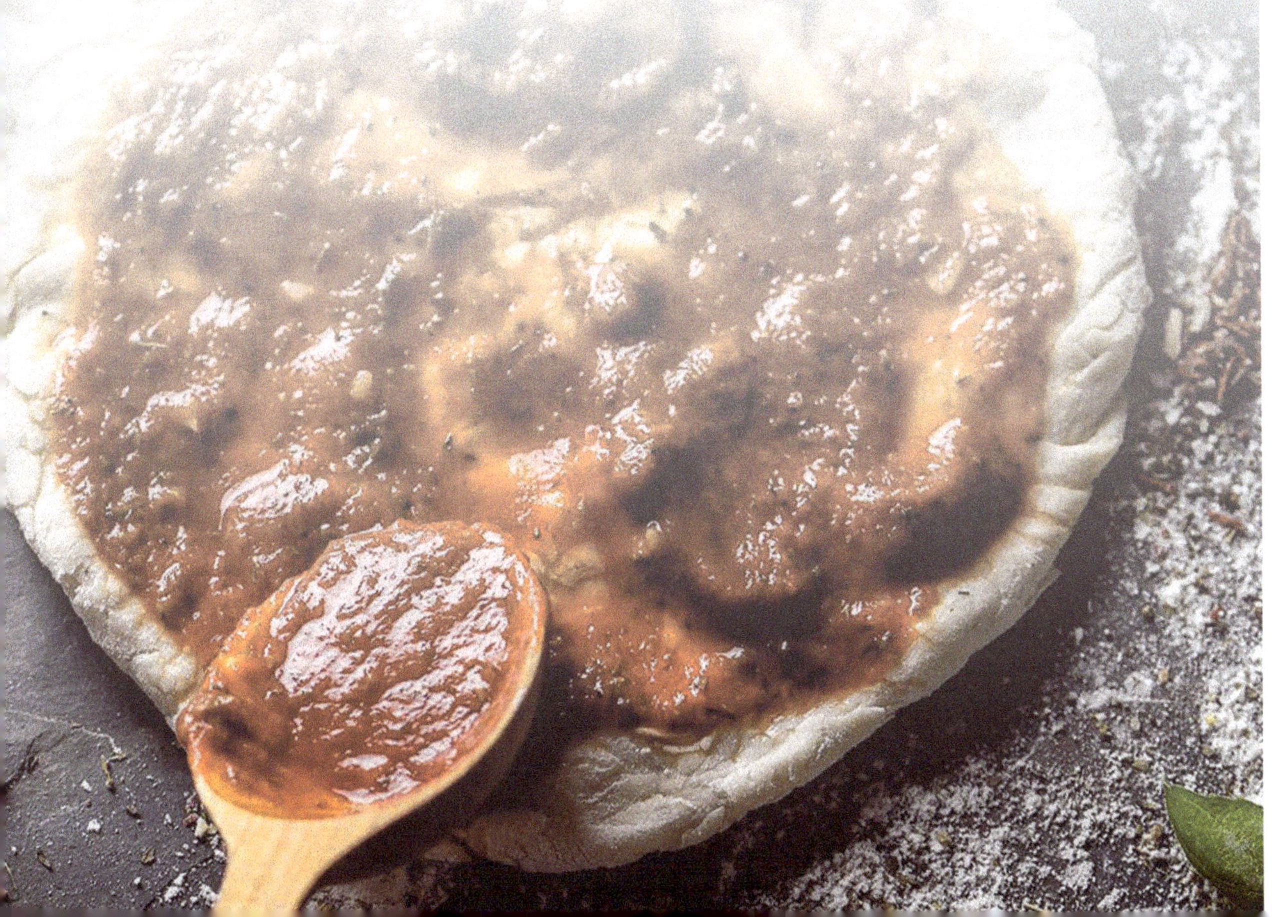

I Won't Back Down Alfredo Sauce

Prep Time: 5 minutes

Cook Time: 10 Minutes

Yield: 8

Everyone has days (and nights) when they feel too overwhelmed and tired to go on—much less cook a healthy dinner. You will be tempted. Do not back down.

Channel your inner Tom Petty, stand your ground and keep this recipe for low-carb alfredo sauce on hand. It's perfect—over zucchini noodles or spaghetti squash, over baked chicken, and in all kinds of casseroles.

1 tablespoon unsalted butter

6–8 garlic cloves minced

1 cup low sodium chicken broth

2½ cups heavy cream

1 teaspoon onion powder

1 teaspoon dried basil

1 teaspoon salt

½ teaspoon ground thyme

½ teaspoon pepper

⅛ teaspoon nutmeg

1 cup Parmesan cheese, grated

Preheat the oven to 350° and grease a large casserole dish.

Grab a large skillet, set the heat on the stove to medium, and melt the butter. Whisk in the minced garlic and cook for 2 minutes, stirring regularly.

Next, turn the heat down to low and whisk in the chicken broth, heavy cream, and the spices: onion powder, dried basil, salt, ground thyme, red pepper flakes, and pepper.

Turn up the heat and whisk until the sauce starts boiling. Then reduce heat to low and simmer for around 8 minutes, stirring occasionally.

Add the cream cheese, onion, and 1 cup of Parmesan cheese and continue to cook until the cream cheese is melted.

To Freeze: Freeze this sauce in a heavy-duty freezer-safe Ziploc bag for up to three months. Make sure you label it with the name of the recipe and reheating instructions: thaw over medium heat on the stove, stirring occasionally. If you thaw overnight in the refrigerator, this will take you considerably less time.

Nutrition Per Serving
(¼ cup = 1 serving)

Calories: 185

Fat: 19.2g

Protein: 2.7g

Fiber: 0g

Total Carbs: 1.2g

Net Carbs: 1.2g

I'll Have What She's Having Basil Pesto with Lemon

Prep Time: 10 minutes

Cook Time: 0

Yield: 12

This homemade pesto takes 5 minutes to put together and is almost as good as, well, you know. You'll use it garnish chicken, pork, steak—and your summer grilling favorites. Pairs well with the diner scene in When Harry Met Sally.

1 cup packed fresh basil leaves

4 garlic cloves, peeled & sliced

½ cup extra-virgin olive oil

¼ cup pine nuts

¾ cup grated Parmesan

¼ cup fresh lemon juice

Salt & pepper to taste

Rinse basil and pat it dry.

Then put basil and garlic into a food processor and process until combined.

Then add olive oil, pine nuts, Parmesan, and lemon juice and process for another 1–2 minutes or until pureed.

Season with salt and pepper to taste and puree for another 30 seconds. Store in an airtight container in the refrigerator for up to one week.

You may want to freeze this—especially if you have a ton of fresh basil you need to use.

To Freeze: Divide the pesto into an ice cube tray and place in the freezer until frozen. Then, pop the cubes into a labeled Ziploc bag and freeze for up to 4 months.

Nutrition Per Serving
(2 tablespoons = 1 serving)

Calories: 91

Fat: 8.6g

Protein: 2.3g

Fiber: 0.4g

Sugar: 0.2g

Total Carbs: 2.2g

Net Carbs: 1.8g

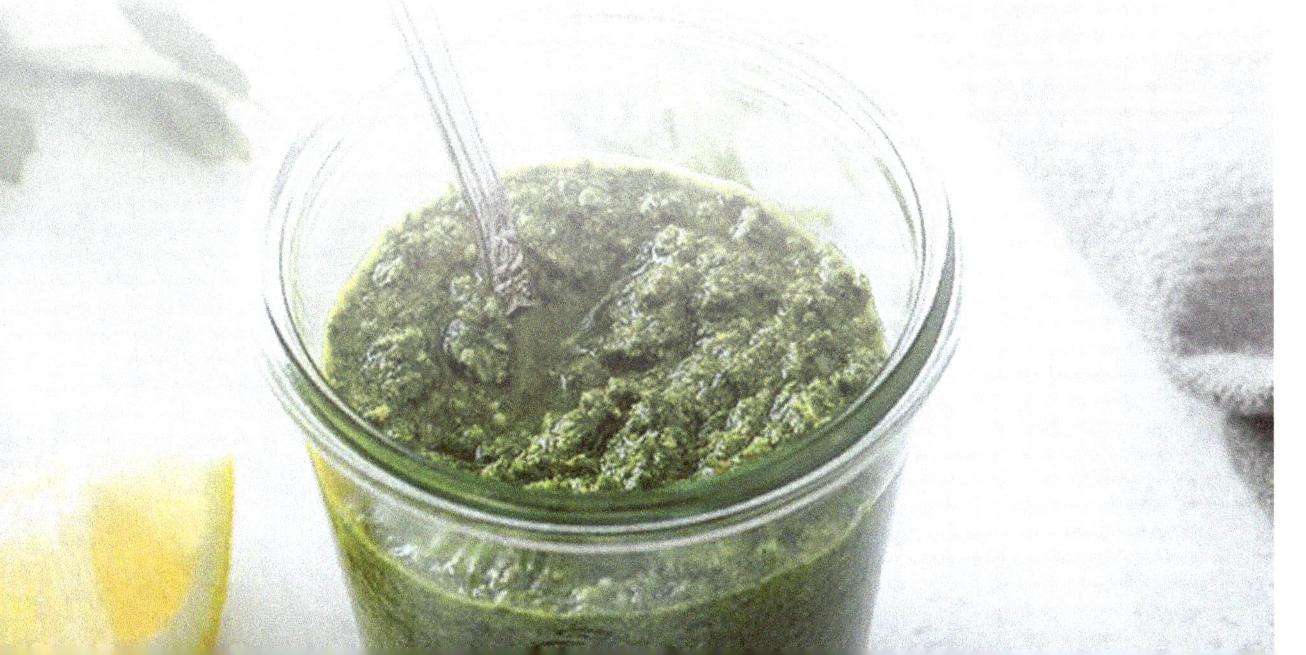

What's The Deal With Gremolata? Green Sauce Recipe

Prep Time: 5 minutes

Cook Time: 2 minutes

Yield: 16

Good question. I'll tell you straight up—gremolata (greh·mow·laa·tuh) is a green sauce that you can use to garnish salmon, steak, or shrimp.

1 cup fresh parsley

½ cup olive oil

2 tablespoons lemon zest

1 tablespoon lemon juice

4 minced garlic cloves

½ teaspoon salt

¼ teaspoon pepper

Rinse and chop parsley.

Then add all of the ingredients to your food processor and pulse until smooth.

Store in an airtight container in the refrigerator for up to one week or freeze for up to 4 months.

To Freeze: Divide the gremolata into an ice cube tray and place it in the freezer until frozen. Then, pop the cubes into a labeled Ziploc Bag and freeze for up to 4 months.

Nutrition Per Serving
(1 tablespoon = 1 serving)

Calories: 63

Total Fat: 6.8g

Protein: 0.2g

Fiber: 0.2g

Total Carbs: 0.6g

Net Carbs: 0.4g

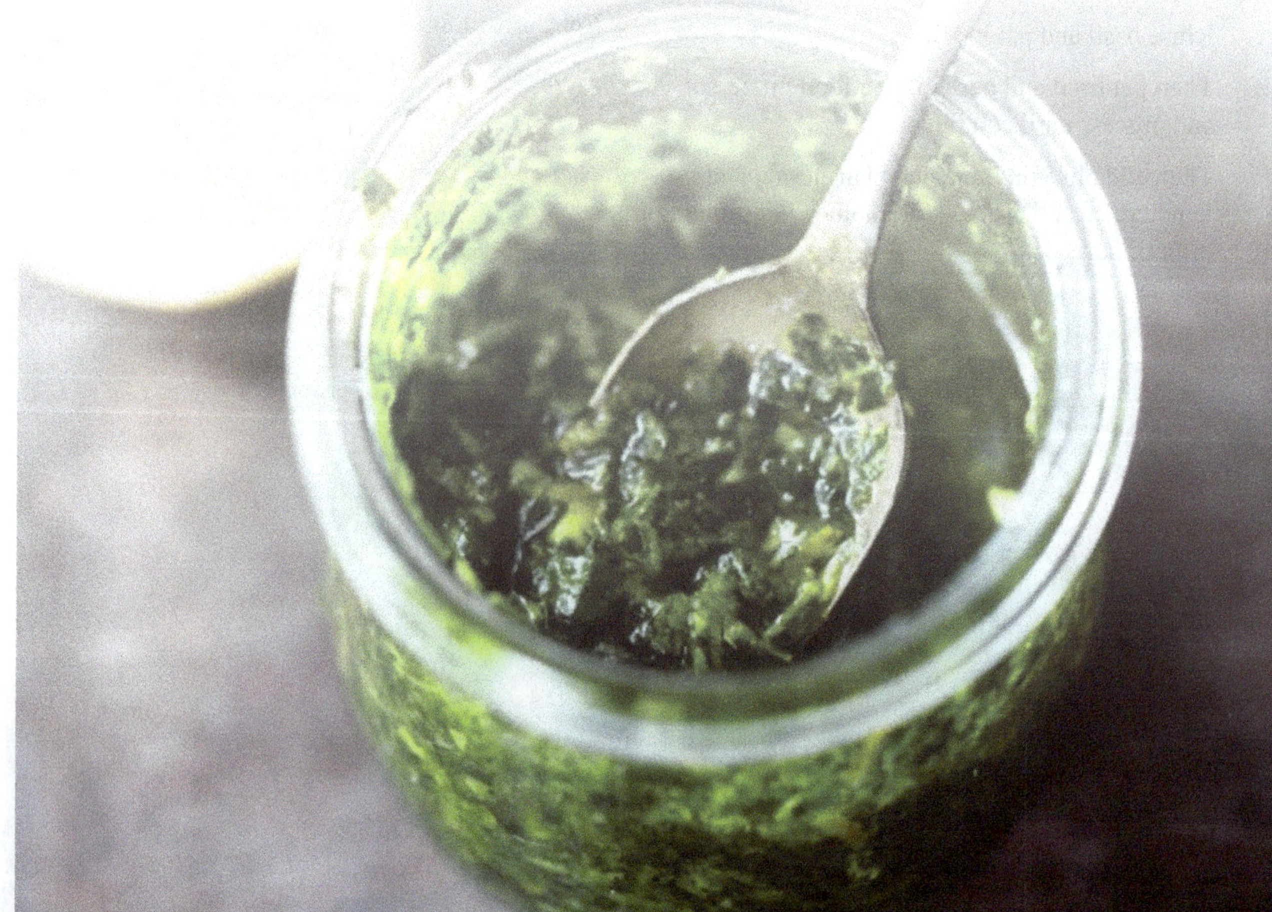

The Great Muppet Caper Butter with Dill

Prep Time: 30 minutes

Cook Time: 1 minute

Yield: 8

That's right; I named this condiment after what may be one of the greatest movies of all time, which is cool because I have always dreamed of using my knowledge of Jim Henson classics.

Anyway, this fabulous compound butter with salty capers, dill, and lemon is a super simple way to dress up salmon and shrimp dishes.

1/2 cup softened butter

2 tablespoons fresh dill

1 tablespoon lemon zest

1 tablespoon capers

Place your softened butter in a bowl.

Add the dill, lemon, and capers and combine them.

Wrap the butter in plastic wrap and store it in the refrigerator until you're ready to use it.

Nutrition Per Serving
(1 ½ teaspoons = 1 serving)

Calories: 102

Fat: 11.5g

Protein: 0.2g

Fiber: 0g

Total Carbs: 0.2g

Net Carbs: 0.2g

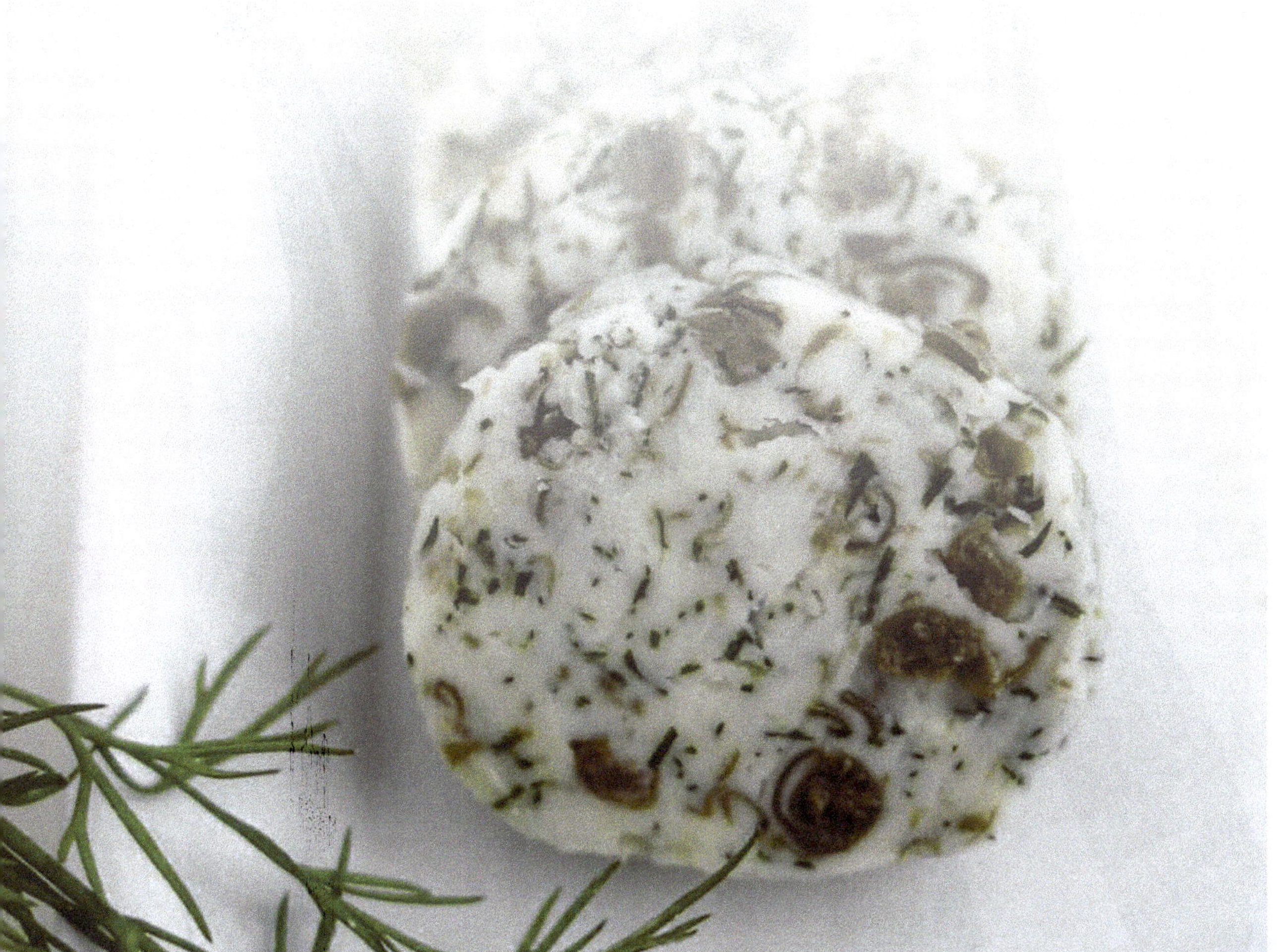

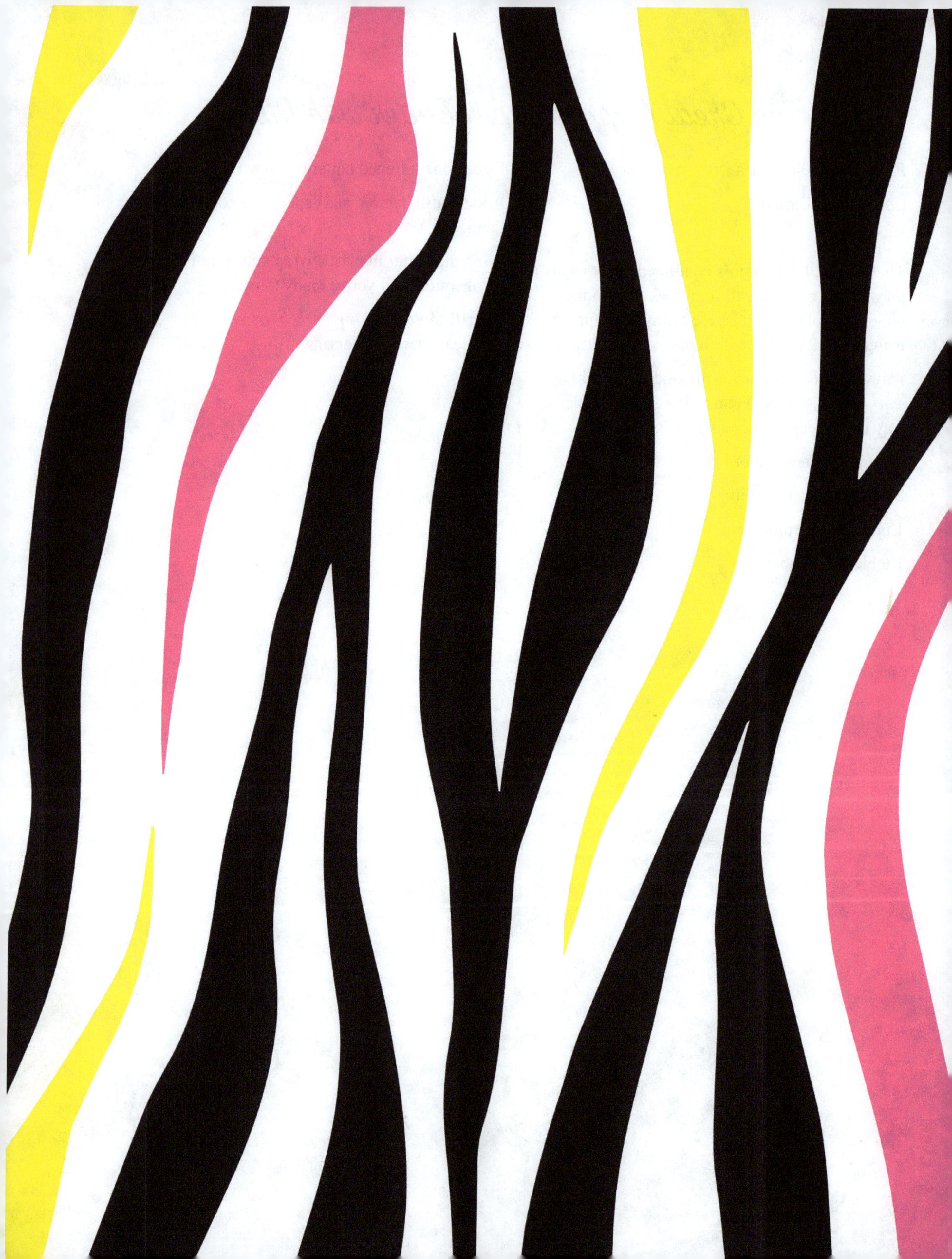

Seasonings

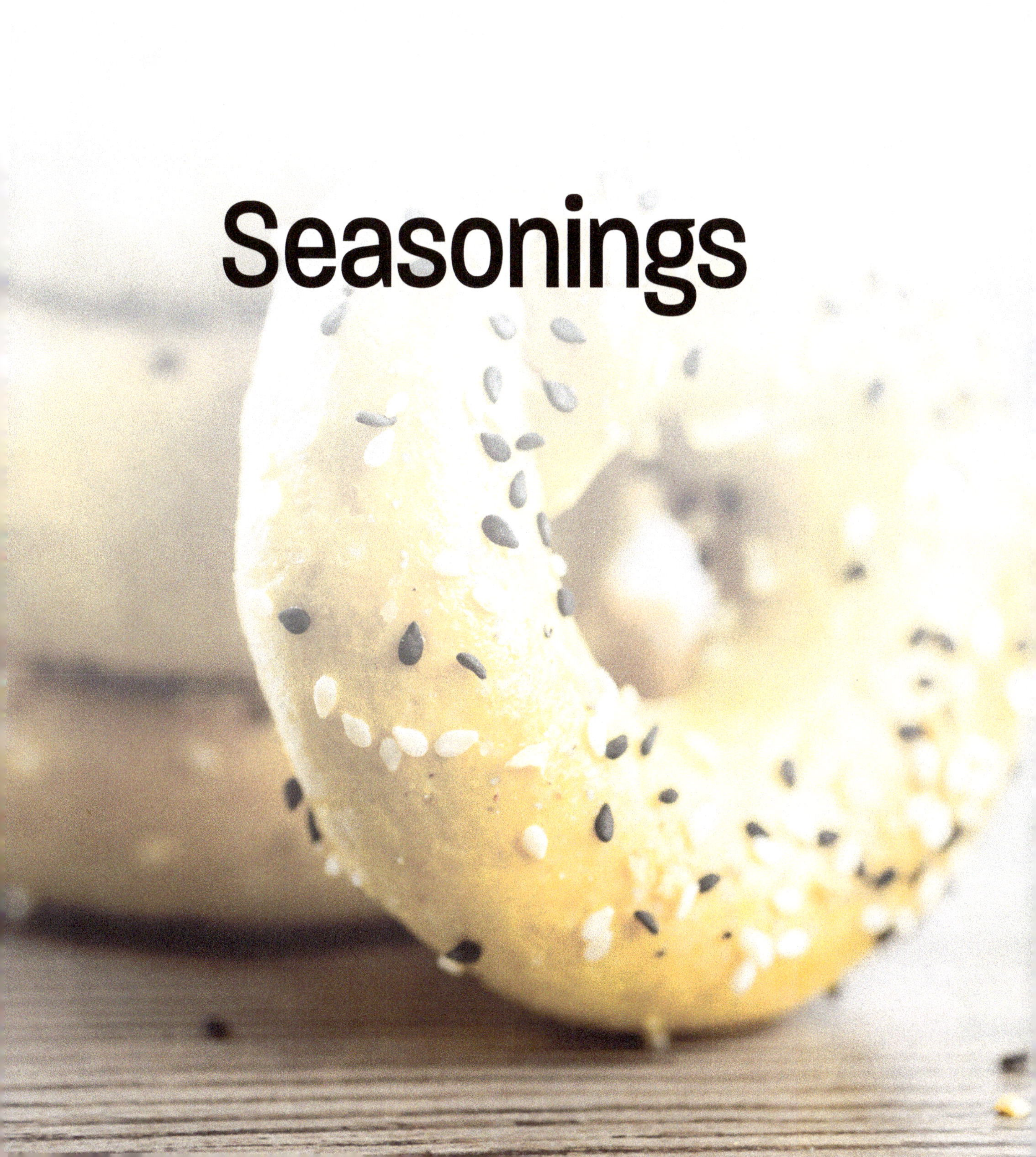

Louisiana Saturday Night Cajun Spice Seasoning

Prep Time: 5 minutes

Cook Time: 0

Yield: 12

This blend of seasonings reminds me of why I love New Orleans style food—it's the perfect combination of salt and spice, and it's preservative and filler-free, which is a big bonus. I'm willing to bet you have everything you need to make this homemade Cajun spice mix in your pantry.

Use this on any meat, chicken, or fish dish that calls for an extra kick.

3 tablespoons smoked paprika

2 tablespoons garlic powder

2 tablespoons kosher salt

1 tablespoon cayenne pepper

1 tablespoon dried oregano

1 tablespoon onion powder

1 tablespoon ground black pepper

1 tablespoon ground white pepper

½ tablespoon dried thyme

Combine all ingredients and store in an airtight container for up to one year.

Nutrition Per Serving
(1 tablespoon = 1 serving)

Calories: 16

Total Fat: 0.3g

Protein: 0.7g

Fiber: 1.3g

Total Carbs: 3.5g

Net Carbs: 1.9g

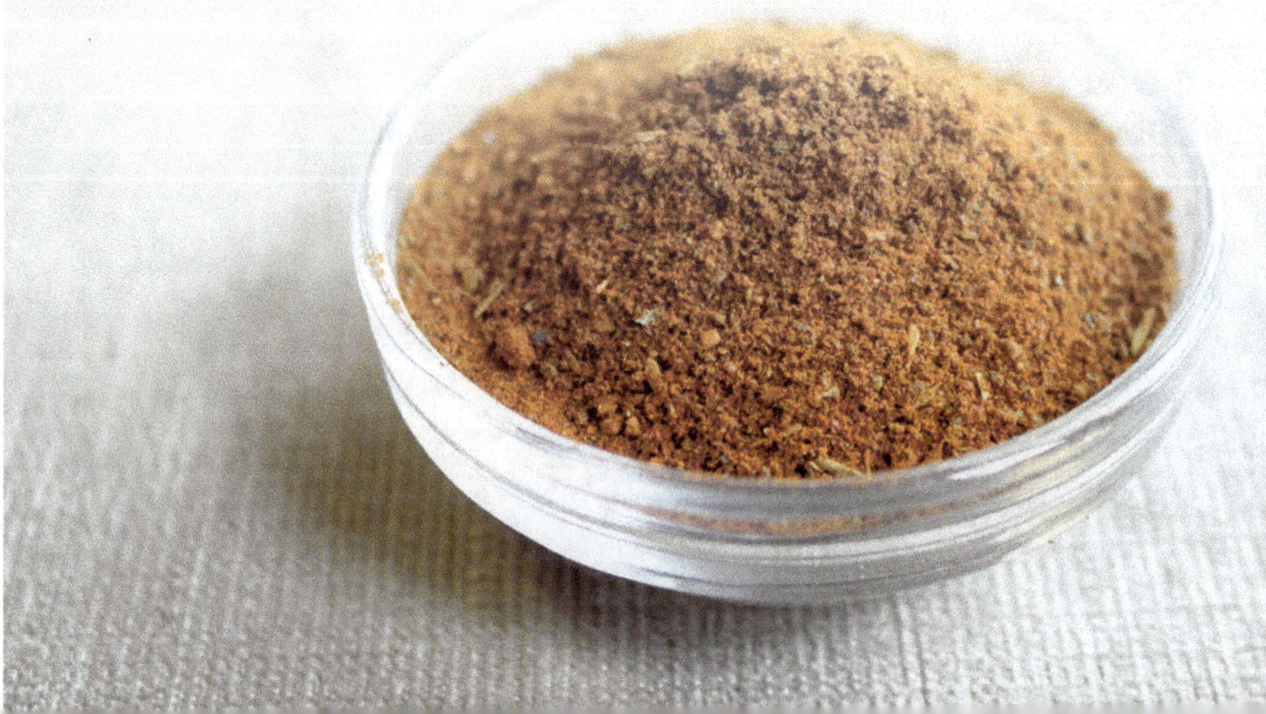

What's Hiding In the Valley Ranch Seasoning

Prep Time: 5 minutes

Cook Time: 0

Yield: 1

2 teaspoons dried parsley

1 teaspoon dried dill

1 teaspoon dried chives

½ teaspoon onion powder

½ teaspoon garlic powder

½ teaspoon sea salt

¼–½ teaspoon black pepper

Combine all ingredients and store in an airtight container for up to one year.

Nutrition Per Serving
(2 tablespoons = 1 serving)

Calories: 16

Total Fat: 0.3g

Protein: 0.7g

Fiber: 1.3g

Total Carbs: 3.5g

Net Carbs: 1.9g

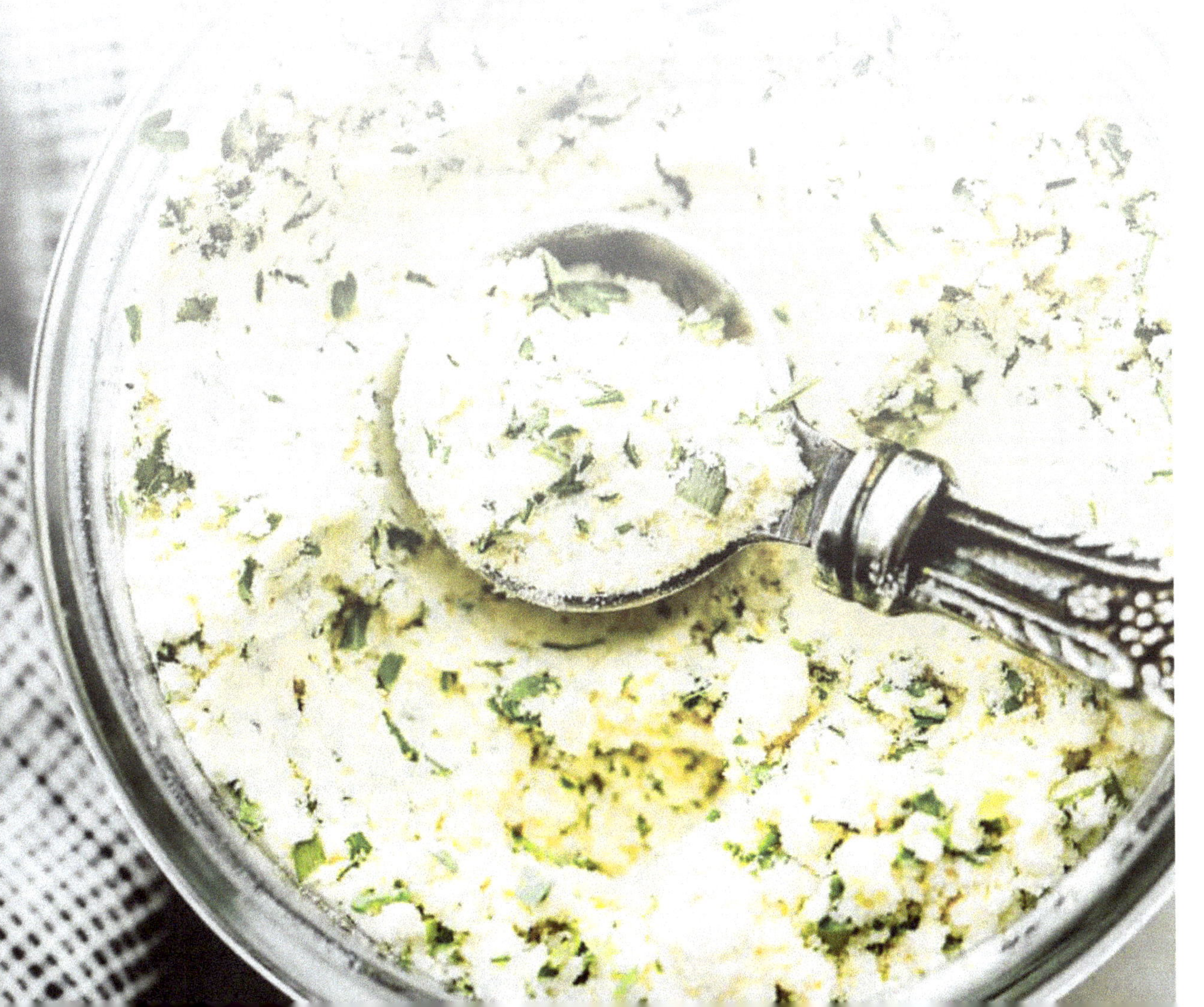

Homemade Everything Bagel Seasoning

Prep Time: 5 minutes

Cook Time: 0

Yield: 16

Trader Joe's Everything But The Bagel Seasoning is a favorite—especially when you're making Everything Bagels. (Duh!) But you can use this for more than bagels. I use it to make eggs and salads a little less boring.

¼ cup poppy seeds

¼ cup sesame seeds

1 tablespoon dried minced onion

3 tablespoons dried minced garlic

2 tablespoons sea salt

Mix ingredients and store in an airtight container. Shake it well before you use it!

Nutrition Per Serving
(1 tablespoon = 1 serving)

Calories: 34

Fat: 2g

Protein: 1.2g

Fiber: 1g

Sugar: 0.2g

Total Carbs: 3.5g

Net Carbs: 2.3g

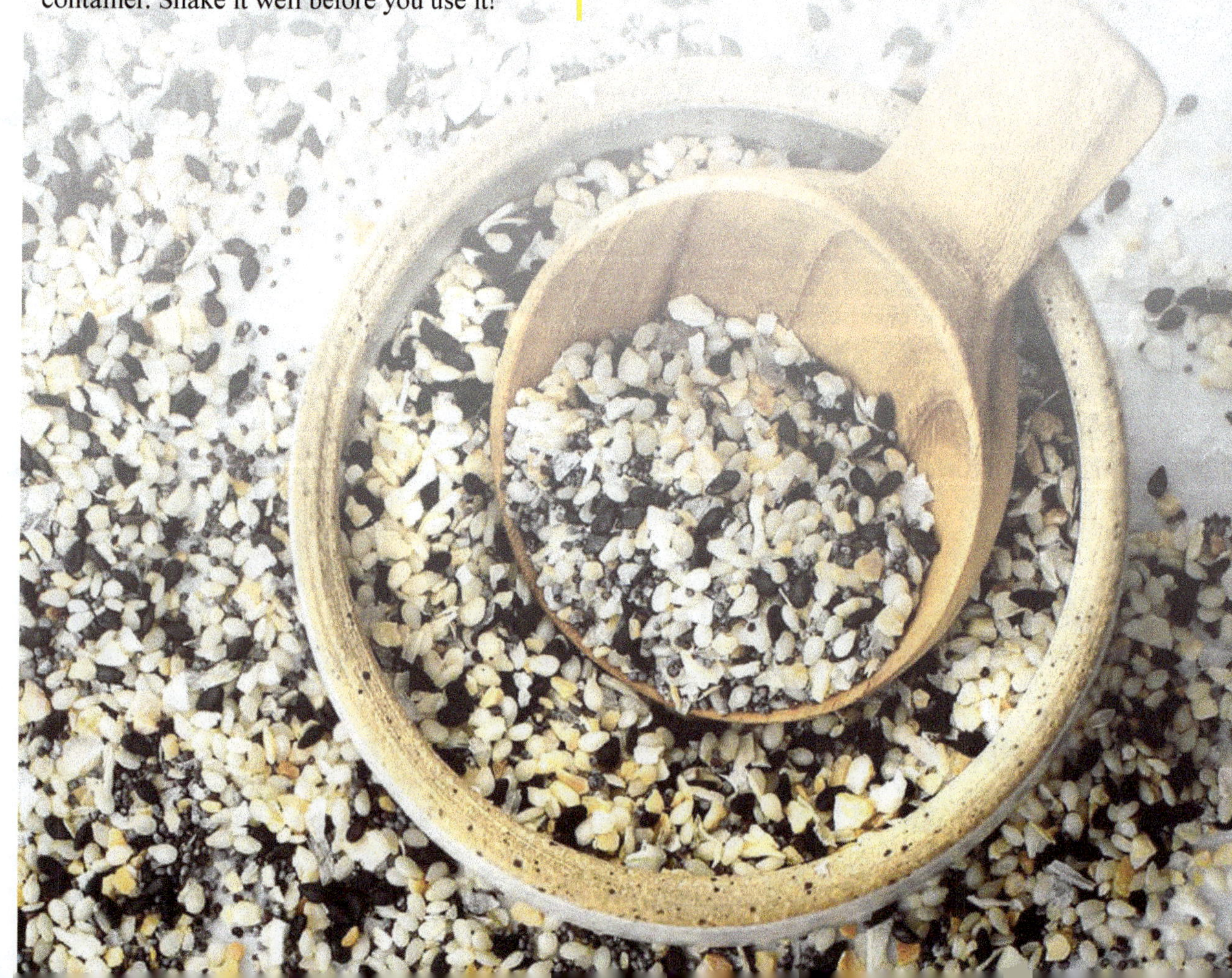

Homemade Taco Seasoning

Prep Time: 5 minutes

Cook Time: 0

Yield: ⅔ cup

¼ cup ground chili powder

2 tablespoons dried oregano

2 tablespoons onion flakes

1 tablespoon garlic powder

1 tablespoon sea salt

1 teaspoon black pepper

Combine ingredients and store in an airtight container.

Nutrition Per Serving
(1 tablespoon = 1 serving)

Calories: 9

Total Fat: 0.3g

Protein: 0.4g

Fiber: 0.8g

Total Carbs: 1.8g

Net Carbs: 1g

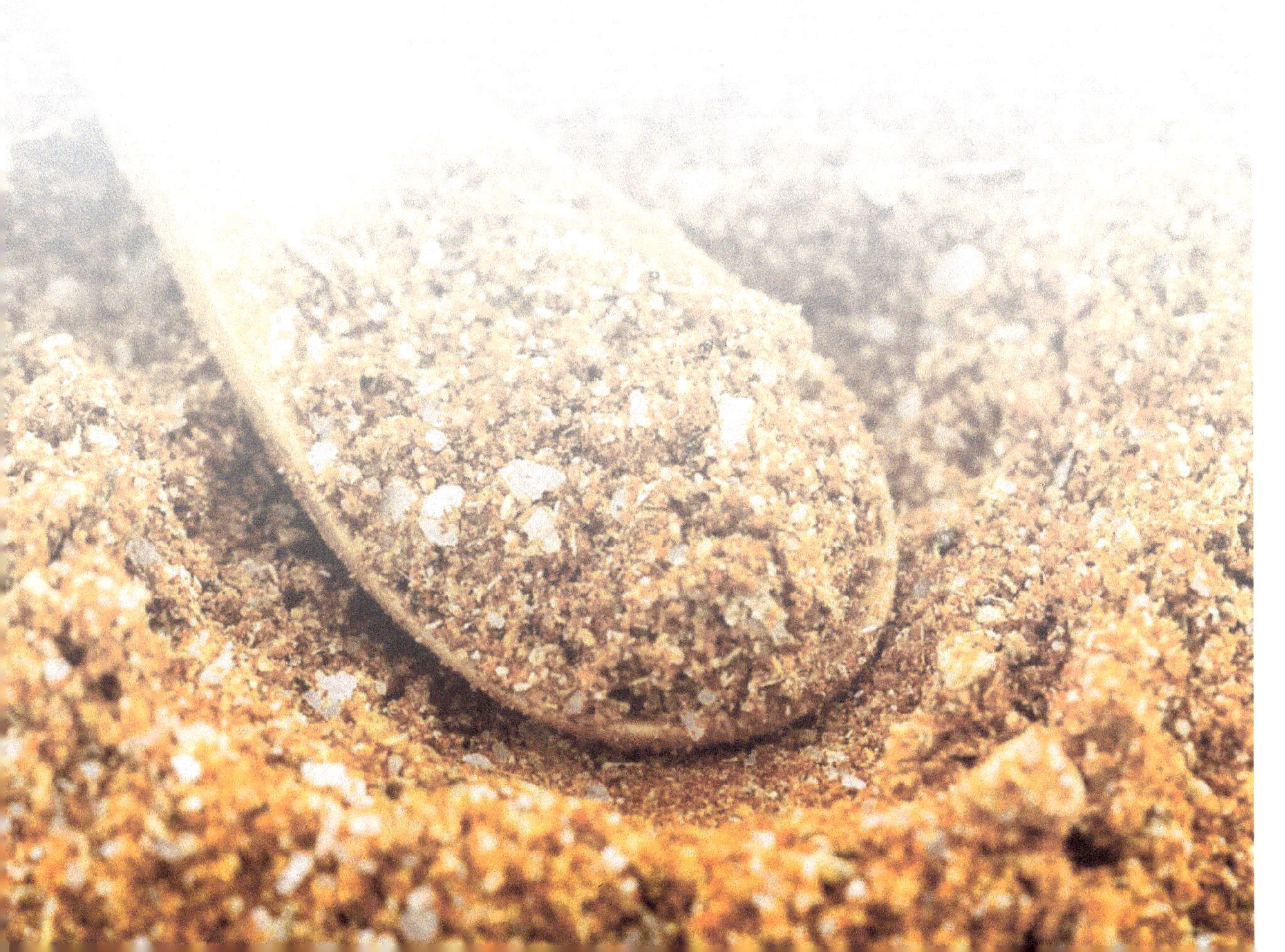

Italian Stallion Seasoning Recipe

Prep Time: 5 Minutes

Cook Time: 0

Yield: 24

Sorry, but I couldn't pass up an opportunity to drop a Rocky reference.

He had the guts, the glory, and the Eye of the Tiger. But Rocky didn't have anything you don't—he just never gave up. If he can do it, you can too.

I use this seasoning combo on all sorts of dishes; to punch up the flavor of chicken, shrimp, or ground beef, on pizza or in pizza sauce, in keto bread, and to season veggies.

1 tablespoon dried oregano

3 tablespoons dried basil

3 tablespoons dried parsley

1 tablespoon sea salt

1 tablespoon onion powder

1 tablespoon garlic powder

1 teaspoon dried thyme

1 teaspoon dried rosemary

1 teaspoon dried sage

¼ teaspoon black pepper

¼ teaspoon chili flakes

Mix all the spices and keep them in a container with a tight lid.

Nutrition Per Serving
(2 teaspoons = 1 serving)

Calories: 6

Fat: 0.1g

Protein: 0.3g

Fiber: 0.6g

Total Carbs: 1.3g

Net Carbs: 0.7g

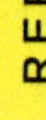

Desserts

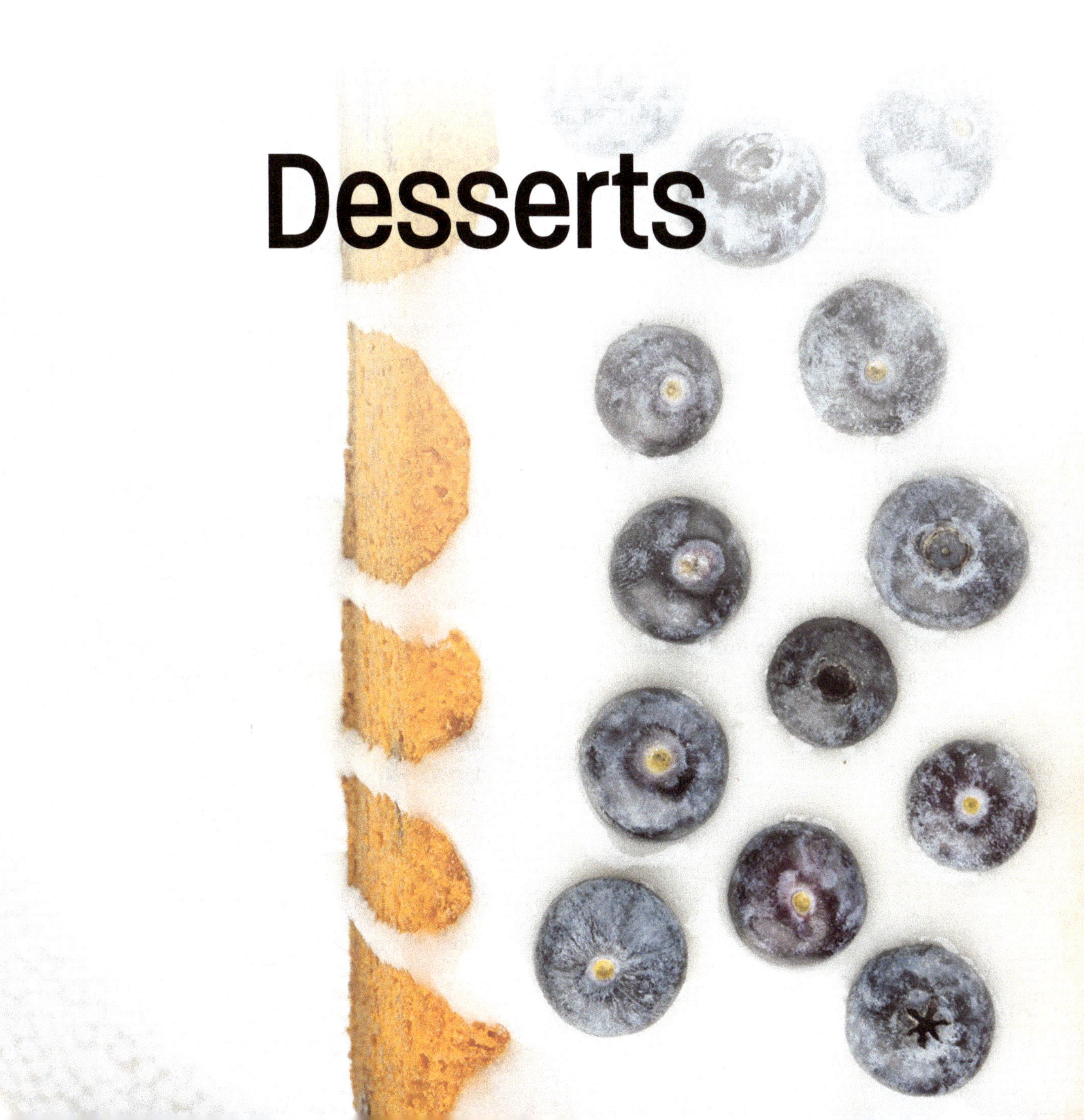

Have Your Blueberry Lemon Pound Cake & Eat It Too

Prep Time: 15 minutes

Cook Time: 50 minutes

Yield: 8 slices

My grandmother always had a pound cake on hand. (It's a Southern thing.) Just as I could count on her pound cake, I could count on my grandfather's running joke: We're going to charge you by the pound, so you better weigh in first.

Of course, he was kidding, and he didn't mean to make me feel conscious of my weight at age 8, but he was right about the poundage of those old school desserts.

Talk about a moment on the lips equals a lifetime on the hips…

THIS pound cake will not put on the pounds thanks to the keto-friendly swap from the OG flour and sugar to almond flour and monk fruit.

You can make it in a loaf or Bundt pan. Either way, it's fabulous.

Note #1: If you're going for presentation, make sure you grease the Bundt pan like your life depends on it. If you don't, be prepared for an epic mess and ugly cake.)

Note #2: You can use frozen blueberries, but if ya do—thaw them first. Otherwise, you risk a watered-down version that will make you sad.

Pound Cake Ingredients:

1 stick butter

1 cup granular sweetener (monk fruit)

4 eggs

1¼ cup sour cream

1 tablespoon lemon zest or ½ tablespoon lemon extract

1 teaspoon vanilla extract

3½ cups blanched almond flour

2 teaspoons baking powder

1 cup blueberries

Lemon Glaze Ingredients

¼ cup lemon juice

2 tablespoons heavy cream

¾ cup powdered erythritol

¼ teaspoon vanilla extract

Preheat oven to 375°

Grease a 9-inch Bundt pan or 9 x 5 loaf pan.

In a medium-sized bowl, combine almond flour and baking powder.

Set aside.

In a separate larger mixing bowl, use an electric or stand mixer to cream butter, monk fruit, and one egg until combined.

Mix in sour cream, lemon zest (or lemon extract), and vanilla.

Slowly add in almond flour combination, ⅓ cup at a time, and the 3 remaining eggs, mixing as you go until you've added all the dry ingredients and eggs to the batter.

Fold in ⅓ cup blueberries.

Transfer the batter into the greased Bundt or loaf pan and bake for 50–60 minutes, or until a toothpick inserted in the center of the cake comes out clean.

Let the cake cool before removing it from the pan.

To make the glaze, combine erythritol, lemon juice, vanilla, and heavy cream-microwave for 30 seconds.

Stir.

When the cake has cooled, remove from the pan—top with glaze, garnish with blueberries and serve.

Dairy-Free Substitutions:

If you're going dairy-free, you have options, but you're entering rogue territory as I can only speak for the original recipe.

Swap butter with ghee or coconut oil

Swap sour cream with almond milk ricotta

Swap heavy cream for almond or coconut milk

Nutrition Per Serving

(1 slice = 1 serving)

Calories: 437

Fat: 39g

Protein: 14g

Fiber: 4g

Total Carbs: 10g

Net Carbs: 6.9g

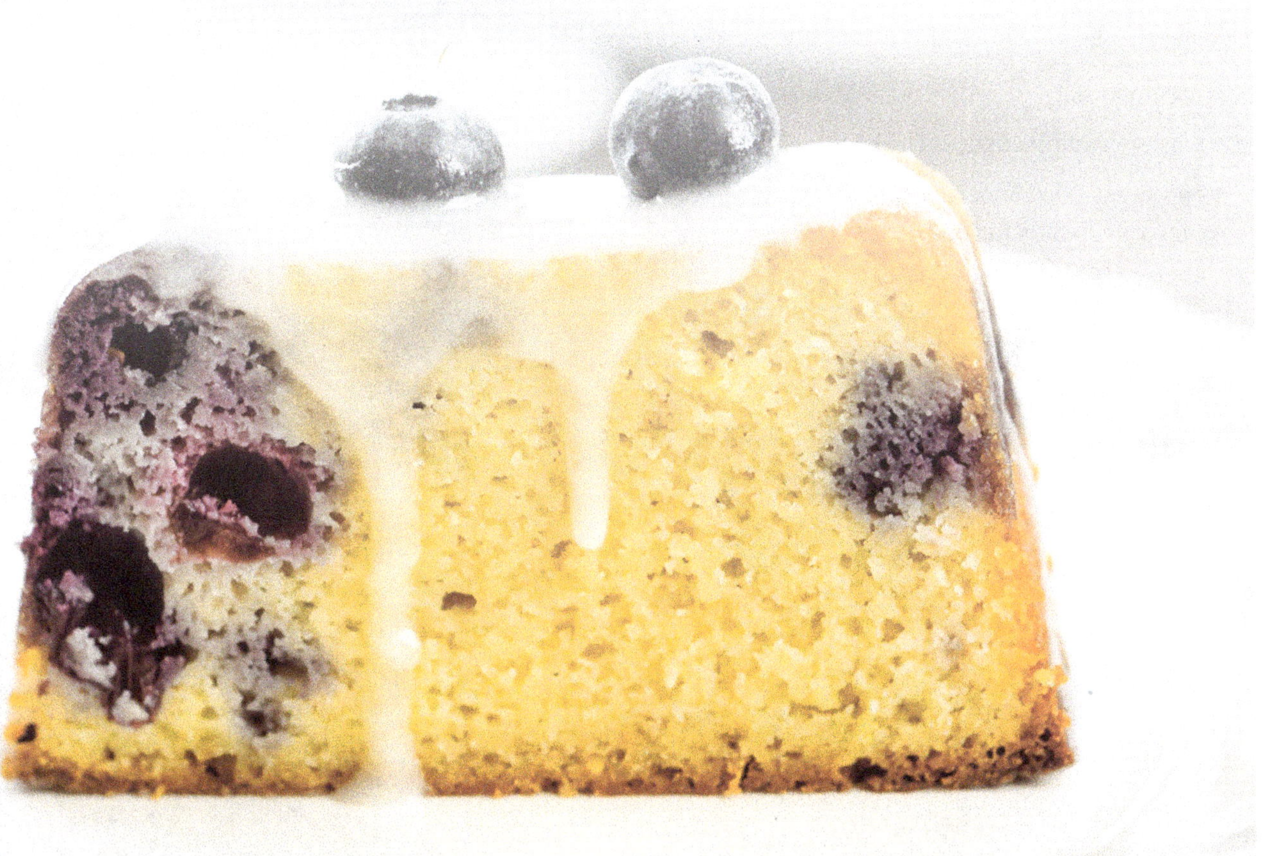

You Dropped A Cookie Dough Fat Bomb On Me

Prep Time: 10 minutes

Cook Time: 1 hour (chill time)

Yield: 14

Drop. A. Bomb.

By the standard definition, fat bombs are small, perfectly portioned snacks or treats loaded with healthy fats, like coconut oil and avocado, that fill you up fast and satisfy any sweet or savory cravings that might sneak up on you.

But if we're keeping it real, they're a metaphor for taking chances, speaking your truth, and being yourself, which is a helluva lot easier to do when you're not 100% that hungry bee-otch.

These fat bombs will be your new favorite when you need something sweet.

1 stick butter, softened

1 8-ounce package cream cheese, softened

½ cup peanut butter

¼ cup Erythritol

¼ teaspoon salt

½ teaspoon vanilla extract (I like Rodelle)

½ cup sugar-free chocolate chips (Lily's is one of my favorite brands for this recipe)

Start by combining room-temperature butter, softened cream cheese, and peanut butter. Stir until smooth.

Add erythritol, salt, and vanilla. Fold in chocolate chips.

Using a cookie scoop or a spoon, scoop 14 balls onto a baking pan. Freeze for two hours until set.

Store in the refrigerator or freezer.

To Freeze: Freeze for up to 3 months in an airtight container.

Nutrition Per Serving
(2 fat bombs = 1 serving)

Calories: 101

Fat: 10.2g

Protein: 1.6g

Fiber: 0.2g

Total Carbs: 3.5g

Net Carbs: 2.5g

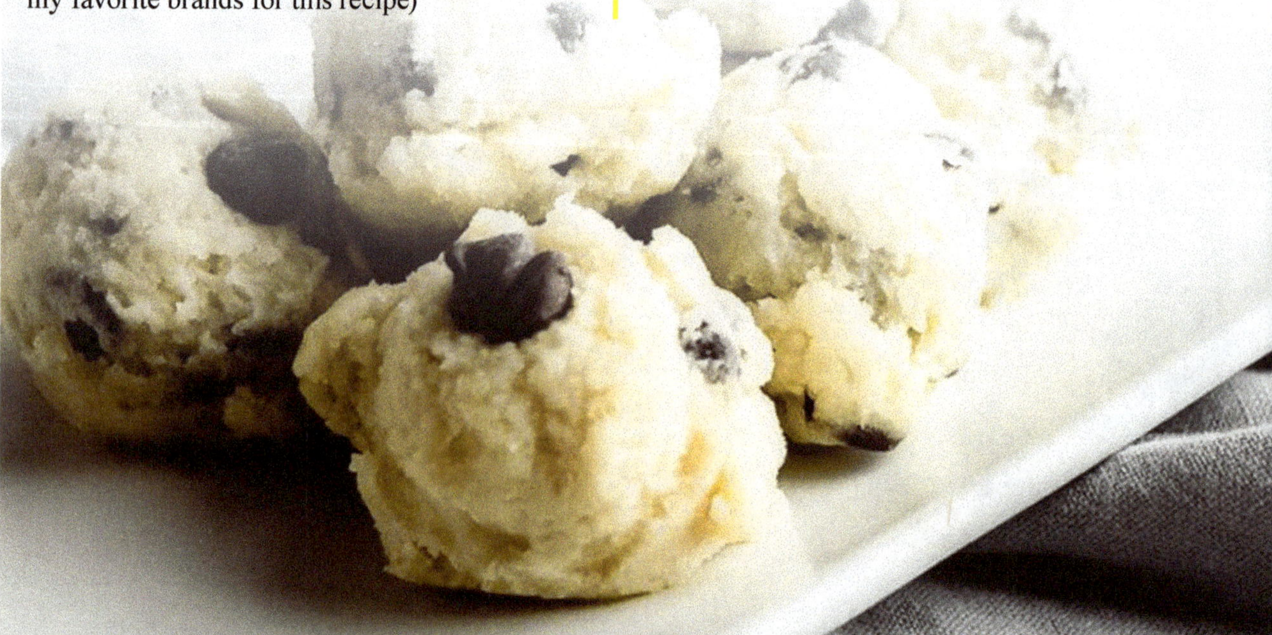

Back In St. Olaf Blueberry Cheesecake Fat Bombs

Prep Time: 10 minutes

Cook Time: 2 hours (chill time)

Yield: 16

You remember Rose from The Golden Girls?

The low-key ditzy blonde played by the high key fabulous Betty White always had a reference to her hometown, St. Olaf, Minnesota, which is a real place.

These cheesecake fat bombs are perfect for a late-night treat with the girls. Pairs nicely with the soundtrack from Miami Vice.

¼ cup butter, softened

¾ cup cream cheese, softened

1 tablespoon powdered Swerve or erythritol

½ teaspoon lemon extract

½ cup blueberries (fresh or frozen)

Cream butter and cream cheese with a hand mixer until smooth. Add sweetener and lemon extract. Fold in blueberries.

Distribute evenly into silicone fat bomb or candy molds. Freeze for 2 hours before serving.

Nutrition Per Serving
(2 fat bombs = 1 serving)

Calories: 66

Fat: 6.6g

Protein: 0.7g

Fiber: 0.1g

Total Carbs: 1.3g

Net Carbs: 1.2g

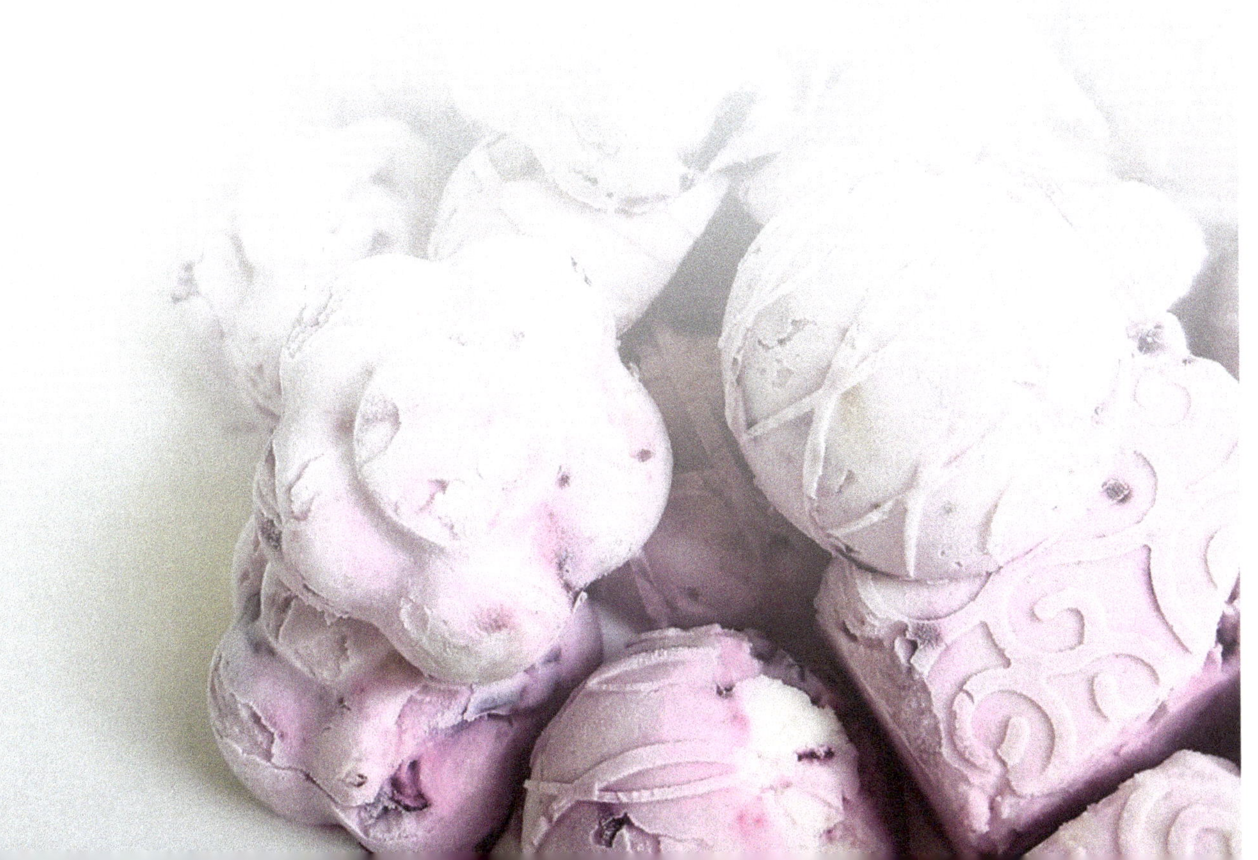

It's The Great Pumpkin. Spice Muffins with Cream Cheese Swirl

Prep Time: 15 minutes

Cook Time: 30 minutes

Yield: 12

Get your pumpkin spice on with these easy keto pumpkin spice muffins with a cream cheese swirl! The best combination of almond flour, pumpkin, and spices that are family and freezer friendly.

Muffins

1½ cups almond flour

1 teaspoon baking soda

¼ teaspoon salt

1 tablespoon pumpkin pie spice

¼ cup butter, melted

¾ cup powdered erythritol or Swerve

3 eggs

1 cup canned pumpkin puree

Cream Cheese Frosting

1 ounce cream cheese, softened

1 egg yolk

¼ cup powdered erythritol or Swerve

2 teaspoons vanilla extract

Preheat the oven to 350° and prep a 12-cup muffin pan with spray or liners.

Find your favorite large mixing bowl and stir the almond flour, baking soda, salt, and spices until they're combined.

Stir in the butter, sweetener, eggs, and pumpkin puree.

Equally distribute batter into 12 muffin cups filling each one ¾ full.

Use a hand mixer and beat the cream cheese until it's smooth. Then add the egg yolk, sweetener, and vanilla, and beat until well combined.

Use a tablespoon to dollop the cream cheese mixture onto each muffin, then "stir" it into each muffin with a toothpick to get the desired swirl effect.

Bake for 15–20 minutes or until a toothpick inserted into the middle of each muffin comes out clean.

To Freeze: Freeze in an airtight container or a heavy-duty freezer bag for up to 3 months.

Nutrition Per Serving
(1 muffin = 1 serving)

Calories: 399

Fat: 33g

Protein: 13g

Fiber: 4g

Total Carbs: 9.2g

Net Carbs: 5.2g

Smooth Operator No-Bake Chocolate Mousse

Prep Time: 10 minutes

Chill Time: 2 hours

Yield: 6

1 ounce cream cheese, softened

3 tablespoons sour cream

1 tablespoon butter, softened

1½ teaspoons vanilla extract

⅓ cup powdered erythritol

¼ cup unsweetened cocoa powder

In a medium bowl, use an electric mixer to combine the cream cheese, sour cream, and butter. Add the vanilla, sweetener, and cocoa powder and blend until smooth.

Place the mousse into cups and store in the fridge for two hours. Serve topped with keto whipped cream—if you want to.

Nutrition Per Serving
(1/2 cup = 1 serving)

Calories: 421

Fat: 41.9g

Protein: 6.03g

Fiber: 2g

Total Carbs: 8.57g

Net Carbs: 6.5g

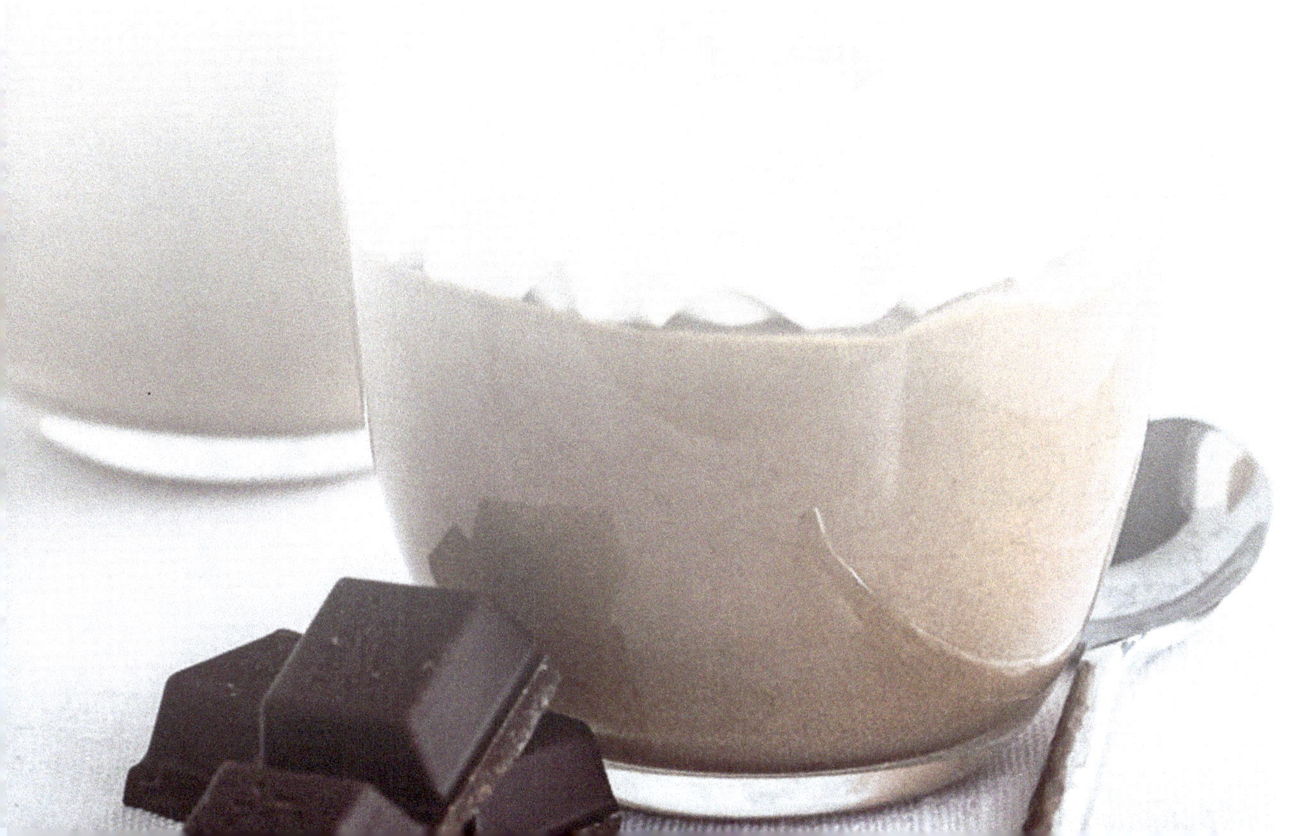

Vanilla Ice Ice 5-Minute Mug Cake

Prep Time: 2 minutes

Cook Time: 3 minutes

Yield: 1

Sure, I could have called this one Robert Matthew Van Winkle mug cake (Vanilla Ice's given name), but it wouldn't be quite as catchy.

No matter what name you put with this easy dessert it will get you through any craving for sweets in under 5 minutes.

1 tablespoon coconut oil

1 tablespoon blanched almond flour

2 tablespoons confectioners erythritol

¼ teaspoon baking powder

½ teaspoon vanilla

1 egg

Pinch of salt

Mix coconut oil (if you're using solid, you'll need to melt it first), almond flour, erythritol, baking powder, vanilla, egg, and a pinch of salt into a microwave safe mug or ramekin.

Microwave for 1 minute, 30 seconds. Boom. You have cake now.

Top with keto whipped cream, cream cheese frosting, strawberries or blueberries, or a little powdered erythritol or nothing because damn, you need dessert.

Nutrition Per Serving
(1 mug cake = 1 serving)

Calories: 361

Fat: 23.2g

Protein: 10.3g

Fiber: 1.1g

Total Carbs: 7.4g

Net Carbs: 4.6g

Lloyd Dobler's Say Anything Double Chocolate Almond Butter Cookies

Prep Time: 10 minutes

Cook Time: 20 minutes

Serves: 16

Remember Lloyd from Say Anything? (He was the hopeless romantic dude who held up the boombox playing "In Your Eyes" to get the attention of the brilliant Ione Skye.) It was quite literally the best '80s movie moment ever.

If you're waiting for your Peter Gabriel-inspired moment in the sun, don't give up. Until then, have a cookie. It will make you feel better.

1 cup natural almond butter

⅔ cup powdered erythritol

2 tablespoons unsweetened cocoa powder

2 tablespoons peanut butter powder

1 teaspoon baking soda

2 eggs

3 tablespoons salted butter, melted

1 teaspoon vanilla extract

½ cup sugar-free chocolate chips

Preheat the oven to 350° and prep a baking pan with parchment paper.

In a large bowl, use a stand or electric hand mixer to combine almond butter and erythritol. Add 2–3 tablespoons of water if needed to manage the dough (it's thick!)

Add cocoa and peanut butter powders, eggs, baking soda, and vanilla. Stir in chocolate chips with a spoon.

Use your hands to roll out 16 evenly shaped balls and place them on a lined baking pan about two inches apart.

Bake for 8–10 minutes.

Cool completely before serving—with or without the 1989 Cameron Crowe film, Say Anything.

Nutrition Per Serving
(1 cookie = 1 serving)

Calories: 115

Fat: 10g

Protein: 4g

Fiber: 2.4g

Total Carbs: 3.9g

Net Carbs: 1.5g

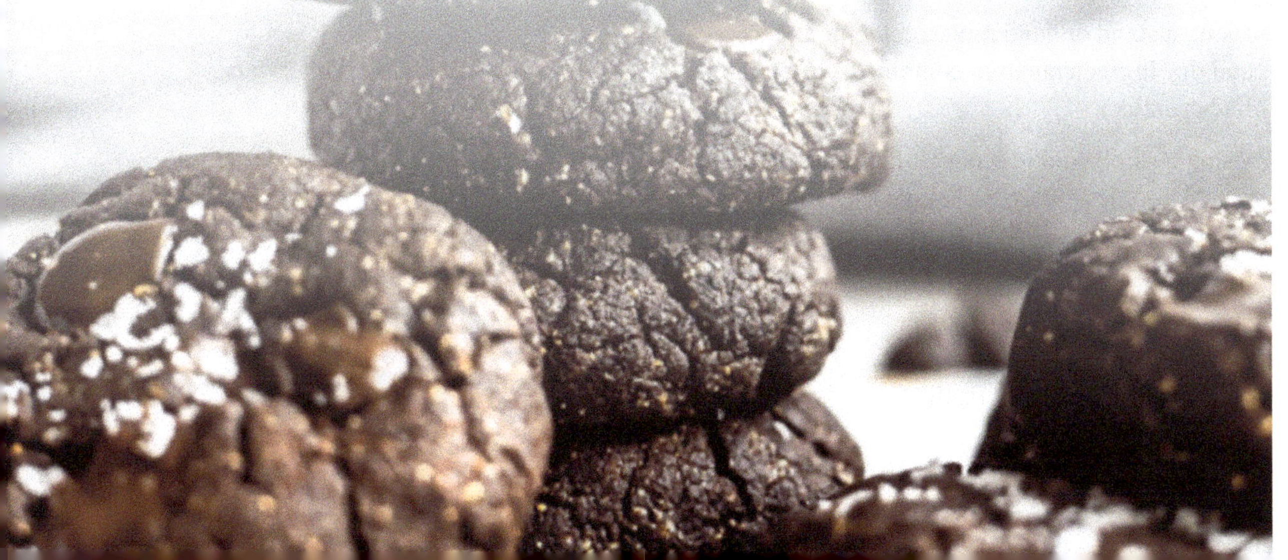

Oh, Snap Ginger Cookies

Prep Time: 10 minutes

Cook Time: 12 minutes

Yield: 24

This cookie recipe may save you from ditching the diet during the holidays or any day you are craving a sugary, spicy flavor combination in the form of a dessert.

2 cups almond flour

1 cup powdered erythritol

2 teaspoons ground ginger

½ teaspoon cinnamon

¼ teaspoon ground nutmeg

¼ teaspoon ground cloves

¼ teaspoon salt

¼ cup butter, melted

3 teaspoons vanilla extract

1 egg

Preheat the oven to 350° and prepare a baking sheet with parchment paper.

In a large mixing bowl or food processor combine the dry ingredients: almond flour, erythritol, ginger, cinnamon, nutmeg, cloves and salt.

In a small bowl, combine the wet ingredients: melted butter, vanilla, and egg.

Using a stand or hand mixer, combine the wet and dry ingredients until combined. (It will look like crumbs.)

Using a small cookie scoop or tablespoon portion out 24 cookies onto your baking sheet about 2 inches apart.

Flatten the top of each with a spoon or spatula. Bake for 10–12 minutes.

Optional: Top with Chai Sugar

⅓ cup monk fruit

2 teaspoons cinnamon

½ teaspoon ground ginger

½ teaspoon all-spice

¼ teaspoon ground cloves

Mix ingredients together and sprinkle liberally on any cookie that will sit still.

Allow cookies to cool before serving.

Nutrition Per Serving
(2 cookies = 1 serving)

Calories: 154

Fat: 14.26g

Protein: 4.66g

Fiber: 2.1g

Total Carbs: 3.72g

Net Carbs: 1.62g

Like Jell-O Pudding Pops

Prep Time: 10 minutes

Cook Time: 5 minutes + 6 hours to freeze

Yield: 8

You remember Pudding Pops, right? Back in the '80s you couldn't watch ten minutes of TV without seeing the famous frozen treat that "always gets the green light from Mommy" because they were made with "wholesome" Jell-O pudding. And moms everywhere bought into the hype.

This version is better for you, doesn't take a lot of work and, big bonus: it's kid-friendly!

1 cup unsweetened almond milk

1 cup heavy cream

⅓ cup granulated sweetener (Swerve or stevia)

⅓ cup unsweetened cocoa powder

¼ teaspoon xanthan gum

1 teaspoon vanilla

Whisk almond milk, heavy cream, sweetener, and cocoa powder together in a medium saucepan. Stir until blended and bring to a boil.

Turn the heat down to low.

Slowly sprinkle in xanthan gum and add vanilla.

Make sure all ingredients are combined, turn the heat off, and let cool for at least 10 minutes. Pour into popsicle molds and freeze until solid (about 6 hours).

Nutrition Per Serving
(1 Pudding Pop = 1 serving)

Calories: 118

Fat: 11.2g

Protein: 1.44g

Fiber: 1.5g

Total Carbs: 3.1g

Net Carbs: 1.6g

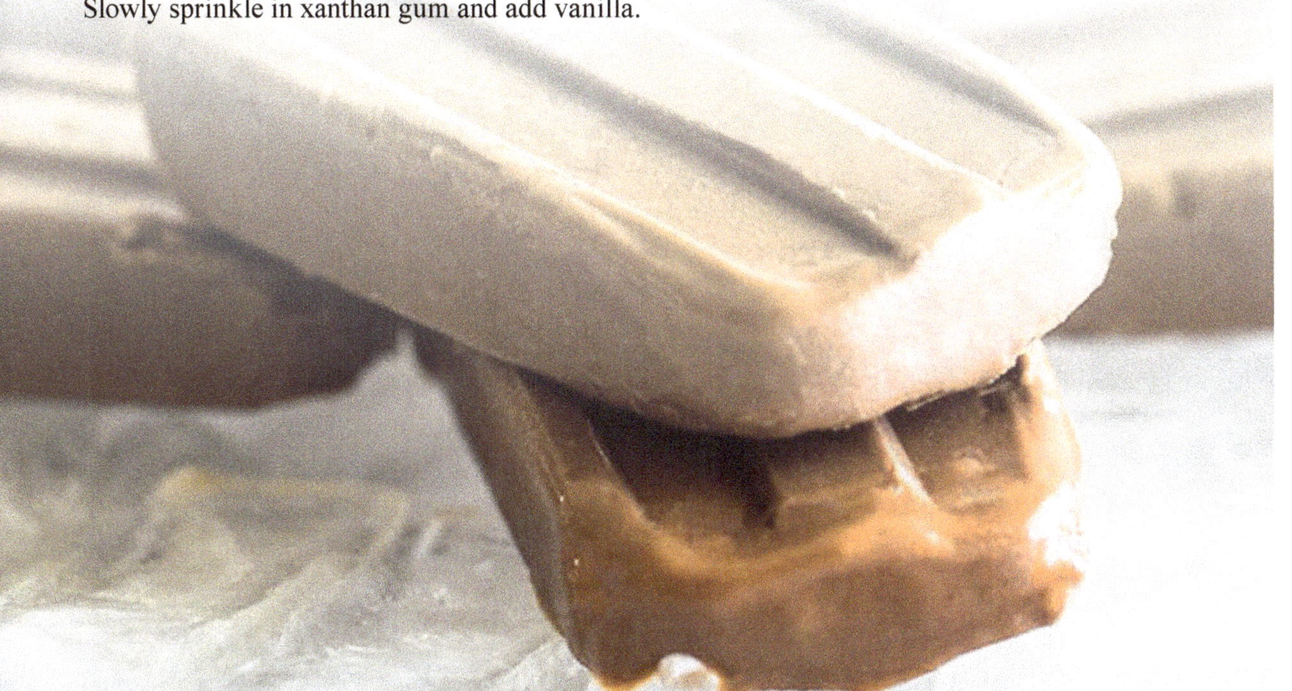

Baked Chocolate Chip Peanut Butter Cookie Bars

Prep Time: 10 minutes

Cook Time: 15 minutes

Yield: 12

1 cup natural peanut butter

¼ cup butter, softened

½ cup granulated erythritol

2 eggs

1 cup almond flour

½ teaspoon baking powder

2 teaspoons vanilla extract

½ cup sugar-free chocolate chips

Preheat the oven to 375° and prep an 8-inch dish with butter or cooking spray. Use an electric mixer to combine the peanut butter and the butter until smooth. Add sweetener, eggs, almond flour, baking powder, and vanilla.

Fold in chocolate chips.

Transfer to a baking dish and bake for 15 minutes. Cool completely before serving.

Store any leftovers in an airtight container for up to 5 days.

Nutrition Per Serving

(1 cookie bar = 1 serving)

Calories: 146

Fat: 12g

Protein: 6.3g

Fiber: 2.8g

Total Carbs: 7.1g

Net Carbs: 4.4g

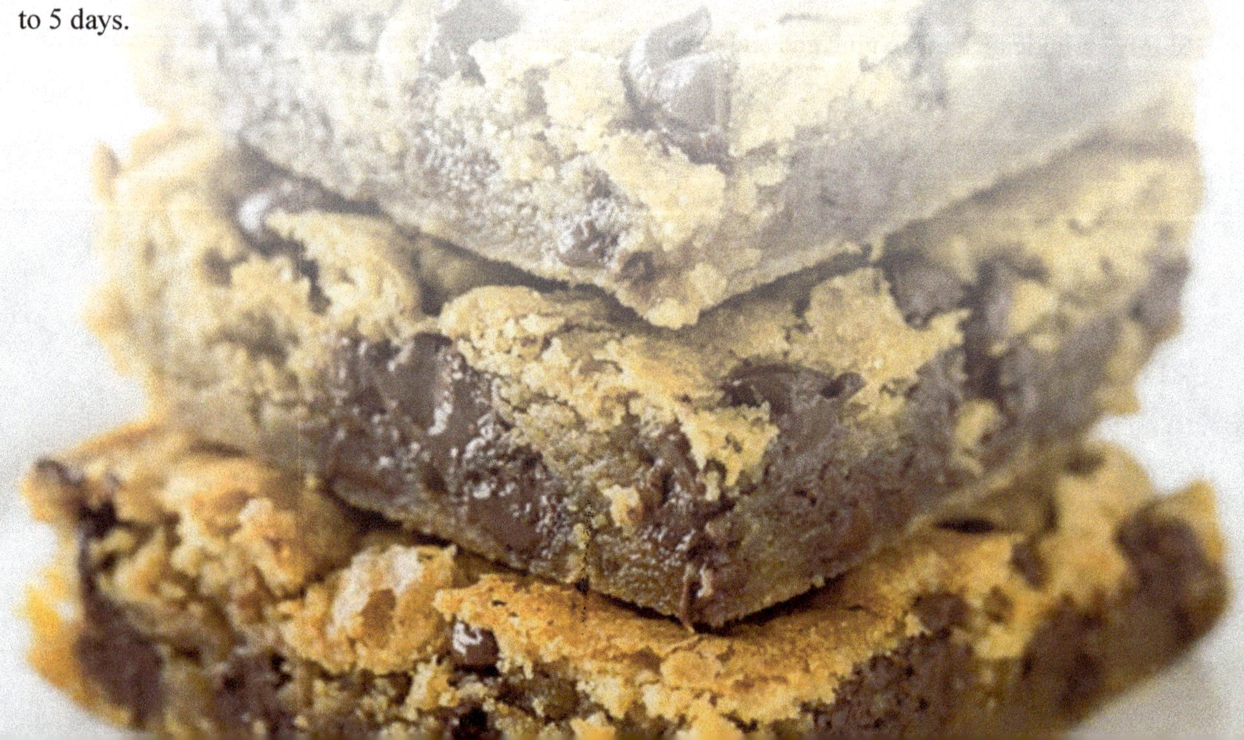

Just Like Heaven & T.J. Cinnamons Roll Chaffles

Prep Time: 5 minutes

Cook Time: 5 minutes

Yield: 4 Chaffles

The first T.J. Cinnamons opened its doors in 1985 at Parkway Shopping Center in Kansas City, Missouri. The massive cinnamon rolls started at $1.25 and were easy to share—which worked out well for me since I had a mall budget of zero dollars. Those melt in your mouth cinnamon rolls would put you in a sugar coma in 5 minutes.

Since we're avoiding all comas, as a rule, I recreated the T.J. Cinnamon's experience by adding a few ingredients to the basic mozzarella chaffle that keeps it sweet, low carb, and just like heaven.

Ingredients for Base Chaffle:

1 ounce cream cheese, softened

2 eggs

1 tablespoon butter, melted

1 tablespoon coconut flour

½ teaspoon vanilla

½ teaspoon baking powder

Pinch of salt

1 tablespoon monk fruit classic

1 tablespoon monk fruit golden

1 teaspoon cinnamon

Ingredients for Buttered Cinnamon Sugar Swirl:

1 tablespoon butter

1 teaspoon cinnamon

2 teaspoons monk fruit classic

Ingredients for Cream Cheese Icing:

1 tablespoon cream cheese, softened

1 tablespoon butter

1½ tablespoon of powdered monk fruit

Combine all ingredients to make base chaffle in a bowl. Set aside.

In a separate bowl, combine Ingredients for Buttered Cinnamon Sugar Swirl. Microwave for ten-second intervals until butter melts and monk fruit and cinnamon have dissolved.

Spray waffle iron with keto-friendly cooking spray and add base chaffle batter, then drizzle the Buttered Cinnamon Sugar Swirl. swirl around on top.

Cook 4 to 5 minutes.

Combine ingredients for Cream Cheese Icing and microwave for ten-second intervals until it has a smooth consistency like icing.

Drizzle Cream Cheese Icing over chaffles and enjoy for breakfast or dessert!

To Freeze: Place each chaffle (without the swirl or icing) in a freezer bag separated with wax paper so they don't stick together. Defrost in the microwave or in your air fryer set at 300° for 2–3 minutes.

Nutrition Per Serving
(2 chaffles = 1 serving)

Calories: 195

Fat: 17.6g

Protein: 5.1g

Fiber: 2g

Total Carbs: 5.6g

Net Carbs: 1.8g

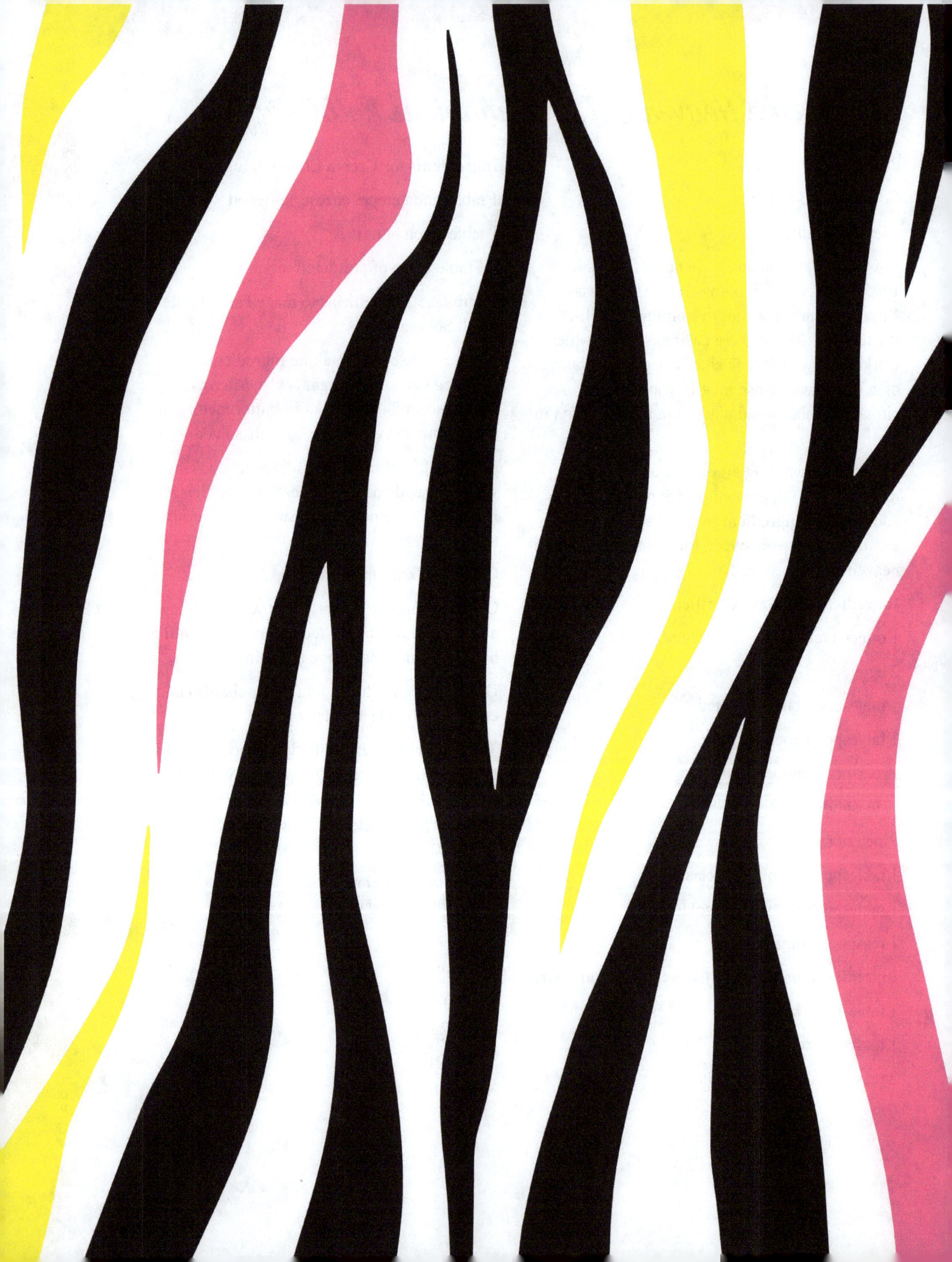

Drinks

Blender Butter Coffee

Prep Time: 5 minutes

Cook Time: 0

Yield: 2

It's a caffeinated butter enriched morning miracle that may or may not make you a morning person. Have a blender on deck!

1 cups of coffee

2 tablespoons butter

1 tablespoon heavy whipping cream

1–2 tablespoons coconut oil or MCT oil

1 tablespoon unsweetened cocoa powder

Brew 2 cups of coffee.

Pour 2 cups of hot water in your blender while coffee is brewing. This will heat your blender and help your drink retain more heat once you've added other ingredients.

Once the coffee is brewed, be sure to empty the water from your blender.

Pour coffee, butter, coconut oil, heavy cream, and cocoa powder into the blender. Blend until combined and frothy.

Additional great idea: Pre-mix your added ingredients (Oil, Butter, Cream, etc.) Pour into silicone ice cube tray. For days when you're short on time, just put your coffee in the blender and pull a cube or two from the freezer.

Nutrition Per Serving

(1 cup = 1 serving)

Calories: 253

Fat: 28g

Protein: 0

Fiber: 1g

Total Carbs: 2g

Net Carbs: 1g

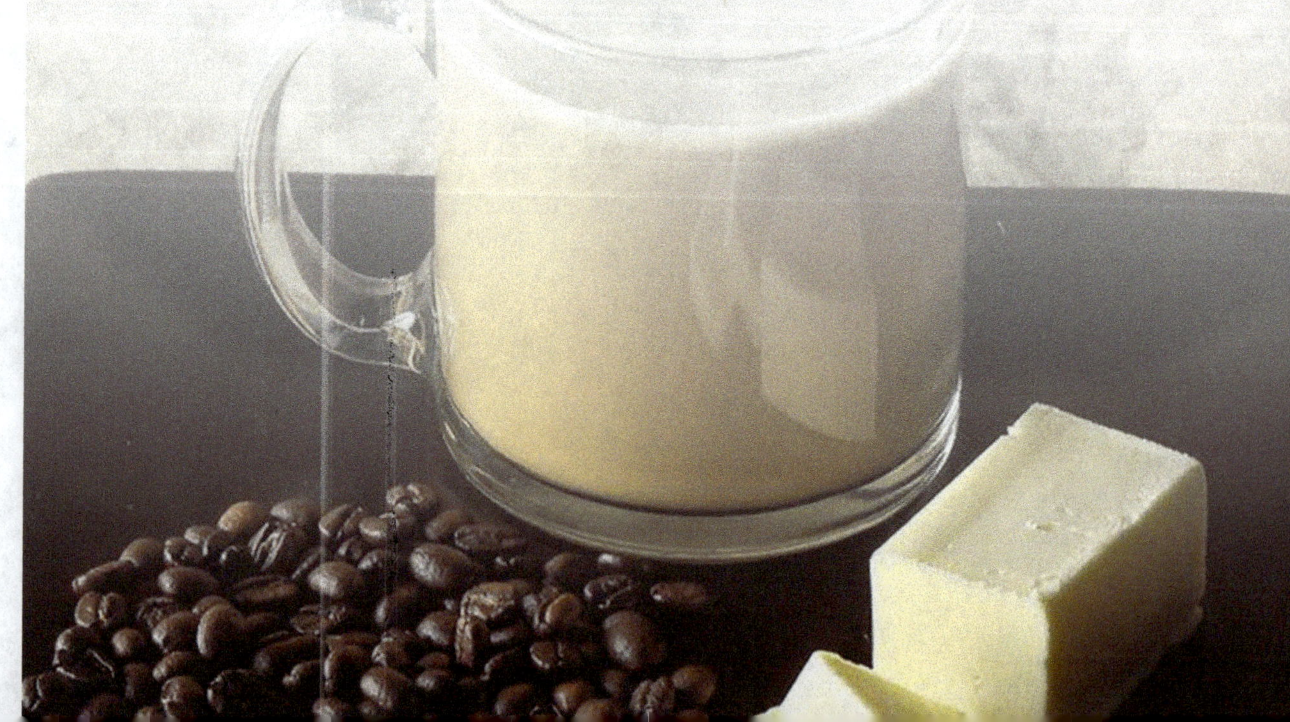

Hippy Hippy Shake Green Smoothie

Prep Time: 5 minutes

Cook Time: 0

Yield: 1

Love a smoothie for breakfast? Or lunch? Or whenever you want one? Here you go! Feel free to swap frozen spinach for fresh, but if you go that route, skip the water, or you'll have a runny smoothie situation.

Pairs well with any Tom Cruise movie, especially Cocktail.

½ avocado, pitted & peeled

½ cup water

½ cup unsweetened coconut milk

1 teaspoon vanilla extract

1 tablespoon MCT oil

4 drops liquid stevia

1 cup spinach

fresh Ice cubes

Place all of the ingredients into your blender and pulse until smooth.

Nutrition Per Serving
(1 shake = 1 serving)

Calories: 504

Fat: 48g

Protein: 5g

Fiber: 9g

Total Carbs: 13g

Net Carbs: 4g

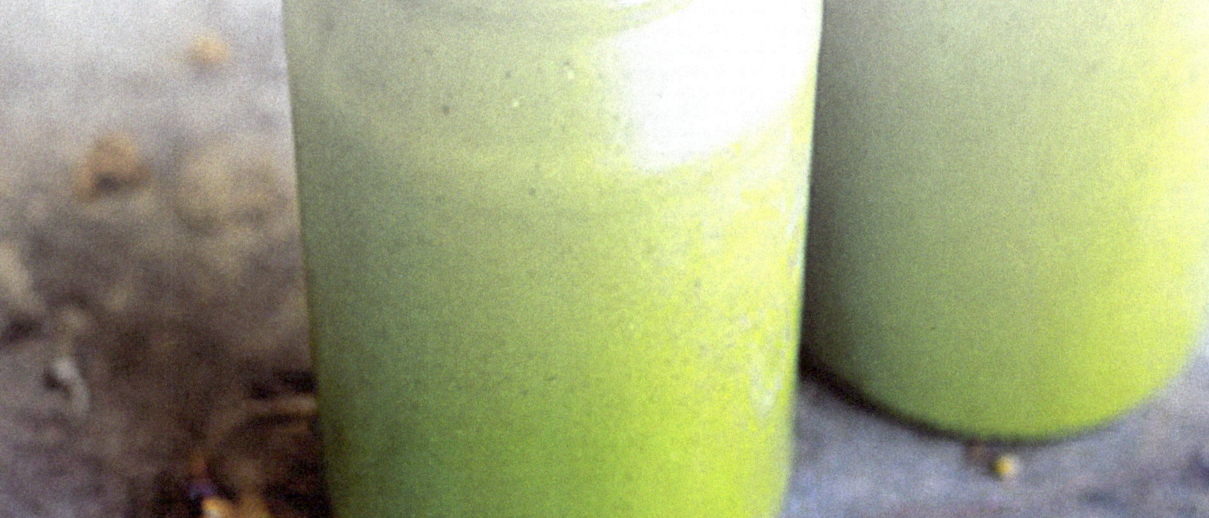

Here's Lookin' At You Kid Key Lime Pie Dairy-Free Smoothie (Vegan-Friendly)

Prep Time: 5

Cook Time: 5

Yield: 3

If you're feeling extra special or you need something to satisfy your Key Lime Pie craving, opt for this smoothie—and feel free to swap the coconut milk for almond milk!

1 cup coconut milk

½ avocado

2 tablespoons lime juice

3 tablespoons lemon juice

1 cup ice

Stevia drops to taste (or your favorite sweetener to taste)

Add all ingredients to your blender and blend until smooth.

Nutrition Per Serving
(⅓ recipe = 1 serving)

Calories: 242

Fat: 23g

Protein: 2g

Fiber: 4g

Total Carbs: 8g

Net Carbs: 4g

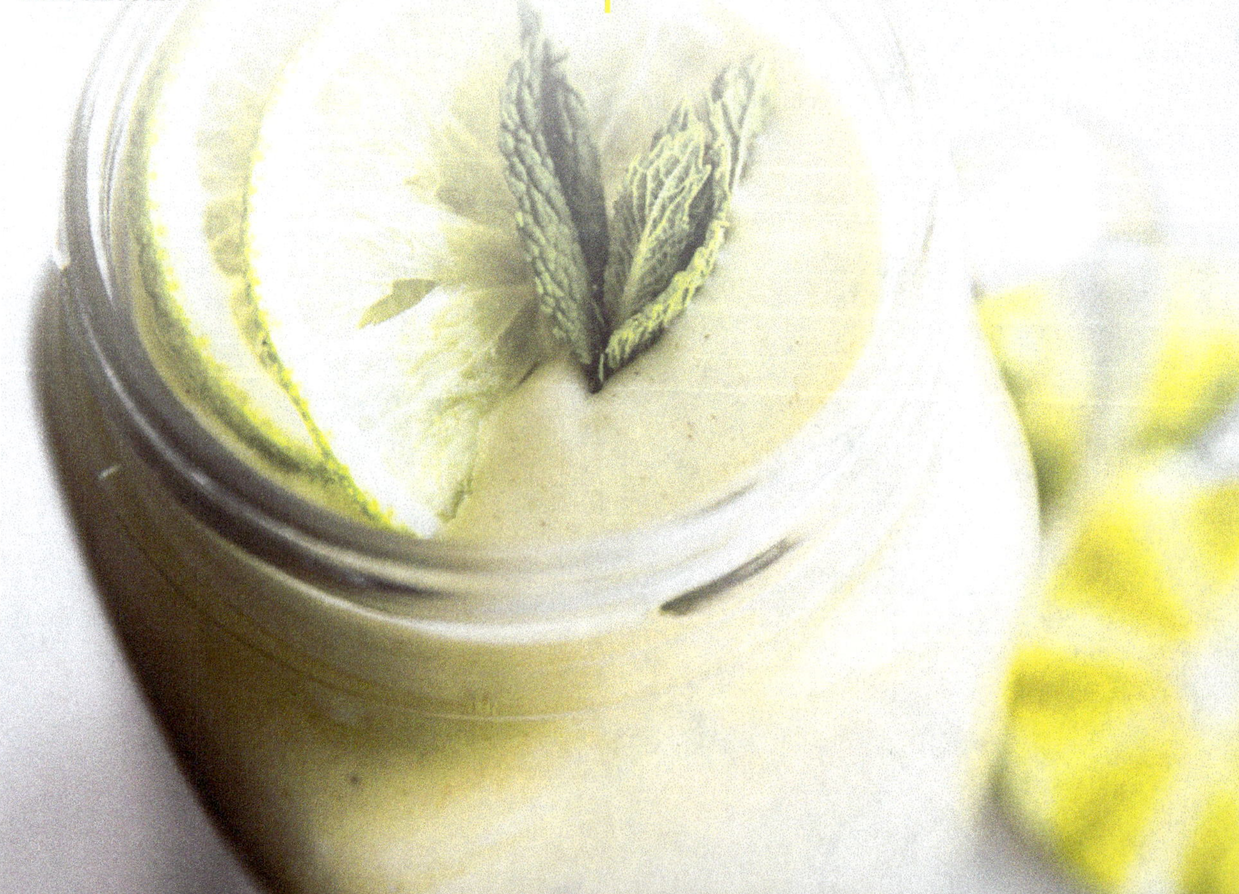

Very Berry Keto Smoothie

Prep Time: 5 Minutes

Cook Time: 3 Minutes

Yield: 1

Blueberries, strawberries, and raspberries all fall into the low carb fruit category—and they're all packed with fiber, which your digestive system will thank you for! Combined with the filling effects of the healthy fats from the avocado and you have a fabulous summer-y smoothie that will keep you full for hours.

¼ cup fresh berries

1 large avocado, peeled and pitted

1 cup unsweetened coconut milk or unsweetened vanilla almond milk

2 scoops vanilla protein powder (I like Bulletproof Collagen)

1 tablespoon MCT oil or coconut oil

6 ice cubes

Blend all of the ingredients in your blender or food processor until smooth.

Nutrition Per Serving

(1 smoothie = 1 serving)

Calories: 331

Fat: 21.9g

Protein: 24.3g

Fiber: 1.1g

Total Carbs: 6.7g

Net Carbs: 5.6g

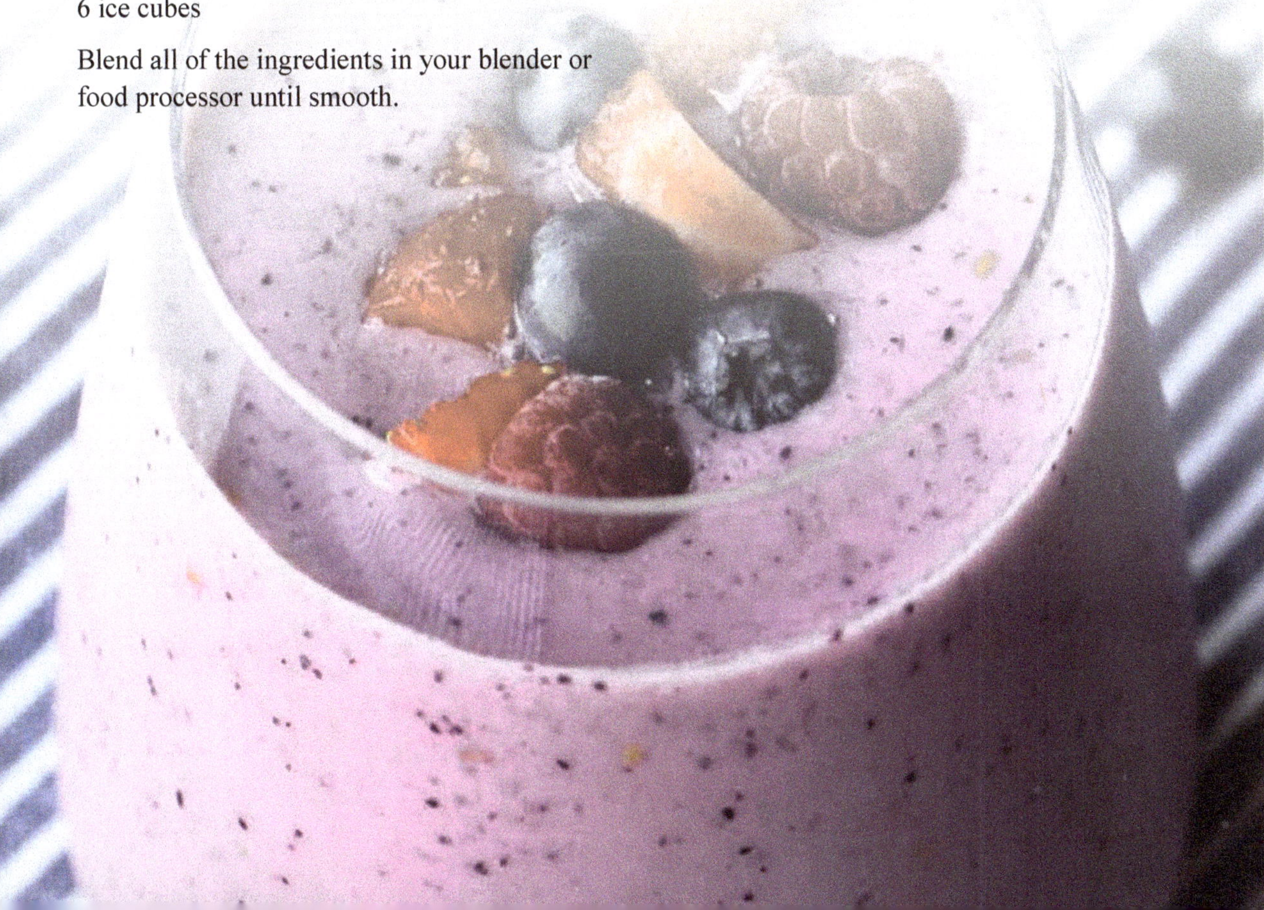

Who Needs Swiss Miss When You Have Keto Hot Chocolate?

Prep Time: 5 minutes

Cook Time: 5 minutes

Yield: 3

We're swapping the standard version's whole milk with almond milk, a little heavy cream (canned coconut milk works if you're avoiding dairy), a dash of vanilla, and a little cocoa powder. We're finishing the job with keto whipped cream and a pinch of cinnamon. If you go for the dark chocolate version and have any chocolate shavings or chips leftover, sprinkle some on top. It looks pretty.

The entire process from start to finish will take you about 10 minutes and will taste so much better than all the Swiss Miss packets in the world. :)

Don't let your pan get too hot, or you will end up with burned chocolate, which may kill your vibe and ruin the hot chocolate.

1 cup unsweetened almond milk

½ cup heavy cream

3 tablespoons unsweetened cocoa powder

½ teaspoon vanilla

2–3 tablespoons granulated sweetener of choice (I use Swerve)

Pinch of salt

Pinch of cinnamon (optional)

Simmer the almond milk and cream over medium heat. Simmer for 5 minutes until smooth.

You may want to whisk your cocoa to de-lump:) Stir it into the almond milk & cream.

Add vanilla and a pinch of salt.

Sip while you gaze into a fire or a candle and contemplate the meaning of life.

Nutrition Per Serving
(1 cup = 1 serving)

Calories: 242

Fat: 23g

Protein: 2g

Fiber: 4g

Total Carbs: 8g

Net Carbs: 4g

Keto Mint Julep

Prep Time: 5 minutes

Cook Time: 5 minutes

Yield: 1

The sugar content in the traditional mint julep will throw your carb count for a loop. The good news is you can dupe that recipe and skip making your simple syrup using Swerve instead.

3 fresh mint leaves

2 teaspoons Swerve

2 ounces + 1/2 teaspoon bourbon

1 cup crushed ice

Mint sprig for garnish

For best results, start with mint julep cups that have been chilled in the freezer.

Take a cocktail shaker and throw in 3 fresh mint leaves, and for the love of all things holy, leave them alone!

Add in 1–2 teaspoons of Swerve. I like 2, but if you're afraid of going too sweet, use 1.5.

Now add in a splash of bourbon. Around 1/2 of a teaspoon; maybe more depending on your mood. Let the bourbon settle for a minute over the Swerve and mint, and then mix it up.

Add in 1 cup crushed ice.

Then pour in 2 ounces of bourbon.

Now shake it until you feel like you've completed a HIIT workout or 60 seconds. Transfer to a chilled mint julep cup and add a sprig of mint as garnish.

Enjoy!

Nutrition Per Serving
(1 Julep = 1 serving)

Calories: 177

Fat: 0g

Protein: 0g

Carbs: 1g

Fiber: 0g

Total Carbs: 1g

Net Carbs: 1g

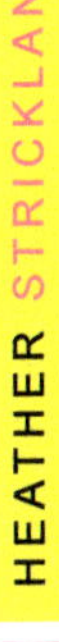

Bloody Mary Is An Urban Legend, But This Drink Is Real

Prep Time: 5 minutes

Cook Time: 5 minutes

Yield: 1

The traditional Bloody Mary that uses tomato juice and Bloody Mary mix contains around ten net carbs per cup. However, you can modify the OG recipe and make it low carb. No lie.

1/2 cup (4 ounces) unsweetened tomato juice or V8

2 ounces vodka

1 ounce beef flavored bone broth

1–2 dashes Worcestershire sauce (Lea & Perrins)

2 teaspoons prepared horseradish

1 teaspoon lemon juice

1 dash tabasco

1 dash Louisiana hot sauce

Dash black pepper

Dash celery salt

Fill a cocktail shaker with ice.

Pour vodka and bone broth into the shaker.

Add tomato juice, tabasco, Louisiana hot sauce, lemon juice, Lea & Perrins, and horseradish. Add pepper and celery salt.

Shake! Shake! Shake!

Transfer to a chilled highball filled with ice. Enjoy!

Nutrition Per Serving
(1 drink = 1 serving)

Calories: 165

Fat: 0.4g

Protein: 1.2g

Fiber: 1.2g

Total Carbs: 7.3g

Net Carbs: 6.1g

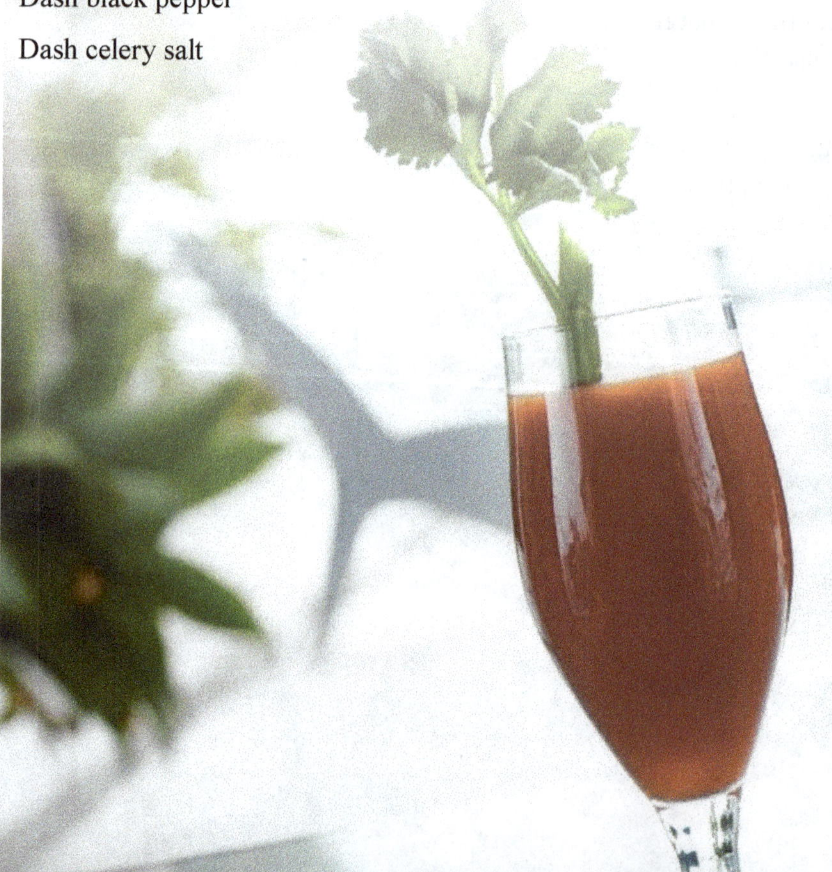

Fizzy Lemon

Prep Time: 5 minutes

Cook Time: 5 minutes

Yield: 1

A refreshing low-carb cocktail to help you power through any summer social event and keep it keto.

6 mint leaves

1 tablespoon lemon juice

2 ounces vodka

1 ounce club soda

1 cup ice

Rosemary sprig (optional)

Lemon garnish (optional)

Muddle mint & lemon.

Mix ingredients in a cocktail shaker.

Shake it like an '80s picture for 30 seconds. Serve in a lowball over ice.

Garnish with rosemary and a slice of lemon. Bottoms up!

Nutrition Per Serving

(1 drink = 1 serving)

Calories: 131

Fat: 0g

Protein: 0g

Fiber:0g

Total Carbs: 0g

Net Carbs: 0g

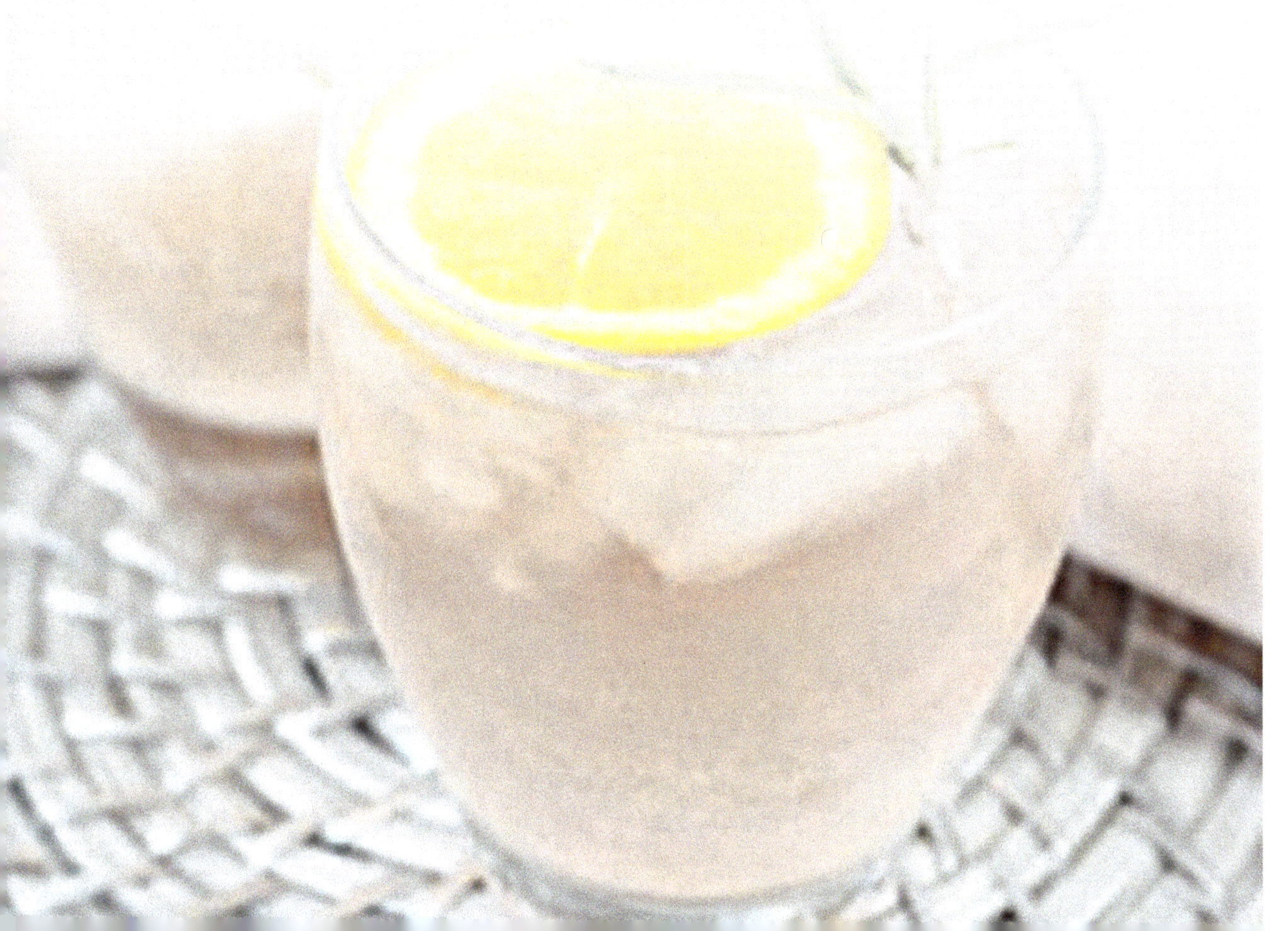

Head Over Heels Spicy Margarita

Prep Time: 5 minutes

Cook Time: 0

Yield: 2

No hassle is required to turn up this sugar-free Margarita!

2 ounces tequila

1 tablespoon fresh lime juice

12 drops liquid stevia

1 jalapeno slices

Ice

Rimmer Ingredients:

Lime

1 teaspoon salt

⅛ teaspoon chili powder

⅛ teaspoon sweet paprika

For the rim: Wet the edge of your glass with the lime. Combine salt, chili powder, and paprika.

Place spice combinations on a plate and dip glass until the rim is well coated.

For the Margarita: Muddle jalapeno slices with fresh lime juice.

Add tequila, stevia, and a handful of ice to a cocktail shaker and shake. Serve over ice. Turn up. Enjoy.

Nutrition Per Serving
(½ recipe = 1 serving)

Calories: 74

Fat: 0g

Protein: 0.1g

Fiber: 0g

Total Carbs: 2g

Net Carbs: 2g

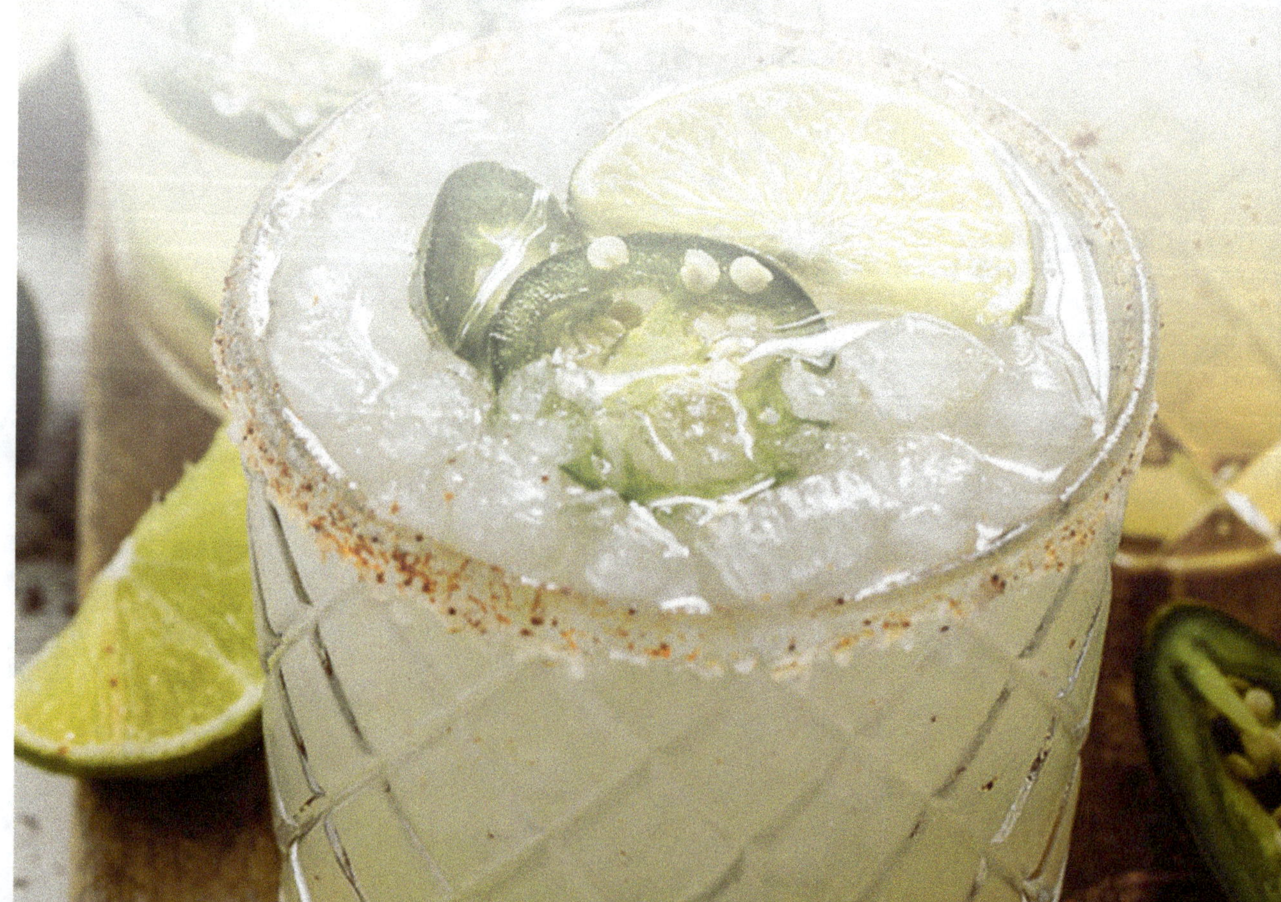

Hit Me With Your Best Three Wise Men Shot

Prep Time: 5 minutes

Cook Time: 5 minutes

Yield: 1

The classic version calls for equal parts Johnnie Walker Scotch, Jack Daniels Whiskey, and Jim Beam Bourbon. Do not ask me who came up with the idea of taking these prudent fellas on excursions to switch up the spirits.

Variations include taking the three men on a hunt by adding Wild Turkey, across the border with a little Tequila, on a tropical vacay with Captain Morgan, and an LSD trip with absinthe. Details are listed below for the classic.

If you're watching carbs, you're covered.

Whiskey has no added sugars and 0 carbs. This 100% whiskey shot is 100% keto: we aren't bringing any sugar-filled mixers to the table.

½ ounce scotch

½ ounce bourbon

½ ounce whiskey

Place shot glasses in the freezer for two hours, or better yet, keep a few in the freezer as a rule. Pour equal parts scotch, bourbon, and whiskey in a cocktail shaker with ice.

Shake! Shake! Shake! Strain and pour into a well-chilled shot glass. Bottoms up!

Variations:

The Three Wise Men Go Hunting – Add 1/2-ounce Wild Turkey (Adds 34 Calories)

The Three Wise Men Cross The Border – Add 1/2-ounce Jose Cuervo tequila (Adds 32 Calories)

Three Tropical Wise Men – Add 1/2-ounce Jack Daniels + 1/2 ounce Jose Cuervo + 1/2-ounce Captain Morgan Rum + a tiny umbrella

Three Wise Men On An Acid Trip – Add 1/2 ounce absinthe (Adds 41 Calories)

Three Southern Wise Men – Add Jack Daniels + Jim Beam + Jose Cuervo (No Johnnie Walker. He was a Yankee.)

Nutrition Per Serving
(1 shot = 1 serving)

Calories: 97

Fat: 0g

Protein: 0g

Fiber: 0g

Total Carbs: 0g

Net Carbs: 0g

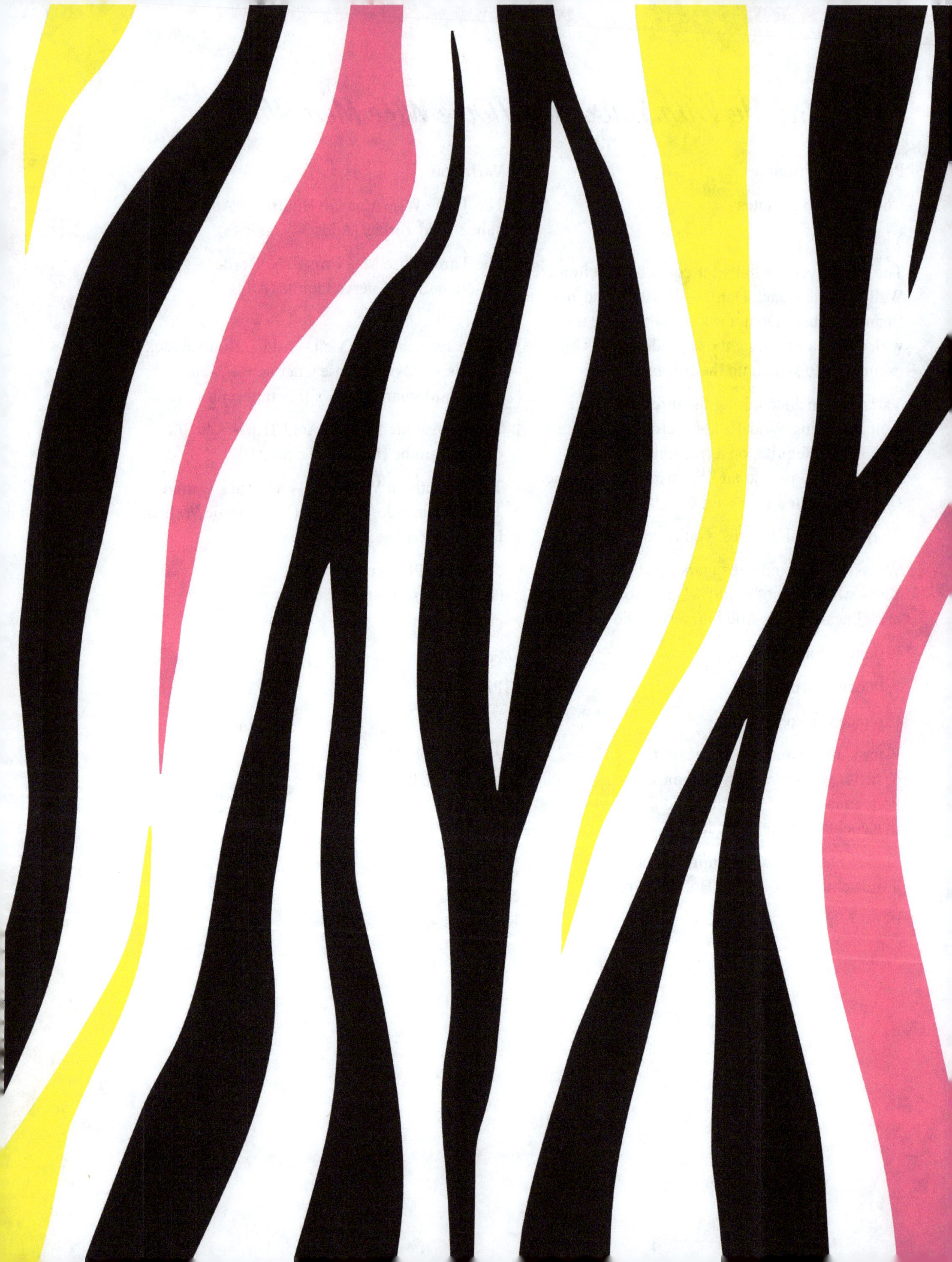

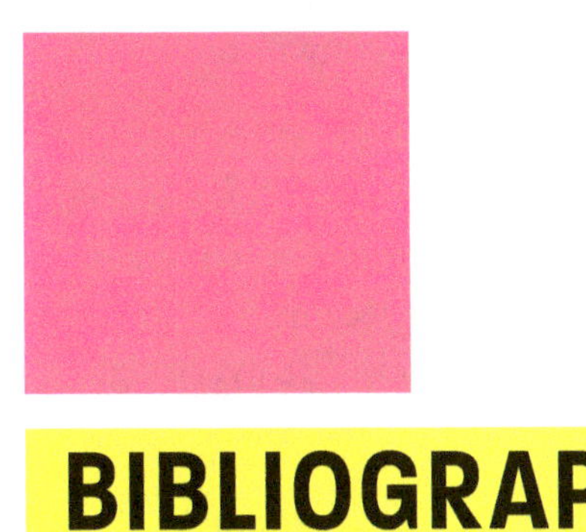

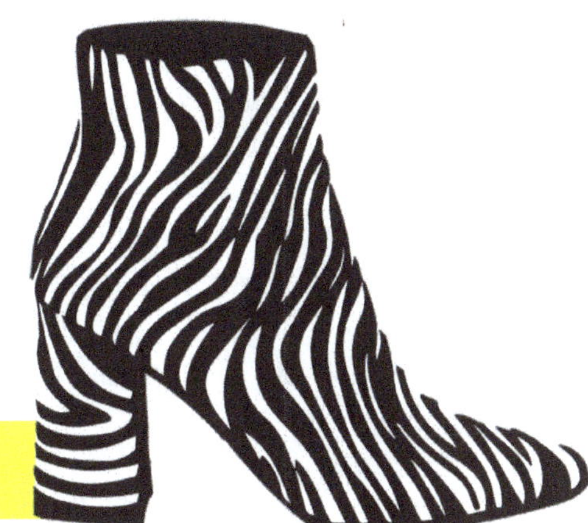

BIBLIOGRAPHY

American Institute for Cancer Research. "Red Meat (Beef, Pork, Lamb): Increases Risk of Colorectal Cancer." 31 March 2021. Accessed August 23, 2021.https://www.aicr.org/cancer-prevention/food-facts/red-meat-beef-pork-lamb/#research.

Astwood, E.B. "The Heritage of Corpulence." *Endocrinology.* 71, Issue 2 (1 August 1962): 337–341, 71.

Aubrey, Allison. "Fresh Research Finds Organic Milk Packs in Omega-3s." The Salt. *NPR.* 10 December 2013. Accessed October 12, 2021. https://www.npr.org/sections/thesalt/2013/12/09/249794467/fresh-research-finds-organic-milk-packs-in-omega-3s.

Brazier, Yvette. "Obesity: What is it, and what causes it?" *Medical News Today.* 26 February 2020. Accessed August 23, 2021. https://www.medicalnewstoday.com/articles/323551.

Britannica, T. Editors of Encyclopedia. "The Coca-Cola Company." *Encyclopedia Britannica.* 21 June 2021. Accessed August 20, 2021. https://www.britannica.com/topic/The-Coca-Cola-Company.

Centers for Disease Control and Prevention. "Adult Obesity Facts." *Overweight & Obesity.* 7 June 2021. Accessed August 23, 2021. https://www.cdc.gov/obesity/data/adult.html#:~:text=The%20US%20obesity%20prevalence%20was,from%204.7%25%20to%209.2%25.

Centers for Disease Control and Prevention. "Heart Disease Facts." 27 September 2021. Accessed October 15, 2021. https://www.cdc.gov/heartdisease/facts.htm.

Centers for Disease Control and Prevention. "Healthy Weight, Nutrition, and Physical Activity: Health Effects of Overweight and Obesity." 17 September 2020. Accessed August 8, 2021. https://www.cdc.gov/healthyweight/effects/index.html.

DiNicolantonio, James J., O'Keefe, James H., and Wilson, William L. "Sugar addiction: Is it real? A narrative review." *British Journal of Sports Medicine.* 2018. 52:910-913. https://bjsm.bmj.com/content/52/14/910.

Freedman, David S. "Obesity --- United States, 1988--2008." *Centers for Disease Control and Prevention.* 14 January 2011. Accessed August 23, 2021. https://www.cdc.gov/mmwr/preview/mmwrhtml/su6001a15.htm.

Fryar, Cheryl D., Carroll, Margaret D., and Afful, Joseph. "Health-E Stats. Prevalence of Overweight, Obesity, and Severe Obesity Among Children and Adolescents Aged 2–19 Years: United States, 1963–1965 through 2017–2018." *Centers for Disease Control and Prevention.* December 2020. Accessed August 20, 2021. https://www.cdc.gov/nchs/data/hestat/obesity-child-17-18/overweight-obesity-child-H.pdf.

Goodman, Martin. "Dr. Toon: When Reagan Met Optimus Prime." *Animation World Network.* 12 October 2010. Accessed August 20, 2021. https://www.awn.com/animationworld/dr-toon-when-reagan-met-optimus-prime.

Hales, Craig M., Carroll, Margaret D., Fryar, Cheryl D., and Ogden, Cynthia L. "Prevalence of Obesity and Severe Obesity Among Adults: United States, 2017–2018." *Centers for Disease Control and Prevention.* February 2020. Accessed August 20, 2021. https://www.cdc.gov/nchs/data/databriefs/db360-h.pdf.

Haskell, William L., Lee, I-Min, Pate, Russell R., Powell, Kenneth E., Blair, Steven N., Franklin, Barry A., Macera, Caroline A. et al. "Physical Activity and Public Health: Updated Recommendation for Adults from the American College of Sports Medicine and the American Heart Association." *Circulation.* 28 August 2007. Accessed August 20, 2021. https://www.ahajournals.org/doi/pdf/10.1161/CIRCULATIONAHA.107.185649.

Howden, Lindsay M., and Meyer, Julie A. "Age and Sex Composition: 2010." *U.S. Census Bureau.* 1 May 2011. Accessed August 20, 2021. https://www.census.gov/library/publications/2011/dec/c2010br-03.html.

Kearns, C.E., Schmidt, L.A., and Glantz, S.A. "Sugar Industry and Coronary Heart Disease Research: A Historical Analysis of Internal Industry Documents." *JAMA Intern Med.* 2016;176(11):1680–1685. doi:10.1001/jamainternmed.2016.5394.

Kosinski, Christophe and Jornayvaz, François R. "Effects of Ketogenic Diets on Cardiovascular Risk Factors: Evidence from Animal and Human Studies." *Nutrients.* 19 May 2017. Accessed August 23, 2021. https://www.ncbi.nlm.nih.gov/pmc/articles/PMC5452247/.

Lenoir, Magalie, Serre, Fuschia, Cantin, Lauriane, and Ahmed, Serge H. "Intense Sweetness Surpasses Cocaine Reward." *PLoS One.* 1 August 2007. Accessed August 23, 2021. https://www.ncbi.nlm.nih.gov/pmc/articles/PMC1931610/.

Leslie, Ian. "The Sugar Conspiracy." *The Guardian.* April 2016. Accessed August 23, 2021. https://www.theguardian.com/society/2016/apr/07/the-sugar-conspiracy-robert-lustig-john-yudkin.

Malkan, Stacy. "Aspartame: Decades of Science Point to Serious Health Risks." *U.S. Right to Know.* 15 November 2020. Accessed November 2, 2021. https://usrtk.org/sweeteners/aspartame_health_risks/.

National Center for Health Statistics. "Table 14. Diabetes prevalence and glycemic control among adults aged 20 and over, by sex, age, and race and Hispanic origin: United States, selected years 1988–1994 through 2015–2018." 2019. Accessed August 20, 2021. https://www.cdc.gov/nchs/data/hus/2019/014-508.pdf.

Office of the Surgeon General (US). "The Surgeon General's Vision for a Healthy and Fit Nation." *NCBI Bookshelf.* 2010. Accessed August 20, 2021. https://www.ncbi.nlm.nih.gov/books/NBK44656/#background.s1.

Passmore, R., and Swindelis, Y. E. "Observations on the Respiratory Quotients and Weight Gain of Man After Eating Large Quantities of Carbohydrates." *British Journal of Nutrition.* 1963; 17: 331-9. doi: 10.1079/bjn19630036.

Peters, Lulu Hunt. *Diet and Health; With Key to the Calories.* Chicago: The Reilly and Lee Co.,1918.

Pirozzo, S., Summerbell, C., Cameron, C., and Glasziou, P. "Advice on low-fat diets for obesity." *Cochrane Database Syst Rev.* 2002;(2):CD003640. Accessed August 23, 2021. https://pubmed.ncbi.nlm.nih.gov/12076496/.

Reuber, M D. "Carcinogenicity of saccharin." *Enivron Health Perspect.* 25 August 1978. Accessed October 27, 2021. https://www.ncbi.nlm.nih.gov/pmc/articles/PMC1637197/.

Rippe, James M. and Angelopoulos, Theodore J. "Relationship between Added Sugars Consumption and Chronic Disease Risk Factors: Current Understanding." *Nutrients.* 4 November 2016;8(11):697. Accessed August 23, 2021. https://www.ncbi.nlm.nih.gov/pmc/articles/PMC5133084/.

Seven Countries Study. "Ancel Keys." Accessed August 23, 2021. https://www.sevencountriesstudy.com/about-the-study/investigators/ancel-keys/.

Spock, Benjamin. *The Common Sense Book of Baby and Child Care.* New York City: Duell, Sloan and Pearce, 1946.

Steele, Tim. *The Diet Hack: Why 95% of diets fail and how you can succeed.* Archangel Ink, 2019.

Shimazu, T., Hirschey, M.D., Newman, J., He, W., Shirakawa, K., Le, Moan N., Grueter, C.A., Lim, H., et al. "Suppression of oxidative stress by β-hydroxybutyrate, an endogenous histone deacetylase inhibitor." *Science.* 11 Jan 2013; 339(6116): 211-4. http://pubmed.ncbi.nlm.nih.gov/23223453

Tate & Lyle., ToxStrategies, Inc. "GRAS Determenation of Allulose for Use as an Ingredient in Human Food." *GRAS Notice (GRN) No. 893, Allulose.* 3 December 2019. Accessed 23 August 2021. https://www.fda.gov/media/136399/download.

The American Society of Sugar Beet Technologists. "Proceedings Eighth General Meeting." 2-5 February 1954;8(1). Accessed August 23, 2021. http://digitalcollections.qut.edu.au/1407/5/American_Society_of_Sugar_Beet_Technologists_1954_Part_1.pdf.

U.S. Food & Drug Administration. "Paws Off Xylitol; It's Dangerous for Dogs." 7 July 2021. Accessed August 23, 2021. https://www.fda.gov/consumers/consumer-updates/paws-xylitol-its-dangerous-dogs.

U.S. Food & Drug Administration. "Use of the Term Natural on Food Labeling." October 2018. Accessed August 23, 2021. https://www.fda.gov/food/food-labeling-nutrition/use-term-natural-food-labeling.

Wilder, RM. 1921. "The effects of ketonemia on the course of epilepsy." *Mayo Clin Bull.* (2): 307-308. https:// www.neslazeno.cz/wilder-1921-the-effect-of-ketonemia-on-the-course-of-epilepsy/.

World Health Organization. "Obesity." 9 June 2021. Accessed August 20, 2021. https://www.who.int/news-room/facts-in-pictures/detail/6-facts-on-obesity.

Yudkin, John. *Sweet and Dangerous: The New Facts About the Sugar You Eat as a Cause of Heart Disease, Diabetes, and Other Killers.* New York City: Peter H. Wyden, 1972.

And Now for The Thank-Yous

This is the part where I send a shout out or say a thank you to the folks who had my back while I was writing this book. While there is no way to acknowledge everyone, Imma do my best because: gratitude.

Thank you, mom and dad, for requiring me to read encyclopedias for fun and for telling me I could do and be anything.

Special thanks to Heather and Emelie Sanders for saving the day in a very red pill way.

Thank you to Leanne Regalia for not straight-up calling me crazy (at least not to my face) after millions of edits.

Thank you to Marsha Stopa for being an evil genius.

Thank you to Bethany McRee of Engagements (in Grenada, MS) for giving me a place to think.

Thank you to the songs, movies, and television shows of the 1980s for shaping the special kind of crazy that I own 100%.

Thank you, ex-boyfriend from high school (who shall remain nameless) for telling me I was no beauty queen and I'd never become anything without him. People don't forget.

Before

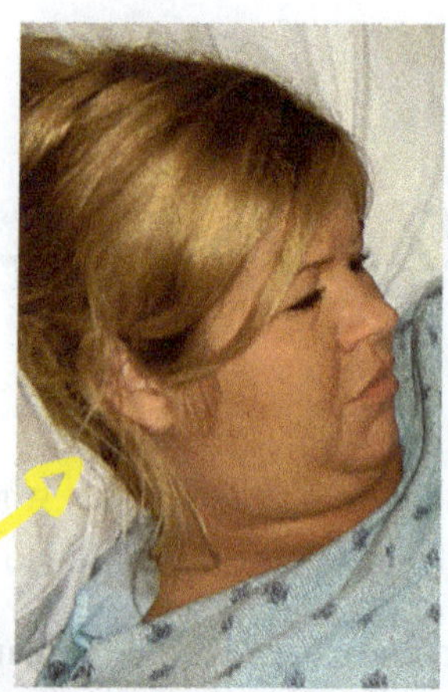

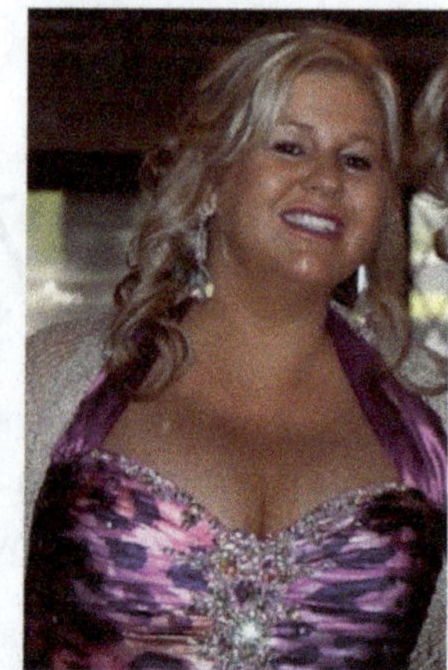

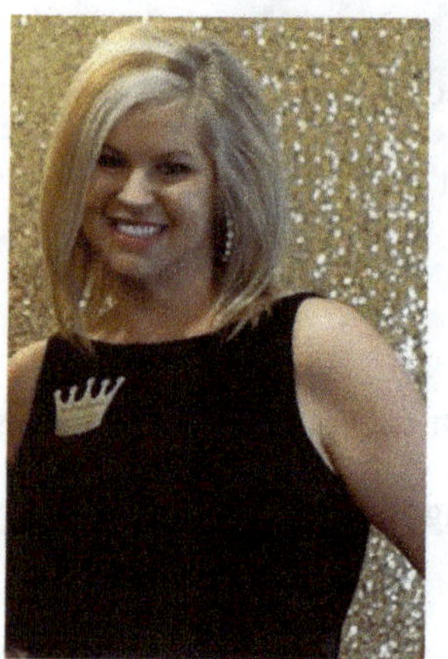

the Middle!

(Because transformation doesn't happen overnight.)

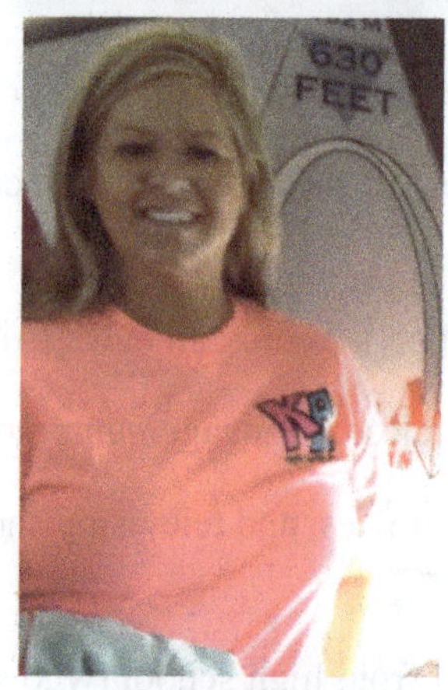

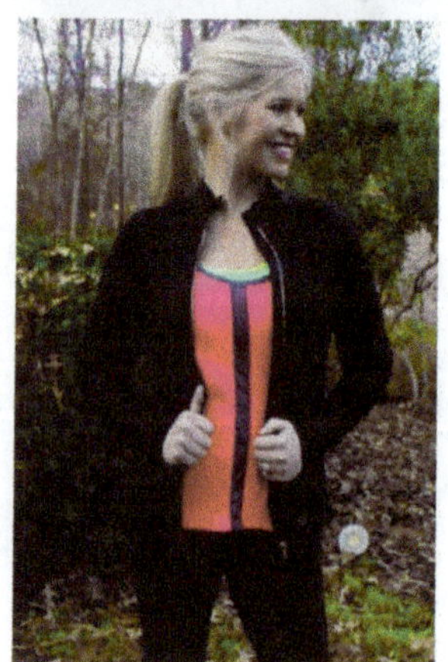

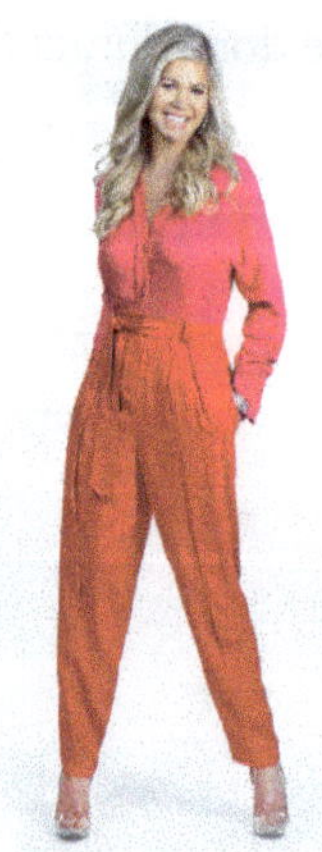

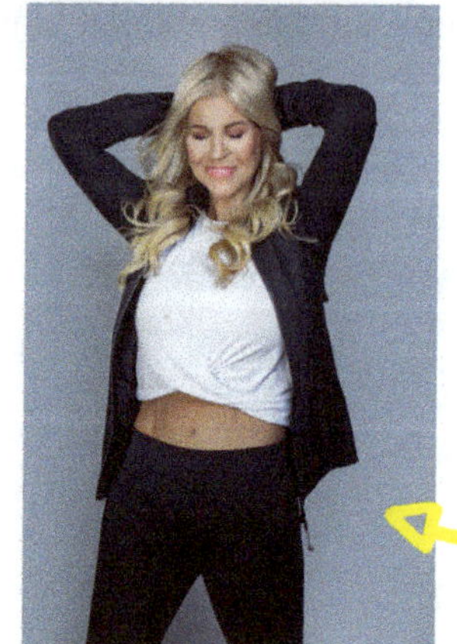

After

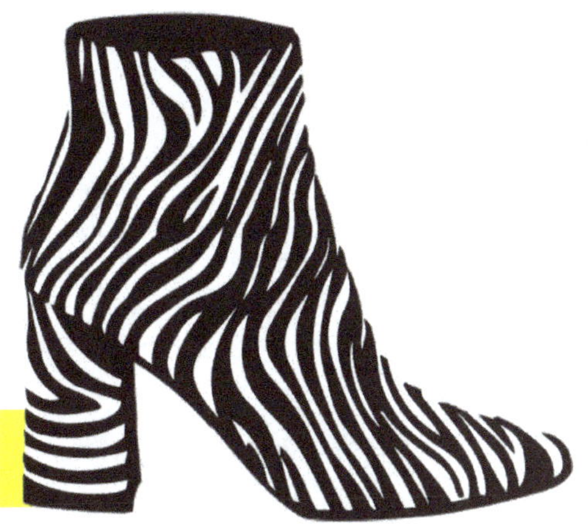

ABOUT THE AUTHOR

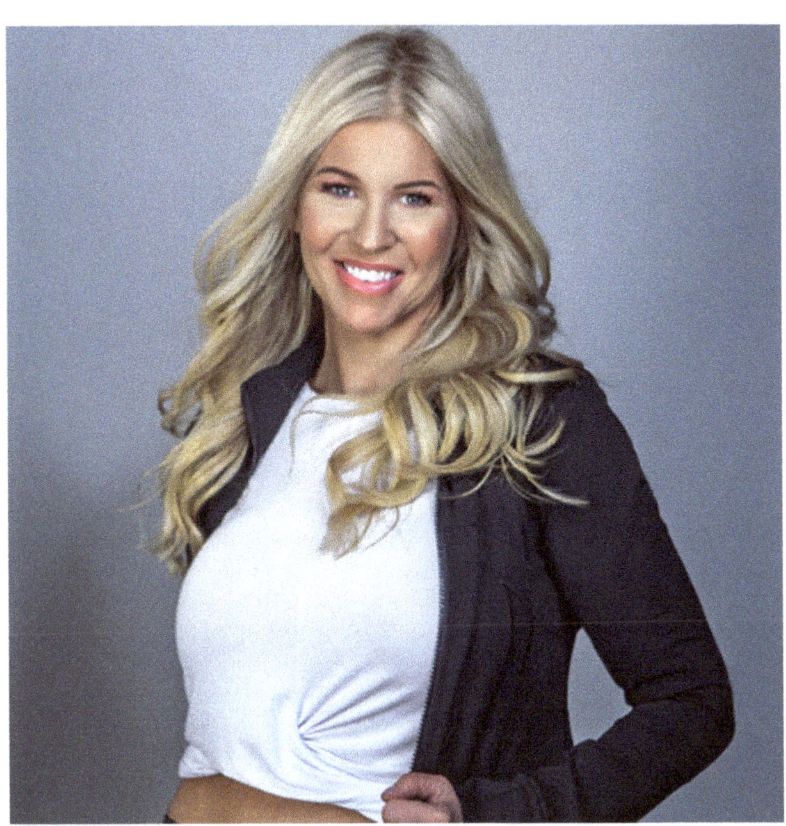

Heather Strickland is a writer, a Certified Health Coach, founder of *Word To Your Mother* Blog, and a woman who knows what it feels like to wake up at 35 and not recognize herself in the mirror. Heather took radical steps to change her health and mind, and now she's on a mission to help other women do the same. She enjoys keeping it real, momming, and dancing like nobody's watching. (Because they're not—they're on their phones.)

www.ingramcontent.com/pod-product-compliance
Lightning Source LLC
Chambersburg PA
CBHW080551270326
41929CB00019B/3263

* 9 7 8 1 9 5 1 6 9 4 6 8 5 *